# Acute Medical Emergencies

*To James, Estelle, Patrick and Desmond*

*For Elsevier:*

*Publisher:* Steven Black
*Project Development Manager:* Katrina Mather
*Project Manager:* David Fleming
*Design Direction:* George Ajayi

# Acute Medical Emergencies

## A Nursing Guide

### Richard Harrison MD FRCP
Consultant Physician, The University Hospital of North Tees,
Stockton on Tees, UK

### Lynda Daly RN RM RHV
Registered Nurse, Middlesbrough Primary Care Trust,
Middlesbrough, UK

**SECOND EDITION**

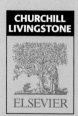

CHURCHILL
LIVINGSTONE

ELSEVIER

EDINBURGH LONDON NEW YORK OXFORD
PHILADELPHIA ST LOUIS SYDNEY TORONTO 2006

# CHURCHILL
# LIVINGSTONE
### ELSEVIER

© 2006, Elsevier Limited. All rights reserved.

The right of Richard Harrison and Lynda Daly to be identified as authors of this work has been asserted by them in accordance with the Copyright, Designs and Patents Act 1988

First published 2001
Reprinted 2002 (twice)
This edition 2006

ISBN 10: 0 443 10048 9
ISBN 13: 978 0 443 10048 2

**British Library Cataloguing in Publication Data**
A catalogue record for this book is available from the British Library

**Library of Congress Cataloging in Publication Data**
A catalog record for this book is available from the Library of Congress

Medical knowledge is constantly changing. Standard safety precautions must be followed, but as new research and clinical experience broaden our knowledge, changes in treatment and drug therapy may become necessary or appropriate. Readers are advised to check the most current product information provided by the manufacturer of each drug to be administered to verify the recommended dose, the method and duration of administration, and contraindications. It is the responsibility of the practitioner, relying on experience and knowledge of the patient, to determine dosages and the best treatment for each individual patient. Neither the Publisher nor the authors assume any liability for any injury and/or damage to persons or property arising from this publication.

Printed in China

The publisher's policy is to use paper manufactured from sustainable forests

# Contents

# Preface

Nursing on the medical wards is becoming dominated by the increasing number of emergency admissions. The average sized district general hospital takes in upwards of thirty acute medical cases per day. This presents a major challenge to the staff and demands the highest level of clinical knowledge and clinical skill.

Most hospitals are meeting this challenge by concentrating resources in Acute Medical Units to which unselected medical patients of all ages are admitted – to be decanted elsewhere after a period, usually 24 hours, of assessment and intensive treatment. Their success depends on the way in which these very sick patients are handled in the first few, crucial hours after they arrive on the Unit. Much of the initial responsibility for this falls on the nurse, who is faced with a daunting flow of patients in terms of both medical complaints and immediate nursing needs. Pre-admission diagnostic labels vary from the specific – 'acute atrial fibrillation' – to the vague – 'off legs and cannot cope' – and the quality of additional information is often poor. From this onslaught of unselected and undiagnosed cases decisions will have to be made:

- Who needs urgent attention and what should this be?
- Who can move off the Unit?
- Who can go home?

To provide this service effectively, there is an increasing overlap between the roles of the nursing and medical teams and it is now becoming commonplace for nurse practitioners to be involved in the assessment, triage and initial management of acute medical admissions. This is a demanding task that requires a detailed understanding of acute medical illness – to make sense of the clinical features; to prioritise emergency treatment; to follow a rational and logical care plan; and, most importantly of all, to recognise the psychosocial demands that these illnesses place on the patients and their families.

The book targets this area of practice in an attempt to bridge the gap between a pure 'nursing' text and a 'medical guide' to emergency admissions. The book assumes that its readers, while already having expert nursing skills, require additional knowledge derived, in part, from the 'medical model' but which is also firmly rooted in the tradition of needs-based nursing. This book therefore aims to:

- describe the common emergency medical conditions

- explain the underlying disease mechanisms
- describe the assessment, observations and management in terms of the disease process
- emphasise the critical role of information gathering in the planning of rational care
- relate the nursing care to the underlying disease
- focus on events within the first 24 hours of admission
- use examples from our practice to put the theoretical information into a practical context

(In the text where patients are referred to as 'he' this should be understood to refer to both male and female patients.)

It is our view that the basis for effective patient care in the critical first 24 hours must be a clear understanding by the nurse of the underlying medical condition. Everything else follows on from this: a logical approach to initial assessment; appropriate monitoring: timely and effective emergency care; and the anticipation of potential complications. This book aims to support this process by actively informing nurses' clinical work and by acting as the catalyst in a reflective assessment of their existing practice.

Stockton on Tees 2001

Richard N. Harrison
Lynda Daly

# Preface to the Second Edition

The Second Edition has been thoroughly revised to incorporate any significant changes in practice and the publication of new guidelines. Two new chapters have been added – an opening chapter that focuses on effective emergency assessment and resuscitation, and a final chapter on the growing threat of emerging new infections and of bioterrorism.

Stockton on Tees 2006

Richard N. Harrison
Lynda Daly

# Acknowledgements

The authors would like to thank the Resuscitation Council for permission to reproduce the text and illustrations relating to life support procedures as described in Chapter 10.

The publishers would like to thank Simon M. Whiteley of St James's Hospital, Leeds for the cover photograph.

# Abbreviations

| | |
|---|---|
| ABCDE | Mnemonic used for primary assessment (Airway, Breathing, Circulation, Disability, Exposure) |
| ACE | Angiotensin-converting enzyme |
| ACEI | Angiotensin-converting enzyme inhibitor |
| ADH | Antidiuretic hormone |
| ADL | Activities of Daily Living |
| AED | Accident & Emergency Department |
| AF | Atrial fibrillation |
| AIDS | Acquired immunodeficiency syndrome |
| ALS | Advanced life support |
| ALT | Alanine transaminase |
| AMI | Acute myocardial infarction |
| AMTS | Abbreviated mental test score |
| APPT | Activated partial thromboplastin time |
| ASO | Anti-streptolysin O |
| AST | Aspartate transaminase |
| AV node | Atrioventricular node |
| AVPU | Mnemonic for assessing consciousness level (Alert, Voice, Pain, Unresponsive) |
| bd | Twice a day |
| BLS | Basic life support |
| BMI | Body mass index |
| BNP | B-natriuretic peptide |
| BP | Blood pressure |
| CABG | Coronary artery bypass grafting |

| | |
|---|---|
| CCDC | Consultant for communicable disease control |
| CCF | Congestive cardiac failure |
| CCU | Coronary Care Unit |
| CJD | Creutzfeldt–Jakob disease |
| CK | Creatinine kinase |
| CNS | Central nervous system |
| $CO_2$ | Carbon dioxide |
| COHb | Carboxyhaemoglobin |
| COPD | Chronic obstructive pulmonary disease |
| CPAP | Continuous positive airway pressure |
| CPR | Cardiopulmonary resuscitation |
| CRP | C-reactive protein |
| CSF | Cerebrospinal fluid |
| CT | Computed tomography |
| CTPA | CT pulmonary angiogram |
| CVA | Cerebrovascular accident |
| CVP | Central venous pressure |
| DC | Direct current (counter shock) |
| DIC | Disseminated intravascular coagulopathy |
| DIGAMI | Diabetic Mellitus, Insulin Glucose Infusion in Acute Myocardial Infarction |
| DKA | Diabetic ketoacidosis |
| DNAR | Do not attempt resuscitation |
| ECG | Electrocardiogram |
| ECT | Electroconvulsive therapy |
| EDTA | Ethylenediamine tetra-acetic acid |

| | | | | |
|---|---|---|---|---|
| EMD | Electromechanical dissociation | | ITU | Intensive Therapy Unit |
| ENT | Ear, Nose and Throat | | i.v. | Intravenous |
| EPAP | Expiratory positive airway pressure | | JVP | Jugular venous pressure |
| ERCP | Endoscopic retrograde cholangio-pancreatogram | | KCCT | Kaolin cephalin clotting time |
| EWS | Early Warning Score | | KCl | Potassium chloride |
| FBC | Full blood count | | LFT | Liver function test |
| FFP | Fresh frozen plasma | | LP | Lumbar puncture |
| GBH | Gamma-hydroxybutyric acid | | LTOT | Long-term oxygen therapy |
| GCS | Glasgow Coma Score | | LVF | Left ventricular failure |
| GI | Gastrointestinal | | MCV | Mean corpuscular volume (size of the red cell) |
| GKI | Glucose-potassium-insulin infusion | | MDAC | Multiple-dose activated charcoal |
| GTN | Glyceryl trinitrate | | MDMA | 3,4-Methylenedioxymeth-amphetamine |
| Hb | Haemoglobin | | | |
| $HbA_{1c}$ | Glycated haemoglobin | | MDTB | Multi-drug-resistant tuberculosis |
| HBeAg | Hepatitis B e antigen | | | |
| HBsAg | Hepatitis B surface antigen | | MEWS | Modified Early Warning Score |
| HBV | Hepatitis B virus | | | |
| $HCO_3$ | Bicarbonate | | MRC | Medical Research Council |
| HCV | Hepatitis C virus | | MRI | Magnetic resonance imaging |
| HDU | High Dependency Unit | | | |
| HIV | Human immunodeficiency virus | | MRSA | Methicillin-resistant *Staphylococcus aureus* |
| HONK | Hyperosmolar non-ketotic diabetic coma | | MSU | Mid-stream urine |
| | | | MTS | Mental test score |
| HR | Heart rate | | NAPQI | *N*-acetyl-*p*-benzoquinoneimine |
| HUS | Haemolytic uraemic syndrome | | | |
| | | | NG | Nasogastric |
| ICD | Implantable cardioverter-defibrillator | | NIDDM | Non-insulin-dependent diabetes (i.e. Type II) |
| ICP | Intracranial pressure | | NIV | Non-invasive ventilation |
| IDDM | Insulin-dependent diabetes mellitus (i.e. Type I) | | NSAIDs | Non-steroidal anti-inflammatory drugs |
| INR | International normalised ratio (test of clotting) | | NYHA | New York Heart Association |
| IPAP | Inspiratory positive airway pressure | | od | Once a day |

| | | | |
|---|---|---|---|
| PACI | Partial anterior circulation infarct | SARS | Severe acute respiratory syndrome |
| PCI | Percutaneous coronary intervention | SCD | Sudden cardiac death |
| $pCO_2$ | Carbon dioxide level (partial pressure) | SHO | Senior House Officer |
| | | SRSV | Small round-structured virus |
| PCR | Polymerase chain reaction | SSRI | Selective serotonin re-uptake inhibitor |
| PE | Pulmonary embolism | | |
| PEA | Pulseless electrical activity | | |
| PERL | <u>P</u>upils are <u>e</u>qual and <u>r</u>eact to <u>l</u>ight | TACI | Total anterior circulation infarct |
| PFR | Peak flow rate | TB | Tuberculosis |
| pH | A measure of acidity (low pH – high acidity) | tds | Three times a day |
| | | TIA | Transient ischaemic attack |
| PND | Paroxysmal nocturnal dyspnoea | TIPS | Transjugular intrahepatic portosystemic shunt |
| $pO_2$ | Oxygen level (partial pressure) | | |
| p.r.n. | As required | U&E | Urea and electrolytes |
| PT | Prothrombin time | UTI | Urinary tract infection |
| PVC | Polyvinyl chloride | | |
| | | VF | Ventricular fibrillation |
| | | VHF | Viral haemorrhagic fever |
| qds | Four times a day | V/Q | Ventilation perfusion (isotope lung scan) |
| RR | Respiratory rate | VT | Ventricular tachycardia |
| rt-PA | Recombinant tissue plasminogen activator | | |
| | | WCC | White cell count |
| | | WKS | Wernicke-Korsakov syndrome |
| SA node | Sinoatrial node | | |

# CHAPTER 1

# INTRODUCTION: IMMEDIATE ASSESSMENT OF THE CRITICALLY ILL

This book is concerned with the recognition, assessment and management of acute medical patients during the first 24 h of admission. The effectiveness of care during this time will have a major impact on both the immediate chances of survival and the long-term outlook. Delays in initiating treatment costs lives; this has long been known in acute myocardial infarction (the familiar issue of 'door to needle' time), but is also the case in other conditions – notably stroke and severe sepsis. The initial care of the critically ill patient has to be targeted and timely.

In order to address this issue, the organisation of the medical care of the critically ill patient has undergone a revolution in recent years. Inter-professional demarcation is being removed, with the development of multidisciplinary teams. The nurses within this team have extended skills in the recognition and management of the acutely ill medical patient. These teams have a number of overriding principles:

1. Core competencies in the management of the critically ill
2. Immediate access to appropriately skilled team members
3. Effective prioritisation – assessing and treating the sickest patients first
4. Emphasis on the immediate identification of patients who are critically ill, who are deteriorating or who are at risk of deterioration
5. The need to initiate appropriate corrective action and to know who to call for help and with what degree of urgency
6. A reduction in duplication of work such as multiple admission clerking

This process has been facilitated by the development of Early Warning Systems based on simple nursing observations. These should identify patients who require urgent intervention and who may need prompt detailed assessment from the medical staff or, increasingly, from a Critical Care Team. Examples of such teams include Medical Emergency Teams and nurse-led Critical Care Outreach Teams.

## ABCDE: IMMEDIATE ASSESSMENT AND INTERVENTION

Immediate survival depends on urgent attention to the safety of the critically ill patient – the *A*irway, the *B*reathing, the *C*irculation. Subsequent progress depends on a more comprehensive assessment – by measuring *D*isability and *E*xposing the patient for detailed examination. This plan of immediate action based on the mnemonic 'ABCDE' is a recurring theme in the book – emphasising the critical importance of urgent and effective resuscitation. Urgent initial treatment may have to proceed in the absence of a definite diagnosis. However, a detailed assessment will be necessary to make a comprehensive diagnosis and to plan subsequent management; to do this requires a history, examination and an understanding of the underlying medical conditions. Each chapter therefore emphasises both the immediate safety of the patient and the nature, mechanisms and management of the underlying disease. The challenge for the nurse is to integrate this very technically demanding work in the critically ill with a humane and caring approach, combining modern clinical expertise with traditional nursing skills.

The first chapter gives an overview of the initial assessment and the early management which will be necessary to ensure the patient's immediate survival. There is a summary of the most urgent nursing observations – matched with the corrective interventions that may be necessary – and page references to relevant sections in the book. Detailed descriptions of resuscitation in specific conditions appear in later chapters.

It is important to develop a structured and systematic approach to immediate resuscitation. The focus should be on two fundamental issues: getting oxygen into the blood (*A*irway and *B*reathing) and getting blood (*C*irculation) to the brain and kidneys. The format for the initial assessment (→ Fig. 1.1) is based on the primary survey performed by first response teams such as the ambulance crew, and is founded on the standard ABCDE system in which the most important observations are performed first and the problems that are identified are rectified before moving on to the next stage. The primary survey is repeated when the patient is admitted to the ward; its structure ensures that the immediate safety of the patient continues to be addressed.

Subsequent progress is monitored from a number of basic physiological measurements obtained using standard nursing observations (the 'vital signs'):

- the respiratory rate
- pulse rate
- oxygen saturations
- blood pressure
- conscious level
- urine output

## EARLY WARNING: TRACK AND TRIGGER SYSTEMS

In response to criticisms that critically ill medical patients are not recognised soon enough and that resuscitative measures are delayed, inadequate, or both, a number of tools have been developed that utilise the observation of vital signs to identify patients who are at risk. These tools, sometimes known as 'Track and Trigger' systems, are used to monitor progress (track) and to provide specific criteria which, when met, trigger a call for assistance with a view to urgent corrective intervention.

*The aim is to prevent any patient passing through an unrecognised yet potentially reversible period of instability and deterioration.*

The most common system in use scores each observation according to its value. For example, in the Modified Early Warning Score (MEWS), a urine output of less than 0.5 ml/kg per hour scores 2 points, whereas between

| Assessment | | | | Possible interventions | Quick reference |
|---|---|---|---|---|---|
| **Airway** | | | | Suction | 338 |
| ☐ Clear | ☐ Partial obstruction | ☐ Obstruction | ☐ Vomited & aspirated | Chin lift/jaw thrust<br>Guedel airway<br>Bag, mask & valve<br>Recovery position | 99 ABCDE<br>107 |
| **Breathing** | | | | | |
| ☐ Present | ☐ Absent | ☐ Rate | | Oxygen | 373 BLS |
| ☐ 1 Normal | ☐ 2 Deep | ☐ 3 Shallow | ☐ 4 Irregular | Bag, mask & valve | 21 LVF<br>68 Asthma<br>73 COPD |
| ☐ 5 Wheeze | ☐ 6 Dyspnoea | ☐ 7 Uneven chest movement | ☐ 8 Unable to talk in full sentences | CPR | 84 Pneumonia<br>251 PE<br>272 Self-harm |
| PFR ☐☐ | | | | Nebuliser | 91 Pneumothorax<br>64 PFR |
| O₂ saturation ☐☐ | | | | Chest drain? | 61 Oximetry |
| **Circulation** | | | | | |
| *Pulse* ☐ Present | ☐ Absent | ☐☐☐ Rate | | CPR | 372 CPR |
| Quality: ☐ 1 Reg | ☐ 2 Irreg | ☐ 3 Strong | ☐ 4 Weak | IV fluids | 68 Asthma<br>41 AF |
| *Capillary refill* ☐ < 2 sec | ☐ > 2 sec | | | | 84 Pneumonia<br>27 Hypotension |
| *Skin* ☐ N | ☐ P | ☐ F | ☐ B ☐ S ☐ C | | 336 Hypotensive<br>collapse |
| *Blood pressure* ☐☐☐ / ☐☐☐ | | | | | 334 Shock<br>182 Acute abdo |
| *BM Stix* ☐ < 2 | ☐ > 30 | ☐☐☐ | | Glucose | 22 Pulse + BP<br>230 Hypoglycaemia |
| *Temp* ☐☐☐ | | | | IV antibiotics | 125 Meningitis<br>159 GI bleeding |
| *Blood loss (GI or haemoptysis)* ☐☐☐ ml | | | | | 361 Acute renal failure |
| *Urine output* ☐☐☐ 1st hr | ☐☐☐ 2nd hr | ☐☐☐ 3rd hr | | Fluid challenge | |

**Fig. 1.1** Scheme for a structured approach to the initial assessment and early management of the critically ill patient.

*Continued*

| Assessment | | | | Possible interventions | Quick reference |
|---|---|---|---|---|---|
| **Disability** | | | | | |
| ☐ A | ☐ V | ☐ P | ☐ U | Secure airway | 99 ABCDE |
| | | | | Correct hypotension (systolic > 100) | 104 AVPU |
| **GCS** ☐ Eyes (4) | ☐ Motor (6) | ☐ Verbal (5) | | Oxygen | 102 GCS |
| | | | | Recovery position | 107 Coma |
| **Eyes** 1. PERL 2. Dilated 3. Constricted 4. Fixed | | ☐ R | ☐ L | Glucose (Beware C-spine) | 230 Hypoglycaemia |
| **Exposure** | | | | | |
| **Abdomen** Pain | ☐ Y | ☐ N | | NG intubation | |
| ☐ 1 Soft | ☐ 2 Rigid | ☐ 3 Distended | | | 155 119 Aspiration |
| **Skin rash** | ☐ Y | ☐ N | | Anaphylaxis ℞ • Adrenaline | 182 Anaphylaxis |
| **CVA/TIA** | ☐ Y | ☐ N | | • Steroids • Fluids | 353 Acute abdomen |
| **New deficit** Speech | ☐ Y | ☐ N | | Antibiotics | 125 Meningitis |
| Facial palsy | ☐ Y ☐ N | ☐ R | ☐ L | Urgent CT | 118 Stroke |
| Weak arm Weak leg | ☐ ☐ Y | ☐ ☐ N | ☐ ☐ R ☐ ☐ L | | |

**Fig. 1.1 cont'd.** Skin: N, normal; P, pale; F, flushed; B, blue; S, sweaty; C, cold. Eyes: PERL, pupils are equal and react to light; R, right; L, left. C-spine, cervical spine. ℞, prescribe

1 and 3 ml/kg per hour scores 0. Scores from each observation are added up, and the total used to determine the level of action. Depending on the total score this will vary, say, from a simple increase in the frequency of observations to an urgent review by middle-grade medical staff. It is

important that there is an explicit protocol to match the score with the action that is required. The nature of the protocol will depend on local circumstances: in some Units, for example, the nurses are authorised to order tests and initiate treatments once a certain level of score is reached, whereas in others the response may simply be based on calling for escalating levels of assistance. In many Units, an important and effective development has been the availability of nurse-led Critical Care Outreach Teams which can react rapidly to deteriorating warning scores by advising and initiating early interventions and liaising with the High Dependency Unit and Intensive Therapy Unit. Once the staff have responded and a management plan is in place, the assessment tools are used to monitor improvement and to provide a mechanism to ensure that patients who fail to improve are identified and re-assessed within explicit time-frames.

It is important, therefore, that any Early Warning protocol should have a time element within it. When every staff member is hard pressed and there are competing clinical priorities, it is vital that there is a clear and mutual understanding of the expected response times; in one system, for example, the maximum response time for a doctor is 1 h for an oxygen saturation of 90% and a systolic blood pressure of 90 mmHg, but 15 min when both values are only 80. Another system specifies the following maximum time intervals: patient first triggering a response and the attendance of the doctor, 25 min for an SHO; if the patient continues to trigger despite intervention, 70 min for the registrar; if there is continuing concern, 120 min for discussion with the on-call Consultant.

---

**Table 1.1    Medical emergency team calling criteria**

The emergency team are called when one or more of the following criteria are reached:

| Acute changes in | Vital signs |
| --- | --- |
| AIRWAY/BREATHING | Threatened<br>All respiratory arrests<br>Respiratory rate <8/min<br>Respiratory rate >25/min<br>Saturations on oxygen <90% |
| CIRCULATION | All cardiac arrests<br>Pulse rate <45 beats/min<br>Pulse rate >125 beats/min<br>Systolic blood pressure <90 mmHg |
| DISABILITY | Patient not responding to voice/GCS 8 or less<br>Sudden fall in level of consciousness<br>(Fall in GCS of >2 points)<br>Repeated or prolonged seizures |
| OTHER | Oliguria: less than 30 ml/h for 3 h running<br>Any patient who does not fit the criteria above, but whom you are seriously worried about |

| Table 1.2 | The Early Warning Score System | | | | | | |
|---|---|---|---|---|---|---|---|
| | | | | Score | | | |
| | 3 | 2 | 1 | 0 | 1 | 2 | 3 |
| HR (beats/min) | | <40 | 41–50 | 51–100 | 101–110 | 111–130 | >130 |
| SBP (mmHg) | <70 | 71–80 | 81–100 | 101–199 | | >200 | |
| RR (breaths/min) | | <8 | | 9–14 | 15–20 | 21–29 | >30 |
| Temp. (°C) | | <35.0 | 35.1–36.5 | 36.6–37.4 | >37.5 | | |
| CNS | | | | A | V | P | U |
| A, alert; V, responds to voice; P, responds to pain; U, unconscious | | | | | | | |

*Examples of 'Track and Trigger' systems*
1. Single-parameter calling criteria (→ Table 1.1)
   This is simpler than a scoring system, but may be less discriminating between those who do and do not need urgent intervention.
2. A multiple-parameter scoring system
   A total score of 3 or more in the Early Warning Score (EWS; → Table 1.2) triggers a contact with the outreach team, and the patient should be re-scored hourly. There is a Modified Early Warning Score (MEWS), which includes an assessment of the urine output and attempts to relate the changes in blood pressure to the patient's normal values.

## CONCLUSION

Whatever assessment tool is used and whatever staff are involved, the fundamental issues are the identification of any patient who is at risk and to ensure that the staff who are giving the care have the appropriate skills in the management of the critically ill. These tools should be seen as an aid to assessment; they do not replace common sense or intuition ('there is something not quite right here'), and they do not acknowledge the need to intervene when there are distressing symptoms or unrelieved suffering. They also do not recognise the critical role of history taking or that of the relatives in recognising change. One of the most telling signs of the at-risk patient is the next of kin who wants to see a doctor because of their increasing anxieties over the deterioration of their relative's condition.

## FURTHER READING

Ball C, Kirkby M, Williams S 2003 Effect of the critical care outreach team on patient survival to discharge from hospital and readmission to critical care: non-randomised population based study. British Medical Journal 327: 1014–1016

Chellel A, Fraser L, Fender V 2002 Nursing observations on ward patients at risk of critical illness. Nursing Times 98 (46): 36–39

**WEBSITE**

NHS Modernisation Agency. Critical Care Outreach 2003: http://www.dh.gov.uk/assetRoot/04/06/35/00/04063500.pdf

# CARDIOLOGY

## INTRODUCTION

Heart disease is the most common single cause for emergency medical admission. The majority of these cases will be the result of ischaemic heart disease and present with a history of chest pain, symptoms of heart failure or non-specific ill health caused by decompensated heart disease. Acute medical wards are neither equipped nor staffed appropriately to deal with patients who have suffered an acute myocardial infarction, in whom the priority is for immediate thrombolysis. Therefore the patient with an obvious myocardial infarction, unstable angina or a serious rhythm disturbance will be admitted straight to the CCU.

In many cases, however, the diagnosis will not be clear-cut. This is particularly true in the elderly, in whom the presentation of acute cardiac problems ranges from sudden confusion to abdominal pain and vomiting. Often, the clinical picture may overlap with non-cardiac conditions. The classical situation is difficulty in differentiating cardiac and respiratory breathlessness in patients with the common combination of COPD and ischaemic heart disease. Other examples include abdominal symptoms in congestive cardiac failure, and cachexia with weight loss in advanced decompensated valvular heart disease.

All these patients will be admitted to the Acute Medical Unit, where the expectation is that they will be assessed, diagnosed and appropriately treated with the minimum of delay. The patients, particularly those who are older than 75 years, frequently have several medical conditions and when admitted are receiving complex treatment regimens. It is often the case that cardiac problems complicate other diseases that themselves were the reason for admission: the patient with anaemia from GI blood loss who develops angina after admission is a typical example.

The task for the nurse is to perform an accurate assessment that takes into account both cardiac and non-cardiac aspects of the patient's medical history. The patient's problems must be prioritised: for example, increasing angina will take priority over a recent change in bowel habit, and attacks of nocturnal breathlessness will be more urgent to address than newly diagnosed but stable Type II (non-insulin-dependent) diabetes.

The management of heart disease must be based on an understanding of the underlying conditions, particularly *ischaemic heart disease* (coronary artery disease), *cardiac failure* and *atrial fibrillation*. There have been important advances in the diagnosis and management of these conditions that have altered our approach to the patients:

● Active management of myocardial infarction
   — the use of troponin-T and other markers for risk stratification
   — immediate thrombolysis/angioplasty in acute myocardial infarction
   — aspirin prophylaxis

— beta-blockers and intensive lipid-lowering therapy with statins to improve long-term outlook
— referral of unstable patients for CABG or angioplasty
● New approaches to cardiac failure
— the use of ACE inhibitors (e.g. enalapril)
— the use of low-dose beta-blockers
— new pacing and electrophysiological techniques
— effective antiarrhythmic drugs: amiodarone and flecainide
● Recognition of the frequency and significance of atrial fibrillation
— increased use of anticoagulation in atrial fibrillation

This chapter aims to provide the basis for this understanding by looking at disease mechanisms and by providing a logical approach to the patient with possible heart disease.

## COMMON CLINICAL PROBLEMS

### Acute severe breathlessness

Acute severe breathlessness is a common problem on the Acute Medical Unit, but there is often a diagnostic dilemma in deciding between pulmonary oedema and asthma or COPD (→ Chapter 3; The breathless patient: the general approach). This chapter looks at the mechanisms and causes of cardiac failure, which will put into context both the clinical features and the management strategy of the patient with pulmonary oedema or congestive failure.

### Chest pain and atypical myocardial infarction

The various clinical problems associated with ischaemic heart disease – infarction, angina and silent myocardial ischaemia – will be described. The chapter aims to clarify the management of chest pain, in particular how to assess the urgency of the situation in a new patient.

### Atrial fibrillation

Atrial fibrillation is the most common arrhythmia encountered on the emergency ward. It causes cardiac failure, syncope and unexplained dizziness, and can complicate any severe febrile illness such as pneumonia or exacerbations of COPD. Atrial fibrillation is a common cause of stroke and is one of the major indications for anticoagulant therapy. The management of atrial fibrillation encompasses the use of a good assessment technique, a working knowledge of modern cardiac drugs, and the ability to recognise and deal with complications such as cardiac failure and angina in an acutely distressed and anxious patient.

### Immediate relevance of heart disease to other acute medical conditions

When assessing an unstable patient with any acute medical condition, it is important to consider the risk posed by any coexisting cardiac problem to the safety of the patient:

- High risk
  — recent myocardial infarction
  — unstable angina
  — cardiac failure
  — rapid atrial fibrillation
  — significant aortic valve disease
- Medium risk
  — stable angina
  — previous myocardial infarction
  — previous cardiac failure
- Low risk
  — poorly controlled hypertension
  — previous CABG, but now asymptomatic
  — angina, but comfortable at a normal walking speed

Any patient within the first category needs to be assessed immediately and with particular care, and there should be no hesitation in involving medical staff if problems arise. In contrast, the cardiac conditions in patients in the medium- and low-risk categories are less likely to be immediately relevant to an acute admission, particularly during the first 24 h of their admission. Box 2.1 lists some key questions that arise in the treatment of cardiac patients.

## CORE NURSING SKILLS

**Application of triage using ABCDE (→ p. 338; primary assessment)** The essential skill of cardiac nursing is to establish the safety of the patient. As with any acute illness, this is based on basic observations of the vital signs. The immediate priority is to establish adequate oxygenation and an effective

---

**Box 2.1 – Critical questions in the cardiac patient**

- Is this chest pain cardiac in origin?
- What is the difference between cor pulmonale and congestive cardiac failure?
- How do I approach acute dyspnoea in an asthmatic with known heart disease?
- The pulse is 135 beats/min: what is the next step?
- Why is this patient cold, clammy and shut down?
- Why are nitrates used to treat angina as well as pulmonary oedema?
- Why can morphine be used for acute LVF but not for treating asthma?
- Does this patient need urgent medical attention?
- How can I make sense of this patient's drug regimen?
- What can I say to the relatives of this patient with acute pulmonary oedema?

circulation. In pulmonary oedema, for example, the patient can be so ill that other nursing considerations are overshadowed by the need to administer opiates, oxygen and intravenous (i.v.) frusemide to save the patient's life.

**Reassurance of acutely distressed and anxious patients** The patient will be acutely unwell, with a combination of unpleasant and frightening symptoms: severe breathlessness, chest pain, rapid irregular palpitations and overwhelming fatigue. Not surprisingly, cardiac patients are among the most frightened and anxious, and this will not be helped by hearing staff talk of heart 'failure' and 'unstable' angina. Anxiety worsens breathlessness, can exacerbate angina and will put an extra load on the heart. Reassurance is vital and this is best provided by nurses who understand exactly what is wrong and why and who can explain the details of their management. It is easy to forget, for example, that patients who are having intensive nursing observations and complex tests carried out may feel very anxious that they are not being told what all this information means and whether they are in fact going to recover.

**Resuscitation skills** Acute cardiac illness is characterised by rapid changes in the patient's condition. The most difficult problems encountered on the Acute Medical Unit are fulminating pulmonary oedema with hypoxia and hypotension and the unexpected cardiac arrest. It is therefore important that all the staff are fully trained in CPR and are familiar with the resuscitation equipment.

**Coordinated care with the medical staff** There is considerable overlap between nursing and medical responsibilities in the care of patients with acute heart disease. The initial nursing assessment will include important diagnostic information: the nature of the predominant symptoms and the identification of ischaemic chest pain are two obvious examples. Subsequently, documentation of the trends in the vital signs, urine output and symptomatic improvement is the main way that the patient's response to treatment is evaluated. It is important that all this information is shared constructively with the medical staff and that the duplication of tasks such as history taking and observations is kept to the absolute minimum, both to save time and to reduce the burden to the patient.

**Anticipating problems**
With experience backed by a good understanding of the underlying disease mechanisms, some problems can be anticipated and often forestalled. Obvious examples include the hypotension that can complicate the use of several cardiac drugs and the development of ischaemic chest pain in a patient who develops rapid atrial fibrillation. It can be extremely helpful to assess the way in which the patient has responded to similar situations in the past by examining the hospital records and noting what the patient and their relatives have to say about it.

# CARDIAC FAILURE

There are two components to heart failure: the primary problem, which damages the function of the heart, and the secondary mechanisms, which are activated to try and compensate for the impaired cardiac function. These are summarised in Fig. 2.1.

## PRIMARY PROBLEMS IN THE HEART

*Heart muscle damage*
The most common cause of chronic heart failure is heart muscle damage from myocardial ischaemia due to coronary artery disease. Most patients give a history of long-standing angina and recurrent myocardial infarctions, but a significant proportion of cases, particularly patients with diabetes, have unrecognised silent ischaemia that presents for the first time as cardiac failure. Hypertension is also an important cause of cardiac failure. The response to long-standing, uncontrolled hypertension is an increase in the bulk and strength of the heart muscle in order to drive blood out of the heart against the increased pressure. In time, however, the muscle fatigues and weakens, leading to reduced cardiac reserve and eventual failure.

Other causes of heart muscle disease are listed in Fig. 2.1. Of these, alcoholic cardiomyopathy is probably the most important, as it is common and will respond to the combination of alcohol withdrawal and thiamine (vitamin B) replacement.

*Valvular disease*
Although not as common as heart muscle damage, valvular disease can lead to chronic cardiac failure that, with correct management, can be alleviated or controlled. Heart valves normally act as one-way doors which ensure that, when the heart contracts, blood can pass in only one direction. To continue the analogy with a door – as a result of damage (e.g. past rheumatic fever or a congenital fault in the valve's structure) the valve can become permanently stuck half open (stenosis), in which case the heart has difficulty expelling blood through it. This has two important consequences: the heart may become overworked, and blood may dam up behind the stenosed valve.

Alternatively, a valve can lose its one-way facility so that, instead of its being normally closed in either systole or diastole (depending on which valve is being considered), blood can pass through it throughout the cardiac cycle; this is known as valve incompetence or valve regurgitation. In valve incompetence/regurgitation, the affected chamber not only has its normal quota of blood to expel each beat, but it also has the added amount that comes back to it as a result of the leaking valve. Thus, in mitral incompetence, during left ventricular contraction blood leaves by the usual route into the aorta, but some blood is also forced back into the left atrium

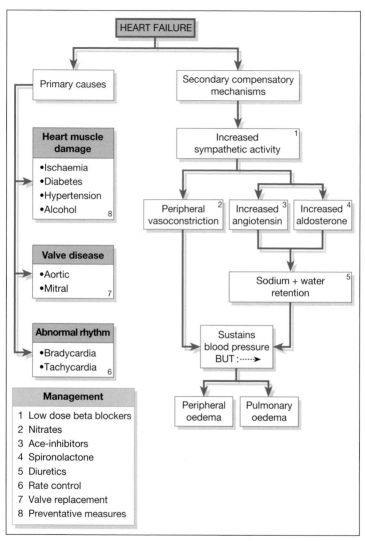

**Fig. 2.1** The mechanisms and management of cardiac failure: an overview. Numbers in management box refer to numbers in the figure

through the incompetent mitral valve. This blood then returns, along with the normal quota of blood, during the subsequent diastole. In aortic incompetence, blood leaks back into the left ventricle during diastole, when the aortic valve should normally be closed. The left ventricle has to deal with this back-flow in addition to the normal amount coming to it from the left atrium. In time the heart muscle fatigues, either because of the extra pressure it has to generate (in, for example, aortic valve stenosis) or because of the extra volume of blood it has to cope with (in, for example, mitral valve incompetence). This fatigue, in turn, in time leads to clinical cardiac failure.

*Rhythm disturbance*
Abnormally slow (bradyarrhythmias) or, more commonly, abnormally fast (tachyarrhythmias) cardiac rhythms can result in heart failure. A slow pulse leads to a fall-off in the cardiac output, simply because the heart beats less often per minute. A healthy heart compensates for a slow pulse by having more time to fill before each contraction; the heart chamber responds to such stretching by producing a more forceful contraction, expelling an increased amount of blood. A diseased heart is unable to respond in this way, so that a reduced heart rate causes a reduced cardiac output. Fast rhythms disrupt the events that occur during diastole – filling of the heart chambers and blood flow down the coronary arteries. Once again, a healthy heart can cope with a rapid rate, but a diseased heart can soon be compromised, particularly if the coronary arteries are narrowed. The most common rhythm disturbance to cause or contribute to cardiac failure is uncontrolled atrial fibrillation, in which the rate is both rapid and irregular. The onset of rapid atrial fibrillation can often trigger acute heart failure.

## SECONDARY COMPENSATORY MECHANISMS IN CARDIAC FAILURE

In response to the basic problem of *reduced cardiac output*, two compensatory mechanisms are activated to try and maintain a normal blood pressure:

1. increased sympathetic nervous system activity (exaggerated stress reaction)
2. activation of the renin–angiotensin–aldosterone hormone system (salt and water retention)

These two mechanisms respectively *increase the narrowing of the peripheral arterioles* and *increase the circulating blood volume* – a strategy designed to keep the blood pressure up and maintain a good blood supply to the kidneys. Although this may work for a while, ultimately it leads to an increased load against which the heart must pump (in the case of the narrowed arterioles) and pulmonary congestion and ankle oedema (in the case of the increased circulating blood volume). Pumping against an abnormally high load eventually leads to heart muscle fatigue, so-called pump failure or 'forward' heart failure (low blood pressure and poor organ perfusion). Conversely, the

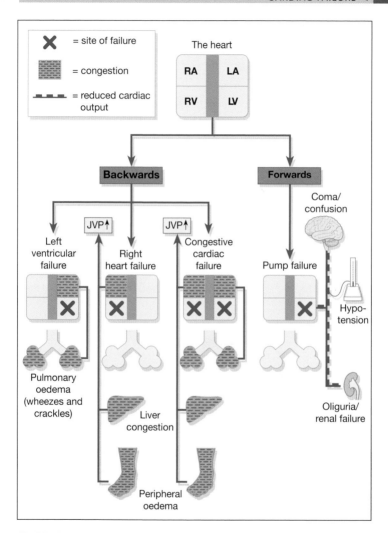

**Fig. 2.2** The two components (backwards and forwards) of cardiac failure. JVP, jugular venous pressure; LA, left atrium; LV, left ventricle; RA, right atrium; RV, right ventricle

congestive component is known as 'backward' failure (pulmonary and peripheral oedema). These two components of cardiac failure are summarised in Fig. 2.2.

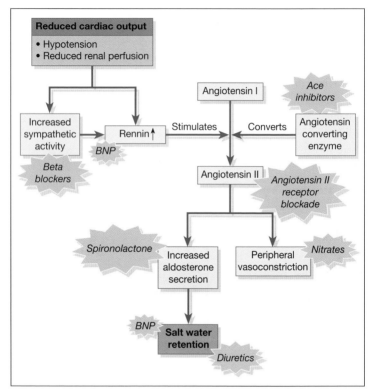

**Fig. 2.3**  Further details of the mechanisms of BNP and of drug treatments in cardiac failure

Modern management of cardiac failure can be understood in terms of reversing these mechanisms by decreasing the resistance against which the heart must pump and unloading the congestion behind the failing heart. As shown in Fig. 2.3, this is achieved by:

- dilating the arterioles (e.g. GTN, isosorbide mononitrate, hydralazine)
- reducing the salt and water retention (e.g. frusemide and bumetanide)
- inhibiting the renin–angiotensin–aldosterone system (ACE inhibitors, angiotensin receptor blockers, aldosterone antagonists)
- reducing sympathetic activity – the cautious use of sympathetic blockade (beta-blockers)

**An important new biomarker of cardiac failure: B-natriuretic peptide**

When the ventricles are put under strain and begin to fail, they release a hormone known as B-natriuretic peptide. BNP enters the circulation and can be measured from a simple blood sample. BNP acts as an 'internal' anti-failure mechanism:

- It inhibits the increased sympathetic drive
- It inhibits the renin–angiotensin–aldosterone system
- It promotes the renal loss of water and salt

There are two important clinical implications. First, the blood test can help diagnose cardiac failure and will become particularly helpful in patients in whom the underlying cause of their acute breathlessness is unclear. Secondly, drugs with the same chemical properties as BNP are being developed to exploit its effects on reversing the underlying mechanisms in cardiac failure.

## TYPES OF HEART FAILURE

### Left heart failure
In left heart failure, the clinical problem is dominated by the build-up of fluid in the lungs, because the failing left ventricle cannot cope with the increased circulating blood volume – blood dams up behind the left side of the heart, producing pulmonary congestion and pulmonary oedema. The symptoms of left heart failure are:

- breathlessness on lying flat (orthopnoea)
- PND
- coughing frothy pink sputum (alveolar oedema)

### Right heart failure
In right heart failure, the right ventricle cannot cope with the increased circulating blood volume and blood dams up in the veins, leading to congestion of the liver, ankle oedema and oedema over the sacrum. The symptoms of right heart failure are:

- swollen ankles
- liver discomfort
- abdominal swelling (ascites)

### Congestive cardiac failure
In congestive cardiac failure, there is a combination of left- and right-sided failure, giving a constellation of symptoms that include:

- breathlessness
- fatigue
- pulmonary and ankle oedema

*Right heart failure and COPD*

Many patients with acute exacerbations of COPD complain about the recent development of ankle oedema that coincided with worsening of their chest symptoms. This is the result of the development of cor pulmonale – right-sided heart failure due to lung disease. The simplest explanation is that the right side of the heart has to do extra work to force blood through pulmonary arterioles that are abnormally narrow because of the low oxygen levels found in COPD.

*Diastolic heart failure*

Diastolic heart failure is a newly recognised condition which may account for a fifth or more cases of cardiac failure. Typically seen in elderly, obese, hypertensive and diabetic women, diastolic failure results from an abnormally hypertrophied and stiffened ventricle, which contracts well enough but in diastole cannot relax sufficiently to accommodate returning blood. The symptoms – pulmonary and peripheral oedema – are the same as in other forms of failure; the diagnosis relies on the characteristic changes on an echocardiogram.

## CLINICAL FEATURES AND MANAGEMENT OF CARDIAC FAILURE

*Characteristics of patients admitted acutely with cardiac failure*

In general, patients with heart failure comprise an elderly group of patients, average age around 75 years, with a strong preponderance of ischaemic heart disease – half will have had a previous infarct. At least half of all these patients will be in atrial fibrillation, and for about a tenth the heart failure will have been triggered by their first attack of atrial fibrillation. One-third will also have COPD and a fifth will be diabetic. In the majority, around 80%, the cause of the failure will be associated with poor heart muscle function; valve problems will only be seen in about 10% of the patients.

It can be helpful to characterise the patient's pre-existing level of disability. The NYHA classification is the one most commonly used:

- **Class I** – no limitations (no fatigue, breathlessness or palpitations)
- **Class II** – slight limitations, fine at rest, but ordinary exertion leads to symptoms
- **Class III** – marked limitations, fine at rest, but symptoms on less than ordinary exertion
- **Class IV** – symptoms at rest

Patients in NYHA Classes III and IV have a poor outlook, with 5-year mortality rates approaching 50%.

*Principles of managing cardiac failure*

1. Management is based first on trying to correct the primary underlying problem:
   — improving the coronary artery circulation (drugs, angioplasty, CABG)
   — correcting any valve abnormality (valve repair and replacement)
   — treating an abnormal heart rhythm (e.g. controlling atrial fibrillation with digoxin).
2. In addition, or as an alternative, the compensatory mechanisms that are responsible for the clinical picture of chronic cardiac failure are addressed:
   — reducing fluid retention (diuretics)
   — reducing the load on the heart (vasodilators)
   — counteracting excessive sodium retention (ACE inhibitors such as enalapril, angiotensin receptor blockers such as losartan)
   — counteracting increased sympathetic activity (low dose beta-blockers).
   *There is an obvious risk in correcting what are supposed to be compensatory mechanisms – in particular, over-diuresis and excessive use of vasodilators can produce hypotension, with a worsening of tissue perfusion.*
3. Device therapy
   In some patients with cardiac failure, delayed electrical activation of the left ventricle (recognised on an ECG by the pattern of left bundle branch block) produces a disjointed and inefficient cardiac contraction. If severely impaired, the contractile state can be resynchronised and improved using a novel permanent pacemaker which, unlike conventional pacemakers, paces the left as well as the right ventricle. This technique, termed dual-chamber pacing, will have an increasing role in selected cases of cardiac failure, although the effects on quality of life surpass those on actual survival.
   Patients with heart failure are at least six times more likely to die suddenly than the general population. In carefully selected patients, ICDs can be fitted to reduce mortality by treating any lethal ventricular arrhythmia.

## Acute left ventricular failure

Acute LVF ($\rightarrow$ Fig. 2.4) is a common cause for acute life-threatening breathlessness (the others being acute asthma, tension pneumothorax and pulmonary embolism). Case Study 2.1 illustrates the typical picture in heart failure due to ischaemic heart disease. Interestingly, the patient did not receive an ACE inhibitor after his infarct; these are now given routinely as post-infarct prophylaxis to lessen the risk of developing heart failure.

*Critical nursing tasks in acute LVF*
**Ensure the patient is adequately oxygenated** Patients in acute LVF die of hypoxia due to pulmonary oedema. Therefore the safest practice is to start with high-flow oxygen or a rebreathing mask, aiming to give the patient at least 60% oxygen. This can be modified in the light of the oxygen saturations

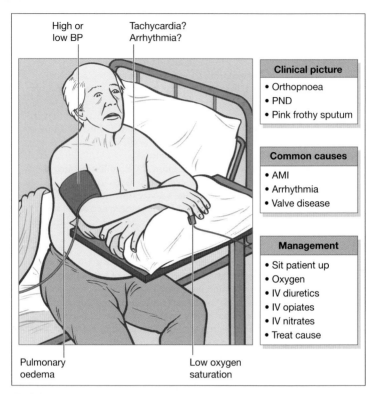

High or low BP

Tachycardia? Arrhythmia?

**Clinical picture**
- Orthopnoea
- PND
- Pink frothy sputum

**Common causes**
- AMI
- Arrhythmia
- Valve disease

**Management**
- Sit patient up
- Oxygen
- IV diuretics
- IV opiates
- IV nitrates
- Treat cause

Pulmonary oedema

Low oxygen saturation

**Fig. 2.4** Acute left ventricular failure. AMI, acute myocardial infarction

or blood gas measurements. Patients must be propped upright – even if they are hypotensive. Their symptoms will improve because pulmonary oedema lessens in the sitting position.

**Measure the patient's blood pressure**

*Hypertension.* Many patients with LVF become acutely hypertensive as a stress response; the blood pressure settles as their condition improves. Less commonly, hypertension is believed to be the cause, rather than the effect, of a patient's LVF. In such cases it is usually severe (e.g. 210/140 mmHg) and persistent, and has to be lowered as part of the patient's immediate management. Fortunately some of the drugs used to treat LVF, such as nitrates and diuretics, have a dual effect: they both eliminate pulmonary oedema and reduce the blood pressure.

*Hypotension.* Hypotension in the setting of LVF is an unfavourable sign, particularly if blood pressure remains low after any abnormal cardiac rhythm

---

**CASE STUDY 2.1**    LVF due to ischaemic heart disease

A 62-year-old man with a previous myocardial infarct was admitted with a 3-week history of increasing breathlessness. He had no other illnesses and was only taking low-dose aspirin. His blood pressure on admission was 180/120 mmHg, the ECG showed heart strain and the chest film showed LVF. Urine testing showed proteinuria. His kidney function was normal.

Initial assessment was of a distressed and overweight man with a resting pulse of 120 beats/min which felt regular, a respiratory rate of 35 breaths/min with an audible wheeze, oxygen saturation on air of 85% and a blood pressure of 180/120 mmHg. His peripheries were cold and clammy and capillary refill time was prolonged. He complained of breathlessness but no chest pain.

The patient was propped upright and given high-flow oxygen; an intravenous cannula was inserted and blood was taken, primarily to check the kidney function, cardiac enzymes, sugar and full blood count. Arterial blood gases were checked. An ECG monitor to identify arrhythmias and an oximeter to confirm adequate oxygenation (saturations more than 90%) were attached to the patient. He was given:

- i.v. frusemide 80 mg
- i.v. diamorphine 2.5 mg
- cyclizine as an antiemetic

Oxygen saturation increased to 94% and the respiratory rate decreased to 25 beats/min; his pulse remained high at 120 beats/min. The patient passed 1 L of urine in the first 1 h of admission, but remained breathless.

An infusion of GTN was started and plans were made for a trial of an ACE inhibitor.

---

has been corrected. It can indicate heart muscle damage, it limits the type and quantity of drugs that can be used – because several cause hypotension themselves – and it can put kidney function at risk. Persistent hypotension is an indication for *inotropic support* (drugs such as dopamine, which improve cardiac performance), particularly if the urine output is inadequate.

*Evaluate the patient's pulse rate* The analysis of the patient's pulse rate is not easy from bedside observation, particularly if the patient is acutely ill, and a monitor and 12-lead ECG will be required. Nonetheless, atrial fibrillation (or its close relation, atrial flutter) is likely to be the cause of any rapid pulse of greater than 130 beats/min.

Occasionally, LVF can be accompanied by, and even caused by, an abnormally slow pulse. Drug treatment, in particular with beta-blockers, can be an important cause of this. The bradycardia resolves once the drug is withdrawn.

# CRITICAL NURSING TASKS IN ACUTE LVF

- **Ensure adequate oxygenation**
- **Measure the blood pressure**
- **Evaluate the pulse**

*Important nursing tasks in acute LVF*

**Does the patient understand and comply with the oxygen therapy?** Ensure that the patient understands the need for continuous (as opposed to symptomatic) administration of oxygen. Is this reflected by appropriate improvements in the oxygen saturation?

**Has the patient responded to the diuretic?** An immediate diuresis is a good prognostic sign, whereas failure to establish a diuresis, especially if it is accompanied by hypotension, suggests a problem with maintaining blood flow through the kidneys. It is important to exclude retention as a cause for a low output, particularly in older male patients. It is common practice to obtain an exact assessment of the urine output in critically ill patients by using a urethral catheter.

**Is the patient less breathless and in a better clinical condition?** As the treatment takes effect, the patient should become less breathless; he will be less distressed and his respiratory rate will decrease.

As the heart picks up the peripheral circulation will also improve: extremities will be less clammy and the feet and hands will warm up – capillary filling should also improve.

Acute myocardial infarction can present as acute LVF and the chest pain may be ignored in the presence of severe breathlessness. It is therefore important to enquire specifically about pain and ensure that appropriate analgesia – morphine or diamorphine – is prescribed.

**Have the blood pressure and pulse returned towards normal?** Stress-induced hypertension should fall. Hypotension, unless it is the inevitable consequence of the drugs that are needed, should improve, either in response to inotropic

## IMPORTANT NURSING TASKS IN ACUTE LVF

- **Ensure compliance with continuous oxygen**
- **Assess the response to diuretics**
- **Look for symptomatic improvement**
- **Demonstrate normalisation of the pulse and blood pressure**

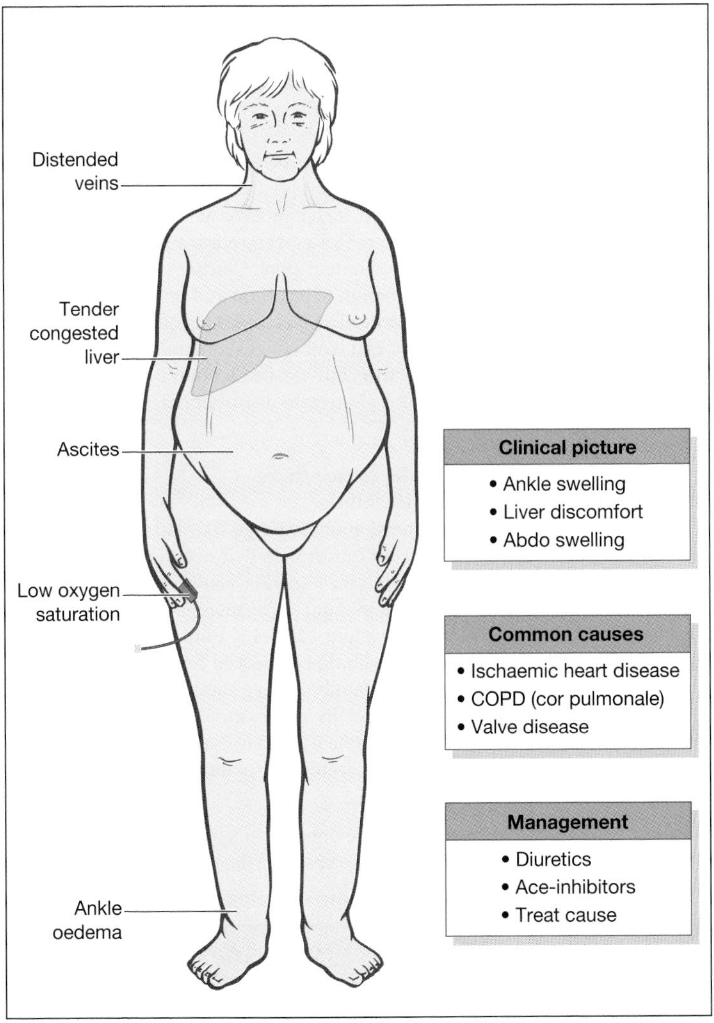

Distended veins

Tender congested liver

Ascites

Low oxygen saturation

Ankle oedema

**Clinical picture**
- Ankle swelling
- Liver discomfort
- Abdo swelling

**Common causes**
- Ischaemic heart disease
- COPD (cor pulmonale)
- Valve disease

**Management**
- Diuretics
- Ace-inhibitors
- Treat cause

**Fig. 2.5**  Congestive cardiac failure

support or spontaneously as the patient's general condition improves. Similarly, a rapid pulse should return towards normal as a result of specific treatment (digoxin, cardioversion, etc.) or as a general response to overall improvement.

## Acute on chronic congestive cardiac failure

The main clinical features of acute on chronic congestive cardiac failure are bilateral ankle oedema, debilitating tiredness and breathlessness on exertion (→ Fig. 2.5). The dominant problem is usually a progressive reduction in exercise tolerance, but in advanced failure there is overwhelming fatigue: patients can be too tired to eat, they cannot cope with personal care and even mild constipation can prove a serious challenge. Patients are often increasingly dependent and depressed, sleep patterns are disturbed (frequent arousals are a consequence of Cheyne–Stokes respiration and paroxysmal nocturnal breathlessness) and the appetite is poor. Cardiac cachexia is a state of malnutrition caused by a combination of anorexia and impaired food absorption in advanced cardiac failure. The weight loss is often accompanied by abdominal pain and swelling due to liver congestion and ascites. Nausea and vomiting can have the same cause, but are also seen in both hypovolaemia and diuretic-induced electrolyte disturbances, particularly hyponatraemia (low sodium).

*Important nursing tasks in congestive cardiac failure*
**Identify possible causes of cardiac failure**
*Uncontrolled hypertension.* Hypertension in the range 160/110 mmHg or higher can lead to cardiac failure, but unfortunately it may have been ignored or inadequately treated. Contrary to earlier views, systolic and diastolic hypertension are equally damaging – treatment is started at sustained levels of 140–160 mmHg systolic or 90–100 mmHg diastolic. If hypertension is identified, the urine should be checked for protein (hypertensive kidney damage) and a family history should be taken to identify familial kidney diseases (especially polycystic kidneys) and unexplained hypertension. Is the patient's hypertension compounded by the presence of the other main cardiac risk factors: smoking, high cholesterol or diabetes? Is there glycosuria?

*Ischaemic heart disease.* A history of a previous infarct, angina or intermittent claudication makes it very likely that the basis for the cardiac failure is ischaemia.

---

**IMPORTANT NURSING TASKS IN CONGESTIVE CARDIAC FAILURE**

- Identify possible causes of cardiac failure
- Establish the *exact* preadmission drug regimen
- Recognise significant hypotension
- Assess the lower limbs and pressure areas
- Assess the fluid balance

*Alcohol-induced cardiac failure.* Chronic alcohol abuse often leads to heart muscle damage. The importance in recognising this lies in the good response that is seen with a change in lifestyle and treatment with vitamin replacements.

*Chronic rheumatic valve disease.* Forty years ago, rheumatic fever with cardiac involvement was common in adolescents in the UK. These patients are now in their 60s and 70s, with ageing valve replacements, chronic cardiac failure, complex drug regimens and extensive hospital notes. Hospital records make extremely interesting reading in these patients and are a useful starting point.

Often, the patient's current problems have been encountered and solved before and will have been documented fully. Examples may include:

- previous episodes of cardiac failure with a documented cause (e.g. attempting to reduce diuretics)
- previous episodes of renal insufficiency triggered by drug interactions (in particular the use of NSAIDs)
- the results of a previous ACE inhibitor trial (in general, the nursing notes give a more detailed account of individual problem episodes during the course of a patient's stay than do the medical notes)
- previous experience with recurrent arrhythmias and their management
- previous problems with anticoagulant control because of intercurrent illness, antibiotic administration or some other drug interaction

**Establish the exact preadmission drug regimen** Patients with chronic heart failure are usually receiving complicated drug regimens that have undergone serial changes as the clinical condition altered. The general practitioner and the hospital clinic may have been adjusting the drugs independently, so that hospital letters and so forth may not reflect the actual situation. Even the instructions on the drug containers may not coincide with what the patient really takes. Important drug toxicity and interactions are common and often unrecognised. Examples include:

- digoxin toxicity, especially in the elderly
- warfarin overactivity due to antibiotic treatment
- electrolyte imbalance from diuretic therapy
- worsening heart failure due to the use of NSAIDs
- dangerous hyperkalaemia with spironolactone, particularly when combined with ACE inhibitors in diabetes

**Recognise significant hypotension** Hypotension is common and important in patients with acute on chronic cardiac failure: a reduced blood flow to the brain and kidneys causes lethargy, near syncope and renal failure. The two most common causes of hypotension are *fluid depletion* and *drug therapy*. Fluid depletion may be caused by:

- over-diuresis
- vomiting and poor intake due to congestion of the gastrointestinal tract and liver

- 'concealed' gastrointestinal bleeding (patients are usually receiving aspirin/warfarin)

Diuretics, nitrates, ACE inhibitors and virtually all antiarrhythmic drugs can induce postural hypotension, as can other classes of drug that may have been 'added in', notably any antidepressant.

In any cardiac patient with a low blood pressure, it is also critical to exclude two other causes: *sepsis* and *acute myocardial ischaemia*. The most common sources of infection are Venflon sites, the respiratory tract (ask the patient to cough and inspect the sputum) and the urine. A rare but serious source of sepsis in these patients is infection of the heart valves (endocarditis). An unrecognised infarct may produce a combination of heart failure and hypotension, which will usually be diagnosed from the ECG and cardiac enzyme results.

**Assess the lower limbs and pressure areas** Oedematous legs and a poor cardiac output are potent causes of poor skin nutrition, soft tissue infection and damage to pressure areas, particularly in the immobile elderly patient. In severe congestive failure, the legs may be blistered and weeping fluid, frequently on a background of chronically inflamed and eczematous ankles and calves. The feet should be examined with care, because the poor blood supply and impaired nutrition can lead to fungal infections between the toes (soggy inflamed looking skin) and even areas of local gangrene. Early dermatological advice can be extremely useful in these situations. Patients who are immobile and oedematous develop oedema over the sacrum and are very susceptible to pressure sores. This area must be assessed with care so that appropriate pressure-relieving measures can be introduced.

**Assess the fluid balance** This is a problematic area of management in patients with cardiac failure, because there is a difficult balance to be maintained between removing unwanted fluid from congested lungs while retaining enough fluid to support the circulation. The acute nursing assessment will help to differentiate fluid overload from diuretic-induced fluid depletion.

- **Symptoms of congestion** – breathlessness, PND, orthopnoea, abdominal discomfort, weight gain
- **Signs of congestion** – increased respiratory rate, ankle oedema, abdominal distension (ascites)
- **Symptoms of fluid depletion** – thirst, nausea, lethargy, postural dizziness, weight loss
- **Signs of fluid depletion** – postural hypotension, poor capillary re-fill, poor urine output

The clinical decision whether to increase or withhold diuretics and whether to restrict or push fluids depends on these basic observations in conjunction with the biochemistry results, particularly the levels of sodium, creatinine and urea. A low sodium is seen with both diuretic-induced fluid depletion and fluid overload, but only in fluid depletion will there be a progressive increase in the urea and creatinine.

## ANSWERING PATIENTS' AND RELATIVES' QUESTIONS IN CARDIAC FAILURE

*What does 'failure' mean?* The heart has been put under temporary strain as a result of infection/angina/blockage of the heart's circulation. As a result, its efficiency as a pump has tired. We are therefore trying to take the strain off the heart with a variety of drugs, bed rest and oxygen.

*What will be the signs of improvement?* The observations such as pulse rate and blood pressure will start to return towards normal. The patient will become less breathless. There will be an increase in the urine output as we get rid of some of the excess fluid on the lungs and in the legs.

*How can we help?* The patient needs complete rest – keep visitors to a minimum to start with. Encourage the patient to keep the oxygen on at all times and to stay propped up in bed. Fluids are likely to be rationed for a time.

*What about the diet and fluid intake once he is discharged?* Salt-rich foods should be avoided and salt should not be on the table or in the cooking. The main salt-rich foods are cheese, crisps, bacon, sausages and processed meat foods such as pies. Fluid intake is not usually restricted unless persistent fluid retention becomes a particular problem.

*What about weight?* If there is obesity, aim for a reduction of around 2 lb (1 kg) or so per week towards a realistic target. Weight gain can be the first sign of fluid retention (worsening heart failure) and regular weighing can be very helpful as part of the patient's follow-up care.

Provide small frequent meals perhaps (with calorie supplements if there is cachexia) and consider water-soluble vitamin supplements (B complex and C). Alcohol may be taken in moderation unless there is an alcoholic myopathy.

*What about smoking?* Smoking must be stopped immediately.

*What about exercise?* Regular non-tiring exercise should be encouraged. 'Reconditioning' with regular graded exercise will help to improve endurance in some patients with cardiac failure. This probably needs to be supervised in some form of hospital-based programme.

**Addressing compliance problems** Lack of compliance is a major factor in triggering readmissions in cardiac disease, especially in the elderly who are often on complex regimens. Side-effects, notably constipation, anorexia and confusion, make the drugs unpopular with the patients and this may be compounded by forgetfulness. It is therefore vital to discuss details of the patient's regimen with the relatives and carers.

# ISCHAEMIC HEART DISEASE

More patients present to the Acute Medical Unit with the consequences of ischaemic heart disease than with any other single condition. Atheromatous narrowing of the coronary arteries leads to cardiac failure, angina, myocardial infarction and cardiac arrhythmias (→ Fig. 2.6). Fortunately, the combination of improved treatment for established disease and the widespread introduction of preventative measures has reduced the mortality from coronary artery disease by 10% in the past decade. However, cardiac ischaemia continues to present major issues for the Acute Medical Unit: recognising its various manifestations (heart failure, chest pain, arrhythmias), dealing with atypical clinical features in the elderly, and identifying those patients who need urgent coronary care.

## CHEST PAIN

### Approach to the patient who has chest pain on the acute medical unit (→ Case Studies 2.2)

*Context*
Chest pain in a patient with a history of angina, previous myocardial infarction or any serious cardiovascular disease should be assumed to come from the heart until proved otherwise. Whereas pain in a young man with a recent chest infection and no risk factors is likely to be pleurisy, in the case of an elderly woman with a recent fall and vertebral collapse, chest pain is as likely to be referred from the back as it is to be angina. The situation in which the pain arises is as important as the nature of the pain in establishing the diagnosis.

Chest pain can be so difficult to describe that it is preferable to be overcautious in your management. After all, if the history was crystal clear, the patient would not be on the Acute Medical Unit in the first place, but in the CCU. This seems to be a particular issue in female patients in whom, for some reason, cardiac symptoms are all too often dismissed as insignificant, leading to diagnostic delays.

*Onset*
Classically, angina builds up over a few minutes into a dull, heavy, central chest ache and spreads into the jaw, upper arm or wrists. It is *not* usually localised to a single spot on the chest or associated with local tenderness; however, so-called 'atypical angina' can be positional, worsened by breathing, and may even radiate through into the back and to the upper abdomen.

Commonly used descriptions in angina include pressure, weight, chest tightness and constriction. Patients often also describe a feeling of breathlessness. Triggers on the ward include showering, temperature changes and strong emotion.

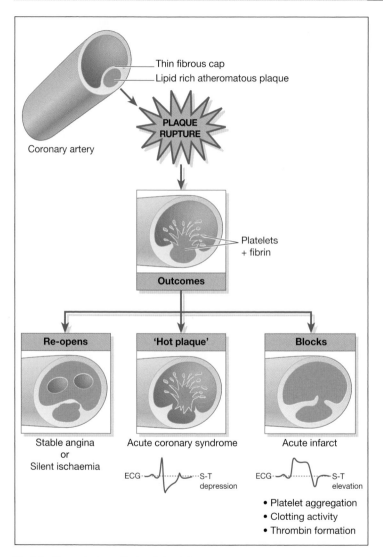

**Fig. 2.6** The mechanisms of ischaemic heart disease

**CASE STUDIES 2.2**  Myocardial infarction on the Acute Medical Unit

## CASE 1

A 75-year-old woman presented with acute sweating, malaise and mild heart burn. She denied chest pain. The ECG was done on admission but not seen for several hours: it showed an acute inferior myocardial infarction. Patients with an atypical history slip through the net. On a CCU the emphasis is on 'door to needle time' in administering thrombolytics with no delay to the true infarcts. In the Acute Medical Unit there will be delays because, by their nature, these patients are atypical. A system of triage is needed.

## CASE 2

A 90-year-old lady awoke with a left-sided stroke. She was alert and denied any chest pain. Her ECG showed a recent inferior infarction and her cardiac enzymes were elevated.

Common reasons for worsening angina on the Acute Medical Unit are:

- anaemia (e.g. recent upper GI bleed, anaemia due to cancer or chemotherapy)
- sudden onset of atrial fibrillation
- stress of acute illness (especially exacerbations of COPD)

*Other important symptoms and signs*
Serious anginal episodes are accompanied by pallor, sweating and hypotension. Prolonged pain, lasting for more than 15 min, especially if it is accompanied by nausea and vomiting, is more in keeping with an infarction than with angina, although the distinction can be difficult, particularly in the elderly.

In the elderly, the symptoms of acute ischaemic heart disease are often atypical and include:

- breathlessness without pain
- acute confusion
- dizziness
- abdominal pain
- syncope

It should be remembered that around one in four acute myocardial infarcts are painless or unrecognised by the patient. This is a particularly common situation in patients with diabetes.

*Why obtain an ECG while the patient is in pain?*
A resting ECG should be recorded during any episode of acute chest pain or discomfort. There will usually be changes during an attack of angina

indicating a temporary reduction in the blood supply to the heart muscle. Persistence of ischaemic changes after the pain has resolved suggests either unstable angina or an actual infarction.

## ENZYME MEASUREMENTS IN CHEST PAIN

The diagnosis of a myocardial infarction is based on three elements: the history, the ECG and measurements of cardiac enzymes in the blood. The CK level increases within 6 h of the infarct, peaks at 24 h and normalises after 96 h. Increased CK concentrations are also seen after falls, with intramuscular injections, in muscle inflammation and after epileptic fits: CK-MB levels can be measured if there is any doubt, as these are specific for cardiac muscle. The AST level shows a similar time course, but is even less specific for cardiac muscle.

Measurement of the troponin T levels has revolutionised the management of patients with chest pain. Even minor cardiac muscle damage (so called micro-infarction) releases troponin T into the blood. Increased concentrations identify a subset of patients who do not have enough damage to warrant immediate thrombolytics but have a risk of death or acute infarct that is four times greater than if they had pain, but normal troponin T levels.

---

**Aggressive intervention in these patients is an urgent priority.**

---

## ACUTE CORONARY SYNDROME (PREVIOUSLY KNOWN AS UNSTABLE ANGINA)

*What is an acute coronary syndrome?*
Myocardial infarction occurs as a result of rupture of an atheromatous plaque, triggering thrombosis, complete arterial blockage and death of cardiac muscle. Instability of a plaque before actual rupture results in rapidly worsening chest pain, termed an acute coronary syndrome. The pattern in an acute coronary syndrome is usually of increasing exertional pain, culminating in prolonged pain at rest. If the troponin T levels are increased, aggressive intervention with antithrombotic agents such as low molecular weight heparin (enoxaparin), the new i.v. glycoprotein IIb/IIIa inhibitors and urgent angioplasty benefit such patients and prevent the progression to myocardial infarction.

*What are the other causes of acute chest pain?*
Pleurisy is severe and stops the patient from moving around the bed or taking a full breath. In the frail elderly, rib fractures and vertebral collapse are common causes of acute severe intractable pain. These are seen after falls, with severe coughing and in osteoporotic patients. Oesophageal pain and

biliary colic can both easily be confused with heart pain. Musculoskeletal pain is positional and is not usually severe. The pain from shingles, however, can be extreme and often appears a day or so before the rash is recognised.

### When to call the medical staff

At-risk patients have cardiac-sounding pain, may be in the convalescent period from a recent infarct, or may have a definite past history of cardiovascular disease. If these patients have rest pain, there should be liaison with the medical staff, particularly if the pain is associated with ECG changes or a decrease in blood pressure. Unstable angina needs active and immediate intervention, probably in a CCU. Such patients, if left on a general ward, do worse in terms of time to thrombolysis, treatment of serious arrhythmias, management of acute haemodynamic changes and their chances of survival from a cardiac arrest.

### When to try GTN

A patient with known angina will be familiar with their pain and can advise you whether any particular episode is unusually severe or prolonged. Their 'usual' angina can be treated with simple sublingual GTN, but the patient must first be assessed for the severity and frequency of their attacks.

### What to say to the patient

'We may have to "nip this problem in the bud" using anticoagulants, i.v. nitrates and so forth. You must report any further chest pain to the nursing staff immediately.'

## ROLE OF THROMBOLYSIS AND ASPIRIN IN ISCHAEMIC HEART DISEASE

A myocardial infarction occurs when an atheromatous plaque suddenly ruptures and triggers local thrombosis, which blocks off the coronary artery completely. Irreversible cardiac muscle death starts within 45 min of the blockage, and the sooner the vessel can be re-opened (re-perfusion) the less the damage and the lower the mortality. The patient should be given aspirin 150–300 mg to chew as soon as there is a suspicion of an acute infarct. Once there is definite ECG confirmation, thrombolysis must be started *without delay*. Maximum benefit is seen in the first 6 h after the onset of pain, but is particularly high in the first (or 'golden') hour. For every hour that passes after the onset of pain, the benefit derived from thrombolysis decreases (→ Fig. 2.7). Intravenous streptokinase is the thrombolytic most commonly used in the UK; the alternative regimen, rt-PA followed by 48 h heparin, is used if streptokinase has been given between 5 days and 2 years previously, as the body will have been primed to produce streptokinase-neutralising antibodies. Except under exceptional circumstances, thrombolytic therapy for

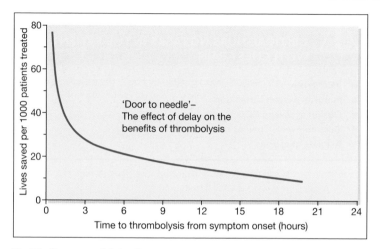

**Fig. 2.7** 'Door to needle': the effect of delay on the benefits of thrombolysis

an acute infarct should be administered on a CCU, where the staff are trained to deal with any complications (re-perfusion arrhythmias, bleeding, allergic reactions) and to assess the response. However, techniques for re-perfusion continue to evolve, and the recent confirmation that urgent PCI involving balloon angioplasty is superior to thrombolysis may well change the approach and organisation of acute coronary care.

Case Study 2.3 illustrates the management of a patient with breathlessness and chest pain.

### Critical nursing tasks in the patient with chest pain

*ABC triage* Chest pain with hypotension and arterial desaturation needs urgent/immediate medical attention. The possible causes in a collapsed patient include a myocardial infarct and a pulmonary embolus; a less common cause is acute aortic dissection.

**Monitor oxygen saturation** Maintain saturations above 90% using high-flow oxygen.

**Obtain a 12-lead ECG** This is useful to confirm a myocardial infarction or unstable angina. A normal ECG is not particularly helpful in ruling out other conditions. The way to gain the most information from an ECG is to compare it with others from the case record.

**Take an overall look at the patient** If the patient is stable, a more measured approach can be used. However, this is not the case if:

## CRITICAL NURSING TASKS IN THE PATIENT WITH CHEST PAIN

- ABC triage
- Monitor oxygen saturation
- Obtain a 12-lead ECG
- Take an overall look at the patient
- Ask key questions

1. the pain sounds anginal and has lasted more than 20 min
2. the patient is also breathless – i.e. pulmonary oedema or pulmonary embolus
3. the blood pressure has dropped
4. the pain is taking place soon after an infarct

Severe angina, myocardial infarction or pulmonary embolus produce a pale, sweaty and clammy patient. A patient who cannot take a full breath because of pain probably has pleurisy. Biliary colic makes the patient roll around the bed in pain.

### Ask key questions

- Where is the pain and where does it radiate?
- What makes it worse (deep inspiration, minor exertion such as showering)?
- What relieves it (e.g. GTN, breathing shallowly)?
- Has it occurred before? Is it like your usual angina/previous heart attack, etc.?

**CASE STUDY 2.3** Breathlessness and chest pain

An 83-year-old man, an independent retired widower, was admitted at 18.00 h with a 4-h history of increasing breathlessness. There had been no response to nebulised salbutamol, which he had tried at home.

He had COPD and, because of an exacerbation, he had been receiving antibiotics and oral steroids for 3 weeks prior to admission.

*Initial assessment.* On admission he was distressed, dyspnoeic and frightened. His oxygen saturations were 87% on high flow oxygen. Respiratory rate 36 breaths/min. His pulse was 120 beats/min and regular. His blood pressure was 170/120 mmHg. There was a severe wheeze and mild ankle oedema. He had been given sublingual GTN and high-flow oxygen by the paramedics. His current medication was:

- uniphyllin (dose unknown)
- inhalers of salbutamol, (Becotide®) and salmeterol
- nebulised ipratropium (Atrovent®) and salbutamol (Ventolin®)

His ECG showed a tachycardia and mild left heart strain. His blood gases on 28% oxygen showed an acceptable $pO_2$ (of 9.4 kPa) and normal $pCO_2$. Chest film showed mild congestion.

### Initial diagnosis

- Exacerbation of COPD
- Possible left ventricular failure

Correctly, the paramedics had considered a cardiac cause for his symptoms and tried GTN. A painless myocardial infarction would have to be excluded with ECGs and cardiac enzymes.

It can be difficult to decide in the emergency situation what is the relative contribution from COPD and the initial management may have to target both conditions. The priority at this stage is:

- to maintain oxygenation
- to correct any reversible underlying cause (LVF, arrhythmia, bronchoconstriction)

*Management.* The patient was propped upright and reassured. 28% oxygen was administered and a cardiac monitor was put in place. He was given:

- i.v. *frusemide* 80 mg
- nebulised *salbutamol* 5 mg (caution is needed if acute cardiac ischaemia is a suspected possible diagnosis as salbutamol can overstimulate the heart – this dose may have been too large)
- i.v. *hydrocortisone* (for presumed bronchoconstriction)
- oral *ampicillin* (if there had been pneumonia on the chest film this would have been given intravenously to a patient as ill as this)

Theophylline levels were checked urgently:

- to guide the further aminophylline doses if they are needed
- to exclude theophylline toxicity as the cause for his marked tachycardia

(continued)

The patient had an immediate diuresis; this was charted and a strict fluid balance chart was started.

**Progress.** At 02.00 h the patient became more breathless and cyanosed. He was sweating profusely and looked extremely unwell. He complained of anterior chest pain that had started 30 min before.

**Assessment.** The patient was severely distressed. His saturations were 75% on 28% oxygen, respiratory rate 40 breaths/min, pulse 140 beats/min and regular, and blood pressure 170/75 mmHg. His abdomen was soft and non-tender and there was no sign of acute urinary retention. (Intra-abdominal catastrophes such as a ruptured aortic aneurysm can present in the elderly with acute sudden cardiovascular deterioration. Acute retention is common in men of this age after i.v. diuretics.)

The ECG had not changed, neither had the chest film. The possibilities at this stage were:

- worsening respiratory failure
- increasing LVF
- possible acute myocardial infarction

The oxygen delivered was changed to 60% (in the acutely deteriorating patient, correcting hypoxia takes precedence over all other considerations). The patient was given:

- i.v. *frusemide* 120 mg i.v.
- i.v. *diamorphine* 2.5 mg i.v. for chest pain and LVF (this must be used with extreme caution in patients with a possible respiratory component to their illness as it will depress ventilation)
- an *aminophylline* infusion was started (the initial theophylline level was in the normal range so a loading dose was not given). Aminophylline has the advantage of working in both pulmonary oedema and bronchoconstriction, although it is not generally used as first-line treatment in either situation.

A decision was made to consider ventilation if the patient did not improve (using information about his previous level of independence and health from the admission assessment). His relatives were contacted and brought in.

The patient's arterial blood gases at this stage showed an acceptable oxygen level but, possibly as a result of the diamorphine, an increasing $pCO_2$. His oxygen mask was changed again to 28% and he was given two further 120 mg doses of

| Table 2.1 Cardiac enzymes from Case study 2.3 | | | |
|---|---|---|---|
| Enzyme level (IU/L) | Day 1 | Day 2 | Day 3 |
| AST | 30 | 129 | 93 |
| CK | 114 | 559 | 354 |

**CASE STUDY 2.3** *(continued)*

i.v. frusemide. By 07.00 h after a significant diuresis there was significant and continued improvement. He was eventually well enough to be discharged back to his home.

Subsequent cardiac enzymes (Table 2.1) showed that he had suffered an acute myocardial infarction, which had presumably caused the sudden deterioration in the early hours of the first morning after his admission.

# SUDDEN CARDIAC DEATH

Sudden Cardiac Death describes a sudden collapse, usually in ventricular fibrillation, ventricular tachycardia or asystole. There are few warning symptoms, perhaps a few seconds of chest tightness, palpitations or weakness. The outlook is variable, with the best survival rates seen in patients experiencing witnessed in-hospital arrests in which the rhythm is ventricular fibrillation or ventricular tachycardia – of whom 20% will leave hospital alive.

Ischaemic heart disease is responsible for 70% of SCDs, and although it may be the first symptom, more commonly it occurs during the first 12 months after an acute myocardial infarction. The use of preventative measures post-infarct, particularly in patients with poor left ventricular function, has had a significant impact on reducing the incidence of SCD. A typical regime in a high risk case would consist of:

- an ACE inhibitor or an angiotensin II receptor antagonist
- a beta-blocker
- spironolactone
- intensive statin therapy
- aspirin

There is increasing interest in preventing SCDs with ICDs. These would be considered, for example, in high-risk survivors of cardiac arrest such as those with poor left ventricular function and in whom electrophysiological testing demonstrates instability of their cardiac rhythm.

# ATRIAL FIBRILLATION AND ARTERIAL EMBOLI

Normally, the heart beats in an orderly fashion and is led in this by the rhythmic activity of the SA node. Each atrial contraction is followed immediately by that of the ventricles. The SA node establishes the heart rate

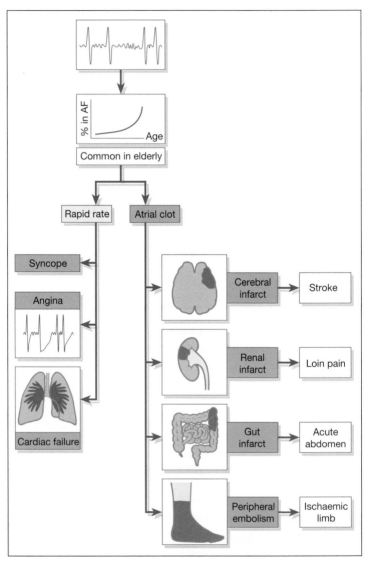

**Fig. 2.8** Atrial fibrillation

through the rhythmic discharge of a small electrical impulse that spreads, wave-like, through each atrium, producing atrial contraction. The impulse then passes through the AV node and continues onwards to initiate ventricular contraction. Thus, if the SA node is firing regularly 75 times per minute, the AV node will in turn be activated at the same rate, leading to a regular ventricular response (and, of course, pulse rate) of 75 contractions per minute.

In atrial fibrillation (→ Fig. 2.8), organised atrial activity is replaced by random electrical impulses which spread chaotically through the atrium. The atrium responds by muscular activity that can be described as a shivering motion (fibrillation), rather than a coordinated contraction. There are two important consequences:

- The atrial 'squeeze', which expels the final 10% of the blood into the ventricle at the end of diastole, is lost. This loss can be important, particularly if the ventricle relies on atrial contraction to ensure it is properly filled, for example when the valve between the atrium and ventricle is already narrowed (as in mitral stenosis).
- The AV node is activated at random by the chaotic atrial electrical activity at rates of anything between 60 and 140 times per minute. The ventricles respond to this random activation accordingly, and produce irregular pulse rates within this wide range. Clearly, an irregular heart rate of 140 beats/min will not be tolerated by the heart for long.

Thus atrial fibrillation reduces cardiac output (→ Box 2.2).

---

**Box 2.2 – Why atrial fibrillation reduces cardiac output**

- Loss of atrial contraction
- Ventricular response too rapid
- Irregular ventricular rate

---

## CAUSES OF ATRIAL FIBRILLATION

Cardiac failure from whatever cause can be associated with atrial fibrillation. The most common situations in which atrial fibrillation is seen on the Acute Medical Unit are:

- the ageing heart (10% of all those older than 75 years old are in atrial fibrillation)
- ischaemic heart disease
- chronic heart-valve disease
- binge alcohol drinking
- atrial fibrillation triggered by hypoxia or infection in COPD

Atrial fibrillation can also be triggered by an acute myocardial infarction and by a pulmonary embolus.

Atrial fibrillation can occur in a normal heart; indeed, this is the case in around 50% of all patients with recurrent attacks of atrial fibrillation (paroxysmal atrial fibrillation). In these patients, such short-lived episodes are extremely unpleasant but relatively harmless; only when they are prolonged is there a risk of embolic complications.

## IMPORTANCE OF ATRIAL FIBRILLATION

### Uncontrolled atrial fibrillation

*Cardiac failure*
Atrial fibrillation itself can cause right and left heart failure if the ventricular rate is excessive. This is particularly the case in elderly patients. More commonly, the onset of atrial fibrillation in someone with pre-existing valvular or heart muscle disease will tip the patient into cardiac failure (→ Case Study 2.4).

*Angina*
Uncontrolled atrial fibrillation can reduce the blood supply to the heart muscle and trigger angina simply because there is not enough time for adequate coronary artery blood flow to occur. The reverse may also occur – an attack of ischaemia can trigger atrial fibrillation – so it is important to take a good history to see which came first, the pain or the palpitations.

*Syncope and near syncope*
The cardiac output may decrease suddenly in acute atrial fibrillation, sufficiently to reduce cerebral blood flow, leading to syncope or presyncope. This is a particular risk if there are existing problems with blood flow because of either aortic valve stenosis or disease in the carotid arteries (→ Case Study 2.5).

---

**CASE STUDY 2.4** Sudden atrial fibrillation in unrecognised mitral stenosis

A 68-year-old woman was admitted severely breathless, coughing up copious frothy pink sputum characteristic of pulmonary oedema. Her pulse rate was 145 beats/min and irregular and her blood pressure was 70/40 mmHg. Her oxygen saturation was 70%.
   The patient was treated with high-flow oxygen and i.v. diuretics. Her atrial fibrillation was controlled with i.v. digoxin (electrical cardioversion was considered but she improved rapidly with initial treatment and it was unclear from the history how long the atrial fibrillation had been present). Subsequent examination and investigation demonstrated tight mitral stenosis. There was no history of cardiac disease but she had had rheumatic fever as a teenager.

> **CASE STUDY 2.5**  Aortic stenosis and paroxysmal atrial fibrillation with syncope
>
> A 68-year-old man was admitted as an emergency with a 4-month history of feeling unwell and collapsing to the floor. Some of the episodes were accompanied by fast palpitations. On the day of admission he had a rushing feeling in his head and collapsed to the floor. His wife said that he was grey and clammy and stayed unconscious for around 10 min. There were no convulsive movements. When he came round he was slightly confused and had been incontinent of urine.
>
> The only finding on admission was a murmur coming from what was thought to be a stenosed aortic valve. The patient's pulse was normal at 86 beats/min. Three hours after admission he suddenly went into rapid atrial fibrillation and felt very faint. His atrial fibrillation stopped without treatment after 2 min but it was followed by a long pause on the ECG during which time the patient felt worse.
>
> He was referred to the cardiologists and urgently transferred to the CCU. A cardiac echo showed severe aortic stenosis.

There are several important issues in Case Study 2.5. The patient's old hospital records showed he had previously been investigated for unexplained blackouts. Some had been associated with transient atrial fibrillation, but his heavy alcohol intake had been blamed for this. The murmur had been heard, but not investigated. Aortic stenosis is a common valve problem and usually results from degenerative calcification of a congenitally abnormal valve. Rheumatic valve disease is a much less common cause of aortic stenosis. The stenosis leads to three symptoms: increasing angina, recurrent syncope and sudden death. All are a manifestation of obstruction to the flow of blood out of the left side of the heart. If undiagnosed, it can eventually lead to LVF. Critical stenosis is potentially lethal, yet easily managed with valve replacement – a diagnosis not to be missed. In this patient, the atrial fibrillation combined with the stenosis led to syncope and the excess alcohol intake may well not have been of immediate relevance, except for obscuring the true nature of the problem.

*Sudden atrial fibrillation causing hypotension during severe illness*
(→ Case Study 2.6)

Acute atrial fibrillation can cause a sudden decrease in the blood pressure and, if this decrease occurs in the setting of a severe illness, it can be misinterpreted as hypovolaemia or sepsis.

In a sick patient, it can be difficult to tell whether a severe tachycardia is the primary cause of a low blood pressure or whether, along with the hypotension, it is one of the effects of the acute illness.

## Complications of atrial fibrillation

*Atrial fibrillation and the formation of left atrial clots*
Unfortunately, blood stagnates in a fibrillating atrium and is liable to clot. A clot that breaks loose can, in the case of those originating in the left atrium, have disastrous consequences: *stroke* as a result of cerebral embolus, *kidney damage* as a result of renal emboli, and *acutely ischaemic limbs* as a result of peripheral vessel emboli.

---

**CASE STUDY 2.6**  Sudden atrial fibrillation

A patient was admitted with severe diabetic ketoacidosis: blood sugar 55 mmol/L, pH 6.85 and an unrecordable blood pressure. His pulse rate was 140 beats/min and was initially misinterpreted as a normal rhythm. He was given aggressive fluid replacement with no improvement in his blood pressure. After 4 h, his heart rhythm suddenly reverted from what was now clearly rapid atrial fibrillation to sinus rhythm. His blood pressure immediately increased to 110/70 mmHg.

---

Of these complications, the risk of embolic stroke is much the most important and is quite common – approaching 5% of patients in atrial fibrillation per year. The risk of stroke is particularly high in those older than 65 years, especially if there are other risk factors present such as diabetes, cardiac failure, hypertension and previous cerebrovascular disease. This group of patients will be considered for anticoagulation as soon as atrial fibrillation has been diagnosed.

## DIAGNOSIS OF ATRIAL FIBRILLATION

Atrial fibrillation causes a chaotically irregular pulse, which can be fast or slow. If the ventricle is contracting quickly and irregularly, the amount of blood expelled with each beat will vary and the very weak beats will not be palpable at the wrist. This produces a deficit between the apical rate (measured with a stethoscope at the apex) and the rate measured by palpation at the wrist.

This is a common pitfall in uncontrolled atrial fibrillation – the pulse can be 80 beats/min at the wrist and 130 beats/min at the apex. *If the pulse feels irregular, measure both the apical and the radial rates.*

## MANAGEMENT OF ATRIAL FIBRILLATION

Unless there is a contraindication, most patients in atrial fibrillation will be started immediately on anticoagulation using low-molecular weight heparin. The choice then lies between:

- observation
- converting the atrial fibrillation to a normal rhythm (cardioversion)
- controlling the atrial fibrillation by slowing the ventricular rate

Management options are summarised in Box 2.3.

> **Box 2.3 – Management options in atrial fibrillation**
>
> - Immediate anticoagulation and observation
> - Immediate anticoagulation and rate control with digoxin (+ other drugs if required)
> - Immediate anticoagulation and cardioversion
> - Immediate anticoagulation and planned cardioversion in 3 weeks

**Observation** This would be appropriate for the first 24 h in a patient with slow atrial fibrillation in whom the rhythm was not compromising cardiac function.

**Cardioversion** It is possible to convert atrial fibrillation to a normal rhythm by using drugs (chemical cardioversion) or by a synchronised shock (electrical cardioversion). In general, in rapid atrial fibrillation of recent onset (less than 48 h), cardioversion is the treatment of choice, particularly if the abnormal rhythm is having an adverse effect on the patient. The sooner that cardioversion is tried, the better the chances of success. Unless the situation is critical, drugs are tried before a synchronised shock is attempted – the two drugs that are most commonly used are i.v. flecainide and i.v. amiodarone.

If atrial fibrillation has been present for longer than 48 h, it is essential to anticoagulate the patient for at least 3 weeks before attempting cardioversion, because of the risk of dislodging a clot from the left atrium. Rather surprisingly, the evidence suggests that patients with well established atrial fibrillation fare just as well from control of the ventricular rate as they do from re-establishing normal rhythm with cardioversion.

**Controlling atrial fibrillation** In many acute situations, the duration of the atrial fibrillation will be unclear, and urgent cardioversion could put the patient at risk from an embolus. As untreated, rapid atrial fibrillation compromises the heart, it is preferable to control the rate using digoxin as first-line therapy, adding other drugs such as beta-blockers if necessary. Digoxin is absorbed rapidly when given orally and will act within hours; however, in acutely ill patients it is frequently given i.v. for an even more rapid onset.

To prevent emboli, once the atrial fibrillation is controlled the choice is between aspirin and warfarin as long-term therapy. Low-risk patients are given aspirin, as their chances of emboli are very small.

- Low-risk patients
  — no previous emboli/stroke
  — non-diabetic

— non-hypertensive
— younger than 65 years
— no valve disease

High-risk patients are treated with warfarin long-term anticoagulation, as there is a high incidence of emboli.

● High-risk patients
— previous emboli
— hypertension
— diabetic
— those with heart failure
— age over 75 years

*Atrial fibrillation in the elderly.* Atrial fibrillation is present in almost 10% of the population over 80 years of age and is associated with a high risk of complications – there is a sixfold increased risk of emboli and atrial fibrillation is implicated in one-third of all strokes in this age group. Although long-term warfarin therapy has dangers in the elderly, particularly in those experiencing confusion and recurrent falls, it also has major benefits, with large reductions in the risk of stroke, provided that there is careful selection of the patient and monitoring of the anticoagulant control.

---

**CASE STUDY 2.7**  Atrial fibrillation induced by alcohol

A 43-year-old man was admitted to hospital as an emergency at 03.00 on a Sunday morning, complaining of palpitations and chest tightness. He had consumed two bottles of red wine and three pints of beer during the course of a dinner party the evening before. He was awoken at 02.00 h with rapid palpitations and chest tightness. The past history was negative but he drank on average, 30 units of alcohol per week and smoked 20 cigarettes per day.

On admission the patient was anxious with an irregular pulse of 110 at the wrist and 140 beats/min at the apex. Blood pressure was 160/90 mmHg and full examination was negative. The chest film was clear and the 12-lead ECG confirmed atrial fibrillation with no evidence of a myocardial infarction.

He and his wife were reassured that this was probably not a heart attack, he was monitored and blood was taken for cardiac enzymes and biochemistry. He was started on subcutaneous low-molecular weight heparin and a decision was made that, as this was a short-lived arrhythmia (and hence there had not been time for a clot to form in the left atrium), it would be safe to try cardioversion, initially with an i.v. infusion of the drug, flecainide. Fortunately, while waiting for the results of his blood tests his monitor showed a sudden return to sinus rhythm with immediate relief of his symptoms. Cardioversion was not needed.

A cardiac echogram was arranged, to look at the heart valves and heart muscle function, and he was discharged home with an appointment for the cardiology clinic. He was strongly advised to moderate his alcohol consumption to prevent any recurrence.

*Atrial fibrillation induced by alcohol.* Case Study 2.7 describes the management of a patient whose atrial fibrillation was caused by excess alcohol intake. The important points from this case study are:

- Alcohol itself can directly trigger atrial fibrillation and is the precipitating factor in up to a quarter of cases of acute atrial fibrillation (it can also eventually damage the heart muscle by causing thiamine deficiency).
- Up to half of all cases of first-time atrial fibrillation will return to a normal rhythm without treatment.
- If the atrial fibrillation is new (less than 48 h old), there is little risk of a clot having formed in the left atrium and cardioversion can be tried without first giving prolonged anticoagulation.
- The alternative to cardioversion would have been to control the rate of atrial fibrillation initially with digoxin, if necessary adding a beta-blocker or verapamil.

### Critical nursing tasks in atrial fibrillation

The aim of the nursing assessment is to document the effect that the atrial fibrillation is having on the patient, and hence to determine the urgency of the situation. If atrial fibrillation is causing angina, hypotension or heart failure, then corrective action is necessary as soon as possible. Slow atrial fibrillation with no acute complication may simply require a period of observation.

**Assess the rate of the atrial fibrillation** Atrial fibrillation at a pulse rate of 80–100 beats/min is unlikely to cause acute cardiac decompensation, whereas at 130–140 beats/min problems will arise. It is important to document both the apical and the radial rate. In uncontrolled atrial fibrillation, not all the apical impulses are conducted to the radial pulse, which leads to a difference between the rates (pulse deficit); this gap narrows as the heart rate comes under control with treatment.

**Identify chest pain** A history of chest pain may mean that the atrial fibrillation has been triggered by an ischaemic episode or even by a myocardial infarction. More commonly, however, rapid atrial fibrillation can cause rate-related anginal pain.

**Look for heart failure** Symptoms of breathlessness, particularly on lying flat, and associated with signs of an increase in respiratory rate and bilateral ankle oedema, suggest that the atrial fibrillation is causing, or contributing to, cardiac failure.

**Document hypotension** Sudden rapid atrial fibrillation can decrease the blood pressure acutely. This can have a critical impact, especially if the atrial fibrillation is complicating further major acute illness such as pneumonia or diabetic ketoacidosis.

**CRITICAL NURSING TASKS IN ATRIAL FIBRILLATION**

- Assess the rate of fibrillation
- Identify chest pain
- Look for heart failure
- Document hypotension

*Important nursing tasks in atrial fibrillation*

**Watch for emboli caused by the atrial fibrillation** The three areas particularly prone to emboli are the brain, limbs and intestine – presenting as stroke-like illness or sudden confusion, acute painful, pale and pulseless limbs and, particularly in the elderly, an acute abdomen.

**Identify factors that could have triggered the atrial fibrillation** Common non-cardiac causes of acute atrial fibrillation are pneumonia, exacerbations of COPD and any source of sepsis, particularly if there is pyrexia.

**Obtain an accurate drug history** The name and doses of all cardiovascular drugs need to be recorded. This is especially important for digoxin (under- or over-treatment can cause problems with uncontrolled atrial fibrillation), oral theophyllines (over-treatment is a potent cause of any arrhythmia) and anticoagulants. Regimens will often need to be cross-referenced with information from relatives and from the GP's surgery.

**IMPORTANT NURSING TASKS IN ATRIAL FIBRILLATION**

- Observe for emboli (brain, limbs, gut)
- Look for non-cardiac triggers
- Obtain an accurate drug history

**ANSWERING RELATIVES' QUESTIONS IN ATRIAL FIBRILLATION**

*What is it and why is it important?*

Atrial fibrillation is a prolonged irregular heart rhythm. It makes the heart pump less efficiently and can cause the blood to stagnate and form potentially dangerous clots. It is often temporary, especially if it has been triggered by some other acute illness.

*How will it be treated?* If it is troublesome, we can slow the pulse down to normal with drugs or try and jolt the heart back into a normal rhythm using either an injectable drug (flecainide/amiodarone) or a small electrical impulse delivered under an anaesthetic ('synchronised DC shock'). While the pulse is irregular, we will keep the blood watered down with heparin/warfarin to prevent it clotting.

# INFECTIVE ENDOCARDITIS

Infective endocarditis is a serious condition in which there is infection of the heart valves, usually the mitral or aortic valve. In the past, only damaged or mechanical valves have been involved, but the increasing incidence of i.v. drug abuse has put even normal heart valves at risk. Other major risk factors are advanced age, diabetes and recent dental, operative and endoscopic procedures, which can result in bacteria entering the bloodstream.

Infective endocarditis is a serious acute medical problem. The affected valve may fail suddenly as it is destroyed by infection. Pieces of infected material can break off and spread via the blood to vital organs, resulting in:

- foci of sepsis, especially in the kidneys
- septic cerebral emboli (stroke-like illness)

## HOW INFECTIVE ENDOCARDITIS PRESENTS

*Pyrexia of unknown origin*
The picture is of severe malaise associated with night sweats and generalised aches and pains. Usually there will be a known valve lesion, valve replacement or previously diagnosed congenital heart defect.

---

**CASE STUDY 2.8**   Endocarditis and intravenous drug abuse

A 45-year-old man with a history of previous drug abuse (which was only obtained 2 days after admission) was admitted with severe pleurisy, haemoptysis and widespread shadowing on his chest film. The provisional diagnosis was multiple pulmonary emboli, and treatment was started with heparin.

The patient's condition deteriorated suddenly and, on the basis that this could be pneumonia, i.v. ampicillin and erythromycin were started. He remained severely hypoxic, deteriorated further and died.

The autopsy finding was a staphylococcal endocarditis involving the tricuspid valve – a typical finding in bacterial endocarditis caused by the use of infected intravenous needles (the infection passes through the veins to the right side of the heart, and when infected particles break off the tricuspid valve, they embolise to the lungs).

*Catastrophic valve failure*

Infection can destroy a cardiac valve and even form an abscess within the heart muscle or in the conducting system. This can lead to devastating cardiac failure, particularly in the case of the aortic valve, and the patient can deteriorate acutely, with sudden pulmonary oedema and hypotensive shock.

*Infected emboli*

The history here is of a recent feverish illness complicated by the acute onset of a stroke (cerebral embolus), ischaemic limb (large vessel embolus) or, in the case of right-sided endocarditis, infected pulmonary emboli as described in Case Study 2.8.

## ROLE OF THE ACUTE MEDICAL UNIT IN SUSPECTED ENDOCARDITIS

**Prompt investigation of any illness accompanied by fever** Infected heart valves shed bacteria into the bloodstream, resulting in positive blood cultures. If endocarditis is suspected, then three sets of blood cultures taken at 5-min intervals on two consecutive days should be taken. The urine should also be cultured.

**Recognition of high-risk patients** These include patients with valve disease or congenital heart disease admitted to hospital with fever or unexplained deterioration, and illicit drug users with breathlessness and fever.

**Appropriate action on finding proteinuria and haematuria** In endocarditis, microemboli of infected material lodge in the kidneys and set up an inflammatory response. As a result, blood and protein appear in the urine. Clearly, in patients with fever, haematuria and proteinuria are more likely to indicate a simple urinary infection; nonetheless, if other risk factors are present this finding can be critical in guiding the medical staff towards the correct diagnosis.

*Principles of management in the first 24 h*
**Ensure the safety of the patient**

- treat cardiac failure
- treat any arrhythmia
- involve the cardiologists and the microbiologists

**Secure the diagnosis**

- identify at-risk patients
- take several blood cultures (avoid the casual use of antibiotics on the ward)
- conduct urine testing and culture
- examine the valves (cardiac echo)

**Initiate antibiotic therapy**

- insert i.v. lines
- monitor antibiotic levels

**Prepare the patient for a 'long haul' of antibiotic therapy (several weeks)**

- take particular care with Venflon sites

**Observe for complications**

- look for antibiotic allergy
- look for left heart failure (breathlessness, respiratory rate, oxygen saturations, pulse, blood pressure)
- monitor temperature
- measure urine output
- look for septic emboli (any sudden event, e.g. confusion, stroke, cold limb)

# DRUGS IN THE MANAGEMENT OF ACUTE HEART DISEASE

*Intravenous frusemide*
*Lasix*

**Indications**
*Acute pulmonary oedema*
*Severe congestive cardiac failure*

- Frusemide is a well tolerated and powerful diuretic with a very wide dose range – from 20 mg to 250 mg or more. Low doses are used in patients not previously exposed to the drug; higher doses are needed with patients taking oral frusemide, patients with renal failure and patients with severe heart failure.
- Diuresis starts within 10 min of the i.v. dose, although it is also a vasodilator and may act even more quickly on pulmonary oedema by causing blood to pool in the peripheries.
- As well as advantages, there are also dangers of a sudden diuresis: this may precipitate acute retention, causing hypovolaemic hypotension and sudden electrolyte changes (predominantly urinary potassium loss).
- For doses greater than 50 mg, the rate of i.v. administration should not exceed 4 mg/min, to avoid the risk of acute hearing disturbance.

*Intravenous nitrates*
*Isosorbide dinitrate (Isoket), glyceryl trinitrate (Nitrocine)*

**Table 2.2 Characteristics of intravenous nitrates**

| Drug parameters | Nitrocine | Isosorbide |
|---|---|---|
| Infusion strength* | 100 µg/ml | 100 µg/ml |
| Starting rate angina | 10 µg/min | 15 µg/min |
| Starting rate LVF | 20 µg/min | 30 µg/min |
| Step up rate every 30 min | 10–20 µg/min | 15–30 µg/min |
| Maximum dose | 100–200 µg/min | 300 µg/min |

* Data sheets must be used with care when preparing the admixture of the drugs and the saline or dextrose vehicle. For example, isosorbide is provided in 0.05% and 0.1% strength ampoules and the examples used in the preparation instructions express the doses in *mg per hour* (2-20 mg per hour). In contrast, the doses for Nitrocine are expressed in *mcg per minute*. Local protocols are invaluable in these situations.

### Indications
*Unstable angina*
*Acute left ventricular failure*

- Nitrates have three important actions: they dilate the coronary arteries, they unload the heart by reducing the load against which it pumps (peripheral arterial dilatation), and they increase pooling of blood in the veins (which unloads the right side of the heart). They are therefore useful in both angina and cardiac failure.
- Patients rapidly develop tolerance to nitrates, so the initial dose may have to be increased repeatedly to overcome this (→ Table 2.2).
- There is a risk of hypotension with i.v. nitrates, particularly when the heart is already in a parlous state. However, this property can be useful in acute LVF associated with hypertension.
- The advantage of the i.v. infusion of nitrates is that the onset of action is immediate and the dose can be titrated continuously to balance haemodynamics (the blood pressure and pulse) with the beneficial clinical response.
- As i.v. nitrates are incompatible with PVC infusion sets (Viaflex, Steriflex) they must be administered through polyethylene or glass containers.

### Digoxin
### Indications
*Atrial fibrillation*
*Cardiac failure*

- The major beneficial effect of digoxin is to slow down the ventricular response to atrial fibrillation and atrial flutter. It does this by slowing the conduction of electrical impulses through the AV node.
- Digoxin increases, albeit to a modest degree, the strength of the heartbeat.
- Rapid control of atrial fibrillation requires i.v. loading:

*0.75 mg to 1 mg of digoxin in 50 ml of fluid over 2 h*

- Lower doses are needed in the elderly, in renal failure and in those who have received digoxin within the past 2 weeks.
- Oral digitalisation can be achieved over 24 h using divided doses of the total loading dose of 1.0–1.25 mg.
- The symptoms of digoxin toxicity (drug levels more than 3 mg/L) are anorexia, nausea, vomiting and an abnormally slow pulse (less than 50 beats/min). Toxicity is more likely if there is potassium deficiency from diuretic therapy.

### ACE inhibitors
*Captopril, enalapril, lisinopril*

**Indications**
*Cardiac failure*
*Hypertension*
*Post myocardial infarct*
*Diabetic renal disease*

- ACE inhibitors have proved an important advance in the treatment of heart failure and hypertension. They improve survival and symptoms in heart failure and after myocardial infarction, and they have a beneficial effect on diabetic renal disease.
- Their use requires close supervision – particularly in the elderly, those with intercurrent illness and those in cardiac failure – because they can adversely affect kidney function through their mode of action, which is to inhibit mechanisms that are normally in place to protect renal blood flow (the renin–angiotensin system).
- First-dose hypotension is a recognised problem, but is usually relieved by lying the patient down. The hypotensive response can be exaggerated in the patient who has severe cardiac failure and is already receiving high-dose diuretics. A small test dose should be given and the blood pressure monitored for 2 h.

### Intravenous amiodarone
**Indications**
*Rapid termination of serious arrhythmias*
*(rapid atrial fibrillation/flutter, ventricular tachycardia)*

- Amiodarone is unusual in that it is an effective antiarrhythmic drug that does not depress the function of the heart. It is therefore relatively safe to use in heart failure, when it is the drug of preference in the critically ill patient with life-threatening arrhythmias.
- The drug causes local phlebitis. Although the loading dose can be given through a peripheral vein, the follow-up 24 h continuous infusion needs a central line.

- The loading dose is 5 mg/kg (usually 300 mg) in 250 ml 5% dextrose over 20 min.
- The infusion dose is 15 mg/kg (usually 1.2 g) in 500 ml 5% dextrose over 24 h.
- Once there is a response, the infusion is replaced, if indicated, by oral amiodarone.
- There are several important drug interactions, notably with warfarin and digoxin, and some potentially serious side-effects on the thyroid gland, lungs and liver. Most of these are associated with long-term rather than acute therapy.

## FURTHER READING

### HEART FAILURE

Lonn E, McKelvie R 2000 Drug treatment in heart failure. British Medical Journal 320: 1188–1192

Millane T, Jackson G, Gibbs CR, Lip GYH 2000 ABC of heart failure: acute and chronic management strategies. British Medical Journal 320: 559–562

Stewart S, Marley JE, Horowitz JD 1999 Effects of a multidisciplinary home-based intervention on unplanned readmissions and survival among patients with chronic congestive heart failure: a randomised controlled study. Lancet 354: 1077–1083

### ATRIAL FIBRILLATION

Lip GYH, Beevers DG, Coope JR 1996 Atrial fibrillation in general and hospital practice. British Medical Journal 312: 175–178

### ISCHAEMIC HEART DISEASE

Edmondstone WM 1995 Cardiac chest pain: does body language help the diagnosis? British Medical Journal 311: 1660–1661

Maynard SJ, Scott GO, Riddell JW, Adgey AAJ 2000 Management of acute coronary syndromes. British Medical Journal 321: 220–223

# RESPIRATORY MEDICINE

## INTRODUCTION

Respiratory emergencies are a major source of work on the acute medical unit. Their management is based on two fundamental clinical issues:

- the assessment and relief of breathlessness
- the prevention and treatment of respiratory failure

This chapter explains the basic principles underlying these two areas and then applies them to the assessment and management of the types of respiratory cases that you will encounter on a day-to-day basis: asthma, COPD and pneumonia.

## THE BREATHLESS PATIENT: THE GENERAL APPROACH

*Is this patient's breathlessness due to his heart or his lungs?*
The two most important and most difficult questions in a breathless patient are always:

- is this cardiac or respiratory breathlessness?
- is this a pulmonary embolus?

Differentiating the causes of breathlessness can be very difficult, and the history and examination will not always provide an answer. Symptoms and signs are shared by many of the common respiratory and cardiac conditions. Thus a patient with LVF and a patient with acute asthma will both have nocturnal breathlessness and severe wheeze. Ankle swelling is characteristic of congestive heart failure, but it can also be a complication of severe COPD. The difficulties are often age related. If a young person presents with a history of intermittent wheeze, breathlessness and cough, the diagnosis is almost certain to be asthma; but what about the obese, wheezy, 70-year-old smoker with previous myocardial infarcts and chronic venous disease in both legs? Why is the patient short of breath? COPD? Pulmonary oedema? Pulmonary embolus?

*What tests will be needed to make the right diagnosis?*
It can be helpful to remember a few ground rules about the investigation of patients with unexplained breathlessness.

- In breathlessness caused by COPD and asthma:
  — the chest X-ray may be normal, it may show overinflation, but it will not show pulmonary oedema
  — the PFR and spirometry will always be very abnormal

- In breathlessness caused by LVF:
  - the chest X-ray will show pulmonary oedema
  - the ECG is abnormal, showing ischaemia, strain or an arrhythmia
  - a cardiac echogram will confirm poor left ventricular function
- In breathlessness caused by pulmonary emboli:
  - the diagnosis is often missed, usually because it is not considered
  - risk factors are usually present (recent surgery, phlebitic legs, etc.)
  - when in doubt, anticoagulate and scan the lungs to confirm later

*Principles of management*
The principles of emergency treatment are set out in Box 3.1 below. It must be recognised, however, that on occasions in a critically ill patient with unexplained breathlessness it may be appropriate to cover a number of diagnostic options until the picture becomes more clear and the results of further tests become available.

| Box 3.1 – Principles of emergency treatment | |
|---|---|
| 1. Correct the immediate and life-threatening problems | |
| —Hypoxia | Oxygen |
| | Ventilation |
| —Acidosis | Correct high arterial carbon dioxide |
| —Hypotension | Fluids ± inotropic support |
| 2. Treat the cause | |
| —Pulmonary oedema | Diuretics |
| | Vasodilators |
| —Bronchoconstriction | Bronchodilators |
| | Steroids |
| —Pulmonary embolism | Anticoagulants |
| —Pneumonia | Antibiotics |
| —Tension pneumothorax | Intercostal drain |
| 3. Prevent further attacks | |
| —Asthma | Education |
| —Pulmonary oedema | Review previous cardiac therapy |
| —Pulmonary embolism | Warfarin |

# RESPIRATORY FAILURE

Normal ventilation is a process in which fresh air is brought through the airways to the alveoli, where it is in intimate contact with blood in the pulmonary capillaries. Gas exchange occurs across the alveolar–capillary interface: oxygen passes from the alveoli into the blood and carbon dioxide passes from the blood into the alveoli. We measure blood gas partial pressures to assess the efficiency of this two-way traffic: the arterial $pO_2$ tells us about oxygenation; the arterial $pCO_2$ indicates how well the lungs are venting carbon dioxide.

Respiratory failure describes a state in which the lungs can no longer oxygenate the blood, and is diagnosed by measuring the arterial blood gases. Conditions that interfere with any part of the process of normal ventilation may cause respiratory failure. Examples from the acute medical unit include: patients who depress their respiratory drive with drug overdosage; patients with progressive paralysis (the most common example is the Guillain–Barré syndrome), in whom respiratory muscles become increasingly weak and ineffective; and, by far the most common causes, acute asthma and COPD, in which there is direct impairment of gas exchange as a result of lung damage.

## TYPE I AND TYPE II RESPIRATORY FAILURE

The lungs are more efficient at venting carbon dioxide than they are at oxygenating blood. As a result, during the development of respiratory failure, problems with oxygenation occur well before carbon dioxide starts to build up. When things start to go wrong, the patient compensates for lesser degrees of carbon dioxide retention by increasing ventilation and blowing off the build-up of carbon dioxide. Thus, if you look at the blood gases in a case of acute asthma, you will find that, in the early stage of an attack, carbon dioxide levels in the blood are often lower than normal.

Unfortunately, this compensatory mechanism does not work at all well for problems with oxygenation. You will find, for example, that arterial oxygen levels decrease early on in an attack of asthma. Several conditions have a similar pattern of *hypoxia without carbon dioxide retention*: this pattern is termed 'Type I' respiratory failure (→ Fig. 3.1 and Box 3.2). (Look at ward blood gas results in some of the conditions mentioned in Box 3.2 – in Type I respiratory failure the arterial $pO_2$ is less than 8 kPa, with a normal or low carbon dioxide at 4 kPa or less. (You need to remember that these figures apply to patients whose gases are measured while they are breathing room air; once oxygen is given to patients with Type I respiratory failure, the $pO_2$ increases.)

With more advanced disease in which the compensatory mechanism of trying to blow off carbon dioxide has 'worn out', *carbon dioxide retention occurs in addition to hypoxia*. This is Type II respiratory failure ($pO_2 < 8$ kPa, $pCO_2 > 6$ kPa while not receiving oxygen; → Fig. 3.1). Examples are listed in Box 3.3; the patient in Case study 3.1 has Type II respiratory failure.

---

**Box 3.2 – Examples of Type I respiratory failure**

- The early part of an attack of asthma
- The thin breathless emphysematous patient
- Pneumonia
- Pulmonary oedema (LVF)
- Pulmonary embolism

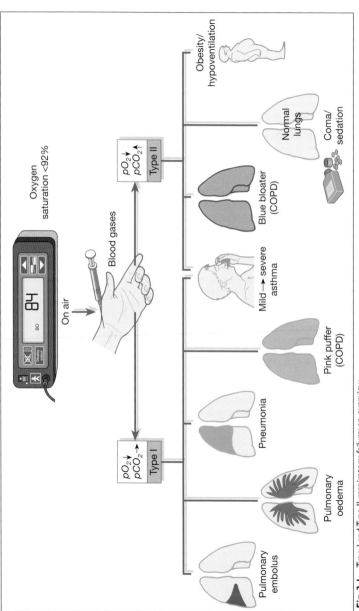

**Fig. 3.1** Type I and Type II respiratory failure: an overview

---

**Box 3.3 – Examples of Type II respiratory failure**

- Severe life-threatening asthma (Type I failure progresses to Type II failure)
- The obese oedematous patient with severe COPD
- Respiratory centre depression in a severe drug overdose
- Obesity/hypoventilation syndrome

---

**CASE STUDY 3.1**   Confusion and falls due to respiratory failure

A 68-year-old non-smoking woman was admitted because of increasing drowsiness following a fall at home. The emergency doctor thought she had probably had a stroke.

She and her husband led 'separate lives' at home but he said that she had become increasingly immobile and had taken to sleeping in an armchair over the previous 3 years. Her only medication was a mild diuretic. After a fall in her bedroom she had not been able to get up and became increasingly difficult to rouse.

On admission she was drowsy and uncooperative; she was morbidly obese and deeply cyanosed. Her respiratory rate was five breaths per minute and she was wheezy; her legs, thighs and abdomen were grossly oedematous. There was no evidence of a head injury or any focal neurological signs. Her chest film was normal. Her arterial gases showed a $pO_2$ of 4.5 kPa, a $pCO_2$ of 16 kPa and a pH of 7.1. A diagnosis of severe Type II respiratory failure due to a combination of obesity/hypoventilation syndrome and asthma was made.

The anaesthetists declined to ventilate her and attempts at NIV (→ p. 0; Ventilatory support in COPD, ) were only partially successful. Intravenous doxapram infusion, 24% oxygen and a combination of twice daily high-dose frusemide and aminophylline were started. With considerable difficulty she was nursed in a sitting position. On this regimen she had a marked diuresis with reduction of her oedema, although with a negative deficit of 10 L she still weighed 150 kg. She became increasingly alert and started to cough up purulent sputum. She slowly mobilised and lost weight over several weeks on the continuing care ward.

---

**Hypoxia and hypercapnia: the blood gases.**   Carbon dioxide is a central nervous system depressant, its build up (termed hypercapnia) leading to a cycle of confusion, lack of cooperation, increasing drowsiness and hence further carbon dioxide retention. Hypoxia impairs the function of the heart, brain and kidneys. The combination of excessive carbon dioxide (hypercapnia) and the tissue hypoxia causes an *acidosis* that produces its own damaging effects on major organ function. (The pH in the blood gas results reflects the degree of tissue acidosis. A pH of less than 7.3 in respiratory failure indicates a major problem and a pH of less than 7.25 requires urgent and aggressive intervention to improve gas exchange.)

*Principles of treatment*

For the treatment of respiratory failure to be effective, it must reverse the process by correcting the cause, which, depending on the disease, may include any combination of:

- airway narrowing
- respiratory muscle weakness
- alveolar damage
- respiratory infection
- impaired respiratory effort

Before vital organ function is compromised, the blood gases must be corrected, at the simplest level by giving additional oxygen and in more complex cases by assisting or even replacing normal respiratory efforts. The introduction of new forms of 'non-invasive' (i.e. the patient does not need endotracheal intubation) respiratory support, now means that selected patients with quite severe respiratory failure can be managed on the acute medical unit with a 'half-way house' type of ventilation. This approach does not have the implications of full ITU treatment with the problems of endotracheal tubes, weaning, hospital-acquired infection and so forth.

**Pulse oximetry.** The oximeter measures the oxygen saturation in the arterial blood. The range of values for a normal saturation is small: thus a saturation of 97% is seen in the healthy population, whereas a saturation of 90% can indicate impending respiratory failure. The pulse oximeter is invaluable in recognising early respiratory failure, particularly when readings are taken on admission, before the patient has been given oxygen. You must remember, however, that the oximeter only measures oxygen saturation – it will tell you nothing about the level of carbon dioxide or the degree of acidosis.

**Why and when do we do blood gases?** Oxygen saturations will be low in all cases of respiratory failure. Only the blood gases will tell you whether this is Type I or Type II respiratory failure. In acute asthma, for example, there is a world of difference between the patient with hypoxia and a normal $pCO_2$ and the patient who is similarly hypoxic but, having passed from acute asthma to near exhaustion, is now retaining carbon dioxide. If you are in doubt about the severity of the patient's condition, examine the blood gases. As a general rule, in Acute Medical Unit patients, arterial blood gases must be checked when the oxygen saturations are less than 92% with the patient breathing room air (you will all see patients with severe Type II respiratory failure who have been given unlimited oxygen on their way in to hospital: the oxygen saturations look wonderful at 97%, but the gases reveal grossly increased levels of carbon dioxide).

## ACUTE SEVERE ASTHMA

Acute asthma continues to be a major challenge to the team on the acute medical unit. The assessment must be quick and accurate, and the treatment has to be tailored to the severity of the attack. The patient's condition can change dramatically and, unfortunately, there is still a significant mortality rate.

### MECHANISMS

*Who gets acute severe asthma and why?*
Any patient with asthma may have an acute attack, but those at a special risk of dying from acute asthma are:

- those who are non-compliant with therapy and follow-up
- those who have previous acute/near-fatal attacks
- those who are poor at recognising the severity of their asthma
- those with a strong history of allergy who are exposed to a high allergic load
- those who normally require regular oral steroids
- those with a history of brittle asthma
- those with serious psychosocial problems

The number of acute exacerbations per year in which asthma treatment has to be intensified is a useful marker of the severity and control of the underlying asthma. The patient in Case Study 3.2 had been getting attacks of nocturnal breathlessness for months, but had not appreciated their significance.

---

**CASE STUDY 3.2**   Acute severe asthma

A 38-year-old man had had asthma for 30 years. Contrary to medical advice his only treatment was occasional inhaled salbutamol. He described chronic sleep disturbance from early morning wheezing, but even the presence of frequent symptoms did not dissuade him from the view that 'normal people like him' should not need to rely on inhalers. His asthma worsened over 2 weeks in spite of oral steroids. After a day of exposure to building dust and grass cuttings he became severely breathless and collapsed. He was admitted after his wife dialled 999.

---

Three major factors narrow the airways in acute asthma:

- airway muscle contraction
- thickening of the airway wall with inflammatory cells
- airway clogging by thickened secretions

**CASE STUDY 3.2** (continued)

The patient was too breathless to speak and unable to tolerate a mask. The peak flow could not be recorded. He was clammy with quiet breath sounds and a pulse rate of 160. He was given high-flow oxygen, nebulised bronchodilators and i.v. steroids. Emergency blood gases with the patient breathing oxygen showed a $pO_2$ of 5.6 kPa, a $pCO_2$ of 16 and a pH of 6.9. A portable chest film showed no sign of a pneumothorax.

Without inhaled steroid treatment, the patient's airways will have been chronically inflamed (→ Case Study 3.2). Uncontrolled airway inflammation in asthma is a potent cause for persistent symptoms and repeated severe attacks.

*What goes wrong during an attack?*
As an attack develops, breathing becomes progressively more difficult because the patient has to drag and push air through increasingly narrow tubes. Air becomes trapped behind the blocked tubes so that the lungs over-inflate, making the work of breathing even harder. There are two consequences as the asthma attack progresses:

- gas exchange worsens
- the muscles used for breathing start to fatigue

The abnormal gas exchange, if uncorrected, goes through two phases.

1. Early in an attack of asthma, a combination of necessity and fear drives breathing sufficiently hard to blow off carbon dioxide. At this point, the levels of carbon dioxide in the blood are normal or low. In contrast, oxygen uptake is impaired and there is hypoxia, even at this early stage.

The patient in Case Study 3.2 had already passed this stage by the time he was admitted to hospital.

2. Later, *as breathing tires*, carbon dioxide builds up, oxygen levels continue to decrease and the patient's condition becomes critical. The increase in carbon dioxide, which can be rapid and dramatic, now causes a sudden and dangerous decrease in the blood pH. If this is unchecked, a respiratory arrest will follow.

The implications for emergency management are to identify the patients who are at risk:

- those who are tiring (history, observation and blood gases)
- those with severe airway narrowing (peak expiratory flow rate)
- those with hypoxaemia (oxygen saturation) and a build-up of carbon dioxide (blood gases)

## ASSESSMENT OF ACUTE SEVERE ASTHMA

**History.** By its nature, acute asthma must be assessed quickly. You must find out from the history whether the patient is in a high-risk group. Four features will warn you of likely difficulties:

- previous severe attacks, AED attendance and hospital admissions with asthma
- patients who are taking, or who have previously needed, steroid tablets
- recent nocturnal attacks (a major sign that the asthma is out of control)
- a history of psychosocial problems, non-compliance, self-discharge, substance abuse

It is unusual for the patient to *over*estimate the severity of their attack. Patients like that in Case Study 3.2 who are panicking and uncooperative are far more likely to be doing so because of impending asphyxia than because of over-anxiety.

**Examination.** The signs of severe asthma must be recognised:

- a pulse rate of more than 110 beats/min
- a respiratory rate of more than 25 breaths/min
- the patient is too breathless to complete a sentence in one breath

A common sequence leading to respiratory arrest is of a desperately breathless patient who becomes ashen, clammy and quietly 'cooperative'. The chest becomes quiet, the pulse slows and respiratory efforts become increasingly feeble. You may have seen patients who are poor at perceiving the severity of their own attacks, and noted how they can pass from the severe to the life-threatening stage with little apparent fuss.

The signs of *life threatening asthma* are any one of:

- oxygen saturations of less than 92%
- cyanosis
- a silent chest with feeble respiratory effort and exhaustion
- increasing confusion or a reduction in conscious level
- a bradycardia or arrhythmia
- hypotension
- PFR less than one-third of their best or their predicted

**Peak flow rate.** The PFR is the simplest and most important objective way to assess acute asthma and to monitor the effectiveness of treatment (→ Fig. 3.2). It must be measured in every case; most patients can produce a reading. However, even the observation that the patient is 'too breathless to do a peak flow' is a clear indication of the severity of the asthma.

It is important to try and find out how the patient is when at their best. There is a world of difference between an admission peak flow of 250 L/min in a steroid-dependent asthmatic patient who never blows better than 275 L/min, and a peak flow of 250 L/min in a previously 'mild' asthmatic

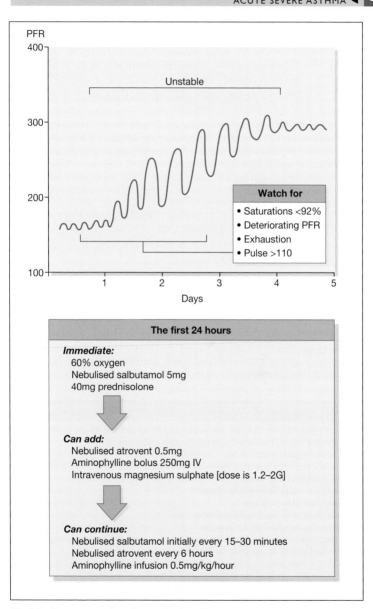

**Fig. 3.2** Acute severe asthma. †Ipratropium bromide

individual who is used to peak flows of 550 L/min. This information may be available in their hospital case notes, GP records and in home peak-flow diaries. *The best ever peak flow* is not necessarily the same as the *predicted peak flow*, but both values are useful to decide the current state of the patient's asthma. To know the predicted PFR you will need a table giving the normal value for a person of the same height, age and sex. These tables should be freely available on the Acute Medical Unit.

- An initial PFR of less than 50% of the predicted value or, if available, 50% of their best ever PFR reading indicates severe asthma. Peak flows down to one-third of these values indicate life-threatening asthma. As a rough guide, acute severe asthma is associated with PFR readings of less than 300 L/min for most males and less than 200 L/min for most females.
- The change in PFR with emergency treatment predicts the likely course of events.
- The subsequent PFR chart shows the level of asthma control and stability. Peak flows seesaw as an attack resolves (Fig. 3.2). Patients are particularly vulnerable during the morning dips in PFR, which occur during the first 2–3 days after an acute attack.

## NURSING THE PATIENT WITH ACUTE ASTHMA

The balance between resuscitation and communication will depend on your initial assessment. A patient with an unrecordable peak flow, a pulse rate of 140 beats/min and an oxygen saturation of 75% will not welcome a discussion on preventative inhalers. He will, however, be terrified by his suffocating breathlessness and will be desperate for your reassurance that he

---

**Box 3.4 – Reassurance for patients with acute severe asthma**

- I will measure your PFR; we will treat you and we will see how it improves.
- The hard work of breathing will lessen with treatment.
- You will regain control of your breathlessness soon.
- We will stay with you until the treatment works.
- We will sort things out for you – try and relax if possible.
- Find your most comfortable position.
- Slow your breathing rate.
- Take deep slow breaths through the mask.
- Allow the nebuliser to do its work.
- If the mask is too claustrophobic we can use oxygen tubing to your nostrils.
- The nurses and doctors will be here near you at all times.
- Call us if your breathing seems to be getting more difficult.
- Don't worry about all the noises from the monitors and drips.
- The oximeter shows that you are getting enough oxygen into your lungs.
- Steroid side-effects will be minimised by the short course that you need.

is not going to stop breathing and die (→ Box 3.4). There will be excellent educational opportunities, before the patient is discharged, and while the attack is fresh in the patient's mind. Your approach will be tailored to the individual patient. There will be an obvious difference between the communication issues in a case of chronic asthma with repeated admissions to hospital and the case of a new asthmatic presenting with their first attack. There will also be sometimes surprising similarities, not least in the most basic of requirements: the understanding and practical use of inhalers.

*Critical nursing tasks during the acute attack*

**Give reassurance and support.** Take the patient through the ways in which each aspect of his treatment acts to bring the attack to an end and enables him to regain control of his breathing (→ Box 3.4).

**Explain.** Explain the importance of effective, continuous oxygen therapy. Show the patient how to use the nebuliser and how to perform a peak flow reading. Explain how the patient can get immediate assistance from the staff.

**Minimise the work of breathing.** Provide effective and timely asthma medication. Sit the patient up in his most comfortable position (this will often involve the patient wanting to sit up, either leaning over a bed table or on the edge of the bed).

### CRITICAL NURSING OBSERVATIONS IN ACUTE ASTHMA

- Pulse rate
- Respiratory rate
- PFR
- Oxygen saturation (preferably before oxygen is started)
- Ability to complete a sentence

### IMPORTANT NURSING OBSERVATIONS IN ACUTE ASTHMA

- Blood pressure (may be increased by anxiety)
- Urine dip stick (for steroid-induced diabetes)
- Sputum colour (wallpaper glue sputum is common in asthma)
- Temperature (a sign of respiratory infection)
- Inhaler technique (critical for future management)

## CRITICAL NURSING TASKS DURING THE ACUTE ATTACK

- Give reassurance and support
- Provide explanations
- Minimise the work of breathing
- Monitor the patient's progress
- Plan to prevent this happening again

**Monitor the patient's progress.** This may need to be continuous for the critical first hour or so. Beware of an increasing pulse rate, decreasing peak flow and a tiring patient. Do not be falsely reassured by a normal oxygen saturation if the patient looks awful. Just before a respiratory arrest, many asthmatic patients become quiet, clammy and cooperative.

**Plan to prevent this happening again.** Identify why this attack occurred. Start a re-evaluation of the patient's long-term management that can be taken over by appropriate follow-up arrangements.

## MANAGEMENT OF ACUTE SEVERE ASTHMA

### Initial emergency treatment

- **Bronchodilators** (to increase airway calibre). Nebulised salbutamol 5 mg combined, if there are life-threatening features, with nebulised ipratropium 0.5 mg.
- **Corticosteroids** (to reduce airway inflammation). Intravenous (i.v.) hydrocortisone 100 mg and/or 40–50 mg oral prednisolone.
- **Oxygen** (to correct gas exchange). High-flow oxygen at 40–60% and oxygen-driven nebulisers.

**Subsequent treatment**  If there is no improvement by 15 min:

- repeat the salbutamol and ipratropium
- consider a single dose of i.v. magnesium sulphate 1.2–2 g over 20 min
- continue to give nebulised salbutamol every 15 min (alternatively use a special nebuliser to give continuous salbutamol at 10 mg/h)
- consider i.v. aminophylline 250 mg over 20 min. Particular care is needed in choosing the doses, especially if the patient has been taking theophyllines as his usual asthma therapy. Start an infusion of aminophylline 750–1500 mg over 24 h. Check daily theophylline levels

**Assessing response**

*Following the PFR and oximetry.* The key to assessment lies in a measurement of PFR. This is done on admission and, while the patient is in the unstable phase, at 15-min intervals. Thereafter, measure the PFR before and after bronchodilator treatment at least four times per day. Oximetry is monitored with the aim of keeping the oxygen saturations above 92%.

*Repeating the blood gases.* During the first few critical hours, you may need to use the arterial blood gases if there is any doubt about the patient's progress. Thus the blood gases should be repeated 2 h after the start of treatment (or earlier) if:

- poor blood gases on admission ($pO_2$ < 8.0 kPa, with a normal or high $pCO_2$)
- saturations cannot be kept above 92%
- the patient's condition deteriorates

*Transfer to Intensive Therapy Unit?* If the patient is tiring, confused or drowsy, if the PFR is deteriorating or unchanged and the patient feels worse, *and particularly if the pCO₂ is increasing and the pH is decreasing*, you should prepare to move the patient to the ITU (→ Case Study 3.2). Respiratory arrest, when it complicates acute asthma, occurs with alarming speed and always poses a major challenge to the resuscitation team. With proper assessment and by monitoring the response to treatment, you can avoid this complication.

---

**CASE STUDY 3.2**   (continued)

The patient was transferred immediately from the Acute Medical Unit to ITU and ventilated for 48 h. His peak flows thereafter slowly improved on 40 mg of prednisolone and nebulised salbutamol. He continued to have early morning wheezing for the next four mornings which required extra nebulisers before his symptoms slowly improved. He was transferred to the chest unit.

---

*A good response to treatment.* In most cases you will see a rapid response to treatment. Salbutamol and ipratropium can be reduced to 4–6-hourly. The PFRs increase and the patient will feel better. However, if you examine the PFR charts of patients who are recovering from acute asthma, you will often see that, despite a trend of improvement, the readings continue to fluctuate for several days. These patients remain at risk, particularly in the early morning when their peak flows are at their lowest. You will find that some asthma guidelines use the degree of variation in PFR between the morning and evening as an indication that the patient is fit to be discharged from hospital.

## EXCELLENT ASTHMA CARE

- Use of British Thoracic Society guidelines for the treatment of acute asthma
- Admission peak flow rates recorded
- Blood gases measured if saturations under 92% and appropriate action taken
- Serial PFRs documented
- The documentation of 'best ever' lung function (PFR or spirometry)
- Referral for follow-up to a respiratory nurse or chest team
- Review of educational needs, compliance and self-management plans for each patient

## ANSWERING RELATIVES' QUESTIONS IN SEVERE ASTHMA

The patient's relatives will have found this as frightening as the patient, and will also need reassurance. You may need to address several issues with them.

*Should we have acted sooner?* Examine their understanding of asthma. Establish if they were aware of a self-management plan. Consider referral to the asthma service or recommend up-to-date written information (e.g. National Asthma Campaign leaflets).

*Was there anything else that we could have done?* Had the patient been underestimating the severity of his asthma? Had there been over-reliance on the reliever medication? What were the methods used to assess the severity of the attack? What about the use of rescue steroid medication?

*The patient has been under stress – is it all nerves?* Provide reassurance about the physical nature of asthma. Any 'nervous' component is almost certainly an effect rather than a cause of the asthma. Ensure that the patient's visitors do not have an adverse effect on his management, particularly in the early stage when cooperation with oxygen therapy, nebuliser treatment and so forth is critical.

*Could any of his other medication upset the asthma?* Examine and list all of the patient's medication. Some drugs such as aspirin, non-steroidal anti-inflammatories and beta-blockers (tablets, or beta-blocker-containing eye drops) can worsen asthma. Assess the patient's compliance with his asthma medication.

## UPPER AIRWAY OBSTRUCTION: NOT TO BE CONFUSED WITH ASTHMA

Upper airway obstruction also produces severe airway noise and breathlessness. Although it can be difficult, a distinction in these cases must be made from acute severe asthma (→ Case Studies 3.3 and 3.4).

---

**CASE STUDY 3.3** Acute epiglottitis

A 35-year-old man had flu-like symptoms for 5 days, culminating in a severe sore throat. For 24 h he could not swallow fluids and had a hoarse voice. On admission he was flushed, pyrexial and breathless. He had a harsh superficial inspiratory and expiratory upper airway noise (*stridor*), which was easily heard at the mouth. He could open his mouth but could not swallow his saliva. His tonsils were inflamed but not particularly enlarged. His PFR was 250. Based on the characteristic history and examination a diagnosis of acute adult epiglottitis with impending respiratory obstruction was made. Intravenous antibiotics were started and he was transferred, accompanied by a competent anaesthetist, to the ENT unit for close observation and upper airway management.

---

**CASE STUDY 3.4** Stridor and haemoptysis due to tracheal cancer

A 55-year-old male smoker was admitted with increasing breathlessness, panic attacks and noisy breathing. On direct questioning he admitted to occasional haemoptysis. He had a virtually unrecordable peak flow. Bronchodilators were ineffective and it became clear his wheeze was in fact stridor. At bronchoscopy his trachea was narrowed to a pinhole at its mid point by a carcinoma. Urgent laser treatment and chemotherapy produced an excellent symptomatic response.

---

# CHRONIC OBSTRUCTIVE PULMONARY DISEASE

## MECHANISMS

*What is COPD?*

The term COPD describes patients who suffer from long-standing airflow obstruction but in whom the response to bronchodilator therapy, no matter how intensive, is either absent or incomplete. The airflow obstruction is predominantly fixed, so most of the patients have symptoms that vary little from day to day or from week to week. Acute exacerbations occur when infection temporarily worsens the airflow obstruction.

**CASE STUDY 3.5** Acute exacerbation of COPD

A 67-year-old man was admitted with breathlessness, general weakness and a productive cough. He had smoked 20 cigarettes a day since his late teens but had given up 3 months previously. He had been 'chesty' for more than 10 years with wheeziness and chest tightness. Colds always went to his chest, leaving him with a prolonged cough with green sputum. He eventually retired in his late 50s because of respiratory problems: a chronic cough, frequent chest infections and increasing breathlessness on exertion. For 2 weeks his cough and wheeze had worsened, he had become weaker and his ankles had started to swell. He had suffered a myocardial infarction 2 years previously and had occasional attacks of angina. He had also been troubled by chronic varicose veins complicated by a venous ulcer. A widower, he lived alone.

COPD embraces a spectrum of cases that range from the steroid-dependent chronic asthmatic patient to the heavy-smoking chronic bronchitic individual with advanced emphysema. The 'mix' in any one patient with COPD concerns how much is asthma (reversible) and how much is irreversible smoking-related damage to both the alveoli (emphysema) and the small airways (→ Case Study 3.5).

There are three elements to COPD, all of which are seen in Case Study 3.5.

1. **Asthma**. This provides the responsive component to the airflow obstruction, which will improve with aggressive bronchodilator treatment. The patient will exhibit wheeze and chest tightness. There will be features of airway irritability: tightness on exposure to cold air and fumes and an early morning wheeze.
2. **Chronic bronchitis**. A smoking-related condition in which there is a long-standing productive cough as a result of the formation of excessive mucus (phlegm) in the lungs. This is usually worse in the winter months. When the mucus becomes infected, the airflow obstruction temporarily worsens.
3. **Emphysema and small airway damage**. These are fixed changes in the structure of the lungs. In emphysema, the alveoli are destroyed and the lung's elastic supporting tissue is lost. Airways collapse through loss of support and the lungs over-inflate to try and hold them open. Patients with over-inflated lungs appear barrel-chested and, to prevent airway collapse, breathe out through pursed lips: a common sign in severe emphysema that becomes particularly obvious during acute exacerbations.

The combination of airway damage and alveolar destruction disrupts the primary function of the lungs: the exchange of oxygen and carbon dioxide between the air and the blood. Too much disruption and the patient becomes hypoxic (blue) and loses the battle to blow off carbon dioxide; a combination described previously and termed Type II respiratory failure.

## COPD complicated by cor pulmonale

Why did the patient in Case Study 3.5 develop ankle oedema, and why is it of such importance to his future management? Patients who are chronically hypoxic eventually develop fluid retention. A major reason for this is the increased strain on the right side of the heart that occurs because the heart has to force blood through abnormal lungs. The first sign of fluid retention, the development of ankle oedema, often occurs (as in the case study) during an acute exacerbation of COPD. The presence of ankle oedema should act as a warning to take a more aggressive approach to the treatment of the underlying lung disease. Right-sided heart failure that occurs as a result of lung disease is known as cor pulmonale. The most common cause of cor pulmonale is COPD, but it can occur in the setting of any chronic severe lung disease.

## Long-term oxygen therapy

Patients with COPD who develop cor pulmonale can be helped by long-term oxygen therapy, which is administered for 15 h per day or more. By correcting the underlying problem, hypoxia, the length and quality of the patient's life can be improved. Once the patient in Case Study 3.5 has recovered from the exacerbation, he should be referred to the respiratory team for possible long-term oxygen therapy.

## Assessment of acute exacerbations of COPD

Patients with COPD who are ill enough to be admitted to hospital during an exacerbation do not fare particularly well. The in-hospital mortality is around 10% and only 50% of the patients will still be alive 2 years after the exacerbation. Information from the initial assessment will help discussions on possible ventilation should the need arise, but such decisions are fraught with difficulty. The patients most in need of ventilation are least able to give a good history. Relatives' information is vital, but may not be objective. There has to be particular caution when a patient such as that in Case Study 3.5 comes in, who is not previously known to the hospital service. Quite often, the patient has been on suboptimal treatment and may do well once the crisis is passed. The prognosis in patients with COPD does not seem to depend on whether they require emergency ventilation, but more on the severity of their pre-existing lung disease.

## History in COPD

Important points in the history are:

- exercise tolerance when the patient is well and during exacerbations (use the MRC breathlessness scale; → Table 3.1)
- the number of exacerbations per year
- previous hospital admissions and their outcome
- any history of ankle oedema
- co-morbidity, especially heart disease
- is the patient using nebulisers?

| Grade | Degree of breathlessness related to activities |
|-------|------------------------------------------------|
| 1 | Not troubled by breathlessness except on strenuous exercise |
| 2 | Short of breath when hurrying or walking up a slight hill |
| 3 | Walks slower than contemporaries on level ground because of breathlessness, or has to stop for breath when walking at own pace |
| 4 | Stops for breath after walking about 100 m or after a few minutes on level ground |
| 5 | Too breathless to leave the house, or breathless when dressing or undressing |

Table 3.1  MRC breathlessness scale

- is the patient on long-term oxygen therapy?
- is the patient still smoking?
- is there evidence of an advanced directive or of the wishes of the patient concerning resuscitation?

**CASE STUDY 3.5** (continued)

On admission the patient was pink, overweight, tremulous and mildly confused. He was receiving oxygen at 6 L/min via a bag and reservoir, which had been started by the paramedics. He had a weak, productive-sounding cough but could not bring sputum up. He was wheezy, tachypnoeic at 28 breaths/min and had quite marked ankle oedema.

The initial assessment must take note of the following:

- Is the patient being given oxygen inappropriately (the patient in Case Study 3.5 was receiving a potentially disastrous quantity of oxygen)? Is the patient confused (confusion suggests $CO_2$ retention)?
- Is the respiratory rate above 25 breaths/min (the patient is already at their limits of reserve)?
- Is the pulse more than 110 beats/min?
- Does oximetry indicate saturations on room air of less than 92%?
- Is the temperature above 38.5°C (indicates severe infection, particularly pneumonia)?
- How long has this attack lasted (is the patient likely to be tiring)?
- Is the cough effective and are there retained secretions?
- Is the sputum purulent?
- Is breathing hard work (pursed lips, the overuse of accessory muscles, patient sitting forwards with arms fixed)?
- How much wheeze is there (bronchodilators and steroids should help)?
- Is there ankle oedema (cor pulmonale)?

### CRITICAL NURSING OBSERVATIONS

- Respiratory rate
- Oxygen saturation (preferably before oxygen is started)
- Is the patient at all confused (possible $CO_2$ retention)?
- Is there an effective cough?
- Is there ankle oedema?

### IMPORTANT NURSING OBSERVATIONS

- Peak flow rate
- Pulse rate
- Sputum colour
- Temperature (a sign of respiratory infection)
- Will the patient cooperate with the oxygen mask?

#### CASE STUDY 3.5 (continued)

The patient's temperature was 37.6°C and he had an irregular pulse, with an apical rate of 125 beats/min. His oxygen supply was changed to 24% by face mask, but his saturations on pulse oximetry decreased to 75%. Immediate physiotherapy helped him to cough up moderate amounts of green sputum and, after an air-driven nebuliser of ipratropium 0.5 mg, he appeared less drowsy. His arterial blood gases on admission, breathing room air, were $pO_2$ 4.5 kPa, $pCO_2$ 10 kPa, pH 7.25. An ECG confirmed atrial fibrillation and a chest film showed overinflation but no evidence of pneumonia.

Analysis of the blood gases of the patient in Case Study 3.5 indicates that he needs urgent and aggressive intervention. Any of the following results needs to be acted on quickly:

- $pO_2$ less than 6.7 kPa
- $pCO_2$ more than 9.3 kPa
- pH less than 7.3

#### Management of acute exacerbations of COPD
In an unfamiliar patient, it can be hard to differentiate a case of end-stage COPD from a case of moderately severe COPD made worse by a reversible factor such as pulmonary embolus, infection or heart failure. If there is any

doubt, it is safer to assume there is a treatable component and to manage the patient aggressively. If all else fails, this may have to include ventilation.

**Controlled oxygen therapy.** Many patients with severe COPD and Type II respiratory failure are in a parlous state with regards to their oxygen needs. During periods of instability there is a fine balance between:

1. the deleterious effects of hypoxia on cardiac, cerebral and kidney function, and
2. the stimulant effects of hypoxia on respiratory drive

If too little oxygen is given, hypoxia damages the function of vital organs. If too much oxygen is given, respiratory drive is switched off, carbon dioxide builds up and as a result the patient becomes acidotic (pH falls), which in itself causes organ damage.

*How much oxygen is safe?* The aim of controlled oxygen treatment is to maintain oxygen saturations above 90% without triggering worsening hypercapnia and a decrease in pH (increasing acidosis). Venturi masks giving 24% or 28% oxygen are safe as an initial step until the arterial gas results are known. Nasal cannulae may give more than 28% and are probably not safe as first-line treatment in the unstable patient, although occasionally patients will not tolerate a mask. Gases should be rechecked 1 h after controlled oxygen is started. A good response sees the $pO_2$ increasing above 7.5 kPa, with no fall in pH or increase in $CO_2$. A poor response sees a falling pH and difficulty in keeping oxygen levels above 6.6 kPa.

If the $pO_2$ can only be corrected at the expense of a decreasing respiratory effort (as indicated by the falling pH and increasing $pCO_2$), then an additional stimulus or aid to respiratory drive may be needed to drive off $CO_2$. Intervention must not be delayed and if, in spite of controlled oxygen, the pH decreases to 7.35 or less, assisted ventilation should be considered. There are three ways to provide respiratory support:

- non-invasive ventilation
- i.v. doxapram – a respiratory stimulant largely replaced by NIV
- formal ventilation on the ITU

*Why measure gases when we have an oximeter?* Pulse oximetry measures oxygen saturation and as such it can be a useful guide to oxygen requirements. It must be clearly understood, however, that oximetry does not measure $pCO_2$ or pH, both of which are critical factors in Type II (hypercapnic) respiratory failure, particularly during the first 12 h of treatment. It is dangerous to rely entirely on pulse oximetry in the unstable patient, in whom blood gases must be measured regularly to evaluate the effect of any change in treatment.

**Bronchodilators in COPD.** The response to bronchodilators is modest in COPD. Nebulised salbutamol 2.5–5 mg 4-hourly should be tried until the patient is well enough to revert to lower dose treatment. Some patients with

COPD probably respond as well or better to nebulised ipratropium (Atrovent) 0.5 mg 6-hourly. For severe exacerbations, the combination of nebulised salbutamol (Ventolin) and ipratropium (Atrovent) is usually given. *If the patient is hypercapnic, the nebuliser must be driven with compressed air and not oxygen. If the patient needs constant oxygen, this can be continued with nasal cannulae during nebulisation.* The driving gas should be stated on the prescription. Intravenous theophyllines can be tried if nebulisers are ineffective, but the response is unpredictable and toxicity may occur. These drugs may have a role with high-dose frusemide when there is resistant oedema in severe cor pulmonale.

**Antibiotics in exacerbations of COPD.** Most exacerbations of COPD are primarily viral in origin. Nonetheless, antibiotics are generally given in patients with COPD who exhibit increasing breathlessness, if the quantity and colour of the sputum are changing. Amoxycillin is the first choice unless it has been given unsuccessfully at home. The emergence of the organisms *Moraxella catarrhalis* and *Chlamydia pneumoniae* as pathogens in some exacerbations of COPD means that other antibiotics such as co-amoxiclav (Augmentin) and erythromycin may need to be considered. Although the choice of antibiotics should be determined by the result of sputum cultures, in most cases these are not available until the patient has been in hospital for several days. If the patient remains unwell with persistent breathlessness, a productive cough and sputum that will not clear, it is justified to try a potent i.v. antibiotic such as a third-generation cephalosporin.

If pneumonia is diagnosed from the chest film, the patient is treated in accordance with the appropriate guidelines.

**Oral steroids in exacerbations of COPD.** Steroids are used in COPD in much the same way that they are given in acute asthma: 30 mg of oral prednisolone daily for 7–14 days. There is some evidence that steroids will shorten the duration of an acute exacerbation. The response will be less marked than in asthma – peak flows will show only modest increases as the patient's symptoms improve. Typical values would be peak flows of around 120 L/min on admission and perhaps 150 L/min before discharge. The question of whether oral steroids should be followed by inhaled steroids will

**CASE STUDY 3.5** (continued)

The inspired oxygen was increased by changing to a 28% mask. This improved the patient's oxygen saturation to 85% but gases repeated after an hour showed a rising $CO_2$ level, and the patient had become more drowsy. It was decided to try non-invasive ventilatory support by assisting his respirations with a tight-fitting nasal mask attached to a portable ventilator (nasal intermittent positive pressure ventilation).

have to be considered at a later stage. In selected, severely affected cases, inhaled steroids reduce the frequency of exacerbations and slow the decline in quality of life. Overall, about 10% of patients with COPD will benefit from long-term inhaled steroids, and they can be difficult to identify during an acute illness. Inappropriate maintenance oral steroids, a common problem in COPD, can only be withdrawn under careful supervision.

**Non-invasive ventilation.** Non-invasive ventilation is the best way to treat patients with acute exacerbations of COPD who remain in Type II (hypercapnic) respiratory failure in spite of maximum medical treatment and controlled oxygen therapy (→ Case Study 3.5). NIV has largely replaced the use of the respiratory stimulant, intravenous doxapram. Patients receiving NIV are less likely to need tracheal intubation, they stay in hospital for less time and are more likely to survive than patients treated conventionally. Success is not guaranteed, however, and before embarking on NIV there must be an explicit decision as to whether or not the patient should be intubated and ventilated if NIV fails – a decision which will be critically dependent on the patient's pre-existing level of dependency, which must be documented in the notes.

> The clearest indication for NIV is Type II respiratory failure with an arterial pH less than 7.35 in spite of maximum medical treatment and controlled oxygen administration.

There must be an explicit record of whether NIV is the ceiling in any management plan, or whether the patient can go on to intubation if NIV fails.

*Ventilator.* The simplest and most popular machine is a Bipap ventilator, which provides two levels (Bi) of *p*ositive *a*irways *p*ressure (pap) – a higher pressure in inspiration (IPAP) to drive air into the lungs and a lower pressure during expiration (EPAP) to keep the bases of the lungs expanded, so helping oxygenation. The machine senses the onset of an inspiratory effort and is triggered to assist the patient by pushing in a bigger breath than would otherwise have been taken. If the machine is not triggered, either because the effort is too feeble or the patient's respiratory rate is too low, the machine takes over and supplies the whole of the breath.

*Masks.* The full face mask is easier to fit than the nasal mask, and it ventilates more effectively, as many patients can only breathe through their mouth. There are established techniques for sizing and fitting the masks, ensuring that leaks are minimised and that the patient is reassured and comfortable.

*Oxygen.* This is fed into the circuit to keep the saturations above 85%; a typical initial flow rate would be 4 L/min.

*The first 24 h on NIV.* Patients who do well settle on the NIV and synchronise with the machine; they struggle less to breathe, use their accessory (neck)

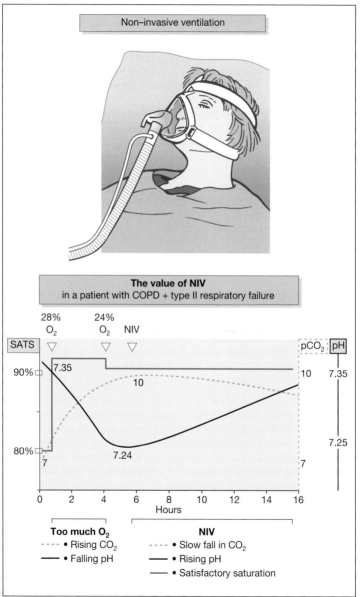

**Fig. 3.3** Non-invasive ventilation

muscles less, their respiratory rate falls and, within 1–2 h, their blood gases start to improve. Patients who do less well show lots of air leaks, they are confused or restless, their chest does not expand well in time with the machine, their vital signs are unstable and blood gases at 6 h are unchanged or worse. For patients remaining on NIV, it should be used for as much of the first 24 h as possible, pausing for physiotherapy, nebulisers and meals. The aim of NIV is to allow oxygenation to take place without an increase in $CO_2$. If it is successful, the $CO_2$ will slowly fall and the pH rise ($\rightarrow$ Fig. 3.3).

Typical signs of success would include:

- respiratory rate falling below 24 breaths/min
- heart rate below 110 beats/min
- saturations more than 90% on oxygen 4 L/min
- pH more than 7.35 (blood gases are checked at 0, 1 and 6 h)

The outlook after ventilation for COPD is surprisingly good: mean survival times are around 3 years. The patients who do well have usually been on suboptimal treatment before their admission to hospital. There is a general view that, in the UK, too few COPD patients with respiratory failure are given the chance of ventilation.

## NURSING THE PATIENT WITH COPD

Patients who are admitted with COPD often have complex nursing and medical needs. Most will have several major health problems besides COPD, and there is invariably a background of increasing disability and dependence. For a number, however, their usual treatment will have been less than optimum and there may be some treatable condition that has tipped the balance and brought them into hospital. As a general rule, therefore, your safest course is to assume that there is a major reversible component in all of your COPD patients. Remember, most of your patients will respond to treatment, they will be discharged with a new and better management plan and will have an improved quality of life. For those who do not improve or for those who deteriorate in spite of maximum treatment, your role becomes one of symptom palliation, but this will not be clear to you in the first 24 h of the patient's admission. Your priorities are therefore to address airflow obstruction, improve gas exchange and prevent respiratory failure. The skill for you as a nurse is to combine this with an understanding of the psychological burden that this condition carries and which colours the patient's physical response to it ($\rightarrow$ Box 3.5).

*Critical nursing tasks during the acute attack*
**Give reassurance and support.** Take a positive approach. Most patients with COPD will have experienced very negative attitudes towards their condition. Some patients will be very fearful that they have reached the terminal phase

---

**Box 3.5 – Reassurance for patients with exacerbations of COPD**

- Your breathlessness and tightness will improve as our therapies start to work.
- You will start to cough up sputum and clear your chest as the treatment takes effect.
- The more you cough up, the better you will feel.
- You can have the nebuliser on frequent occasions during the first few days.
- Because you are getting oxygen through the mask you do not have to fight for breath.
- Try not to panic on the mask, it needs to stay on to boost your oxygen levels.
- The oximeter reading is more than 80% so you are getting plenty of oxygen into your lungs.
- Your ankle swelling is due to fluid retention; it will improve slowly with treatment. It is not a sign of heart weakness.
- Find your most comfortable position even if it means sitting out in the chair.
- You will start to eat again as the infection clears and your oxygen levels improve.
- We will work hard on your chest for the next 24 h and you can rest after that.
- You will get some sleep once things improve; a sleeping tablet would be dangerous.
- We will give you your other medications just as you were having them at home.

---

## CRITICAL NURSING TASKS DURING THE ACUTE ATTACK

- Give reassurance and support
- Provide explanations
- Minimise the work of breathing
- Monitor the patient's progress
- Prepare the patient for possible active intervention

---

of their illness. Reassure them about the new techniques and approaches to treatment that we are now using.

**Explain.** Despite its inconvenience, the mask *must* be kept on, because it is not there simply to relieve breathlessness – it is part of the continuing treatment. Take some time to familiarise the patient with the mask and to ensure it fits comfortably. Prepare the oedematous patient for the effects of the diuretics. To a severely breathless patient, asking for, and using, a bottle or bed pan will be a major undertaking.

**Minimise the work of breathing.** Many of your COPD patients will be bordering on panic. Prop the patient up with pillows or allow them to rest on pillows across a bed table. Obese and oedematous patients will be nursed

## EXCELLENT CARE FOR COPD

- Documentation of existing exercise tolerance and quality of life
- Attempts to identify the patient's wishes regarding active treatment and resuscitation
- Documentation of discussions with the patient's family
- Chest film report in the notes
- Evidence that old hospital notes have been reviewed
- Appropriate use of blood gases
- Safe oxygen prescribing
- Documentation of inspired oxygen at the time arterial gases were measured
- Statement of treatment aims (e.g. 'To maintain saturations above 92%')
- Availability of NIV
- PFR chart or regular spirometry

best sitting out or resting with their legs over the side of the bed. One close relative can be very helpful in ensuring cooperation with masks and so forth: any more than this is counterproductive.

**Monitor the patient's progress.** The first 12 h are critical. Keep oxygen saturations around 85–92%. Patients who are becoming drowsy or confused need a detailed reassessment, including blood gases. Fluid balance becomes critical if diuretics are being used. Monitor the pulse: your patient is at risk from arrhythmias, particularly if they are hypoxic, are receiving aminophylline or have a cardiac history.

**Prepare the patient for more active intervention if there is no improvement.** Explain about the possible need for nasal ventilation. Many patients will feel relieved that the work of breathing is going to be taken from them. It is helpful to give some warning about the need for ITU ventilation if this looks like becoming an option.

## ANSWERING RELATIVES' QUESTIONS IN COPD

The patient's relatives are likely to have witnessed the effects of the progressive loss of lung function at first hand. They will be anxious about the immediate outcome and will often express strong views about the patient's existing quality of life. While these are important, they are subjective and will not necessarily mirror those of the patient. When discussing prognosis, you can emphasise the positive benefits of re-examining aspects of the patient's long-term management, particularly when combined with cessation of smoking. Bear in mind, however, that the hospital mortality in COPD with respiratory failure is as high as 10%, so reassurance must be tempered with caution.

*Is this asthma or emphysema?* The lay view is that emphysema is untreatable and often fatal. Explain that, in most cases of COPD, there is a mixture of asthma and emphysema, and that our aim is to correct the asthmatic component. Emphasise the role of smoking cessation in preventing further deterioration.

*Why is he so depressed and lacking in energy?* This may be caused by chronic lack of oxygen, and we can look into this after this episode is over. There may also be a true depressive element or an anxiety state. If you suspect this, note it down for future action.

*Why does he keep coming back in so quickly?* You may have to accept that your patient has reached a stage where there is no further respiratory reserve. However, readmissions can also be due to social factors: loss of confidence, fear and isolation. These issues should be noted and tackled later. Social work and occupational therapy input is likely to be helpful here.

*Is the heart affected?* Patients with COPD often have coexisting heart disease, simply because they share the main risk factors: age and smoking. More often than not, however, ankle swelling is due to cor pulmonale rather than to congestive cardiac failure. Reassure the relatives that, as the lungs improve, the ankle oedema should resolve.

*Can we get a nebuliser or oxygen for him?* There are guidelines for nebulisers and home oxygen in COPD. These are best applied after specialist assessment by the respiratory team.

*What can we do when he panics at home?* Stay with him, give him a nebuliser – followed, if it is available, by oxygen. Wait to see the effect. If he deteriorates, particularly if he appears to be drowsy, or more blue than normal or confused, ask for help.

# RESPIRATORY INFECTIONS AND PNEUMONIA

Respiratory infections are a common cause for admission to the Acute Medical Unit (→ Case Study 3.6). Most occur in a setting of pre-existing lung disease, usually COPD, or some other debilitating condition. An infective exacerbation of COPD is characterised by an increase in cough, an increase in the volume and stickiness of the sputum, and a change in sputum colour to green. There may be a fever and the infection may precipitate respiratory

---

**CASE STUDY 3.6**  A bad case of flu or severe pneumonia?

A 54-year-old fit man had been unwell for 8 days. His symptoms progressed from generalised flu-like symptoms to severe malaise and confusion. On admission he was pyrexial and unwell with a respiratory rate of 30 and a blood pressure of 80/40 mmHg. His chest X-ray showed a solid upper lobe in the right lung. His blood count showed a very low white cell count (polymorphs $0.2 \times 10^9$), a raised urea of 25 mmol/L and a low albumin of 19 g/L. The bacterium *Streptococcus pneumoniae* was grown in both sputum and blood. The pneumococcal antigen was positive in the urine.

The patient was treated with i.v. benzyl penicillin, oxygen and aggressive fluid replacement, combined with careful monitoring of the urine output. His temperature settled over 4 days and he slowly improved.

---

failure or cor pulmonale. In a frail, debilitated patient, a respiratory infection may simply cause a general deterioration with nothing more in the chest than a fruity-sounding cough and an increase in the respiratory rate. Major risk factors for the development of respiratory infection are mouth sepsis, a weak and ineffective cough, and associated conditions such as stroke or coma that increase the risk of aspiration.

## PNEUMONIA

Pneumonia is a type of respiratory infection that leads to consolidation of part of the lung. Consolidation impairs gas exchange and is visible on the chest X-ray. Even in a previously fit person who acquires pneumonia outside hospital, it can be a clinical challenge and there are still a substantial number of deaths. The mortality rate in cases of pneumonia admitted to hospital is 10%, but this increases to 50% in patients who are ill enough to need ITU care.

### Signs and symptoms of pneumonia
The clinical features of pneumonia are due to a combination of lung involvement and sepsis:

- breathlessness
- cough and sputum
- cyanosis
- chest pain (usually pleurisy)
- marked tachypnoea
- fever
- systemic illness

In severe pneumonia, there are signs of systemic upset, including myalgia (muscle pains), diarrhoea and, in extreme cases, restlessness and shock. Even without pre-existing lung disease, pneumonia can cause severe Type I respiratory failure. Any two of the following key features are associated with a mortality rate of 20%:

- respiratory rate more than 30 breaths/min
- diastolic pressure less than 60 mmHg
- blood urea more than 7 mmol/L

*Assessment of pneumonia*
The history will identify patients who are particularly vulnerable to the development of pneumonia:

- over 65 years of age
- chronic lung disease, especially in heavy smokers
- underlying ill health or alcohol abuse
- patients who are immunosuppressed (recent chemotherapy, AIDS, myeloma, etc.)

*The severity score in pneumonia: CURB-65*
CURB-65 (→ Table 3.2) is a simple five-point scoring system based on nursing observations and a blood test. It is used to assess the severity of the pneumonia and is a fundamental part of the initial assessment. Severe

## CRITICAL NURSING OBSERVATIONS

- **Respiratory rate**
- **Blood pressure**
- **Conscious level (particularly confusion)**
- **Oxygen saturation**
- **Pulse (rate *and* rhythm)**

## IMPORTANT NURSING OBSERVATIONS

- **Temperature**
- **Sputum colour**
- **Presence of pleuritic pain**
- **Evidence of mouth sepsis (including oral candida)**
- **Evidence of existing airways disease**

**Table 3.2 CURB-65**

| CONFUSION | New-onset disorientation for time, place or person/MTS 8 or less | SCORE 1 |
|---|---|---|
| UREA | Greater than 7.0 mmol/L | SCORE 1 |
| RESPIRATORY RATE | Greater than 30 breaths/min | SCORE 1 |
| BLOOD PRESSURE | Systolic less than 90 mmHg or diastolic less than 60 mmHg | SCORE 1 |
| 65 | Over 65 years of age | SCORE 1 |

SCORE 0–2 = mild   SCORE 3–5 = severe;   SCORE 4–5 = move to HDU/ITU

pneumonia is defined as a score of 3 or more; a score of 4 or 5 carries a high mortality rate, and these patients should be considered for early transfer to an HDU/ITU bed.

### Finding the cause of pneumonia
In order to identify the likely cause of pneumonia, and therefore to choose the most appropriate treatment:

- note the history (AIDS, recent travel, etc.)
- culture blood, sputum, urine, pleural fluid (if an effusion is present)
- send the blood and urine for immunology (Legionnaire's, *Pneumococcus*, atypical pneumonia) and arrange for convalescent samples to be sent for comparison at 10 days. There should be an urgent testing and reporting service for Legionnaire's urinary antigen that should be used for patients with severe pneumonia

### Assessing the effect of pneumonia on the patient
A few simple tests will give you an accurate measure of the impact that the pneumonia is having on the patient:

- the extent of shadowing on the chest film
- an ECG, particularly to look for atrial fibrillation, a common complication in severe cases
- the degree of hypoxia ($pO_2$ less than 8 kPa)
- the degree of acidosis (pH less than 7.3)
- WCC either less than 4 (marrow depression in severe sepsis) or more than $20 \times 10^9$/L
- blood urea more than 7 mmol/L (indirect evidence of hypovolaemia and potential kidney damage)
- low serum albumin (albumin less than 35 g/L) as a result of the toxic effect of severe infection on protein manufacture

*Management of pneumonia*
If the assessment indicates features associated with a high risk of death (respiratory failure, shock, acidosis, disseminated intravascular coagulopathy) and particularly if the CURB-65 score is 4 or more, the patient should be managed where ventilation is available at short notice. The key to treatment lies in:

- fluid balance
- oxygenation
- appropriate antibiotics

**Basic aims of treatment**
*Fluids.* Suitable fluids are administered:

- to maintain a blood pressure of more than 90/60 mmHg
- to maintain a urine output of more than 20 ml/h (crystalloids such as normal saline are preferable to colloids such as polygeline [Haemaccel]). Fluids may need to include inotropic support

*Oxygen.* Sufficient oxygen is administered to maintain saturations of more than 92%. In the absence of COPD, patients with pneumonia are not at risk from a worsening of $CO_2$ retention by receiving too much oxygen. A high-flow mask should be used. NIV or CPAP should be used in pneumonia only in an HDU/ITU setting, as at least half the patients who reach this stage will need tracheal intubation and ventilation of the lungs.

*Antibiotics.* Appropriate antibiotics are administered to cover the likely causative organisms. These are based on the 'best guess' for the likely organism within the context of local antibiotic guidelines. The choice of antibiotics may have to be modified once results of cultures and blood tests become available.

**Which antibiotic for which patient?** Examples of suitable initial regimens pending microbiological results include the following:

- Non-severe pneumonia
  — oral amoxycillin 1 g tds
  *plus*
  — oral erythromycin 500 mg qds or clarithromycin 500 mg bd
- Non-severe pneumonia, but intolerant or allergic to first-line drugs
  — oral levofloxacin 500 mg od
- Severe pneumonia
  — i.v. co-amoxiclav (Augmentin) 1.2 g qds and i.v. erythromycin 500 mg qds or i.v. clarithromycin 500 mg bd
  *or*
  — i.v. cefuroxime 1.5 g qds and i.v. erythromycin 500 mg qds or i.v. clarithromycin 500 mg bd

- Severe pneumonia with other problems
  — i.v. cefotaxime 1 g qds and i.v. clarithromycin 0.5g bd
  *or*
  — i.v. ceftriaxone 2 g od and i.v. clarithromycin 0.5 g bd
- Intravenous rifampicin 600 mg bd can also be added in very severe cases

Intravenous antibiotics are a major burden for the acute medical unit in terms of both time and expense, so patients should be transferred to oral antibiotics at the earliest opportunity. The current recommendation is to switch the i.v. regimes to oral co-amoxiclav 625 mg tds and either erythromycin or clarithromycin. Antibiotics can usually be stopped after 7 days, except in particularly severe cases of pneumonia.

### Pleural effusion and pleural empyema

One of the most common complications of pneumonia is the development of a pleural effusion. If the fluid in an effusion becomes infected, an empyema (pus in the pleural cavity) will develop.

Empyemas are seen in the elderly and debilitated, particularly when the treatment of a pneumonia has been delayed (→ Case Study 3.7). An empyema should be suspected if there is persistent fever associated with weight loss, pleuritic pain and weakness despite appropriate antibiotics. The treatment of an empyema involves clearing the infected fluid from the pleural cavity by intercostal drainage.

## NURSING THE PATIENT WITH PNEUMONIA

The patient with pneumonia combines the challenges of uncontrolled sepsis with the management of threatened or actual respiratory failure (→ Case Study 3.7). For many patients, the pneumonia will be complicating pre-existing medical conditions, so your assessment will need to be both comprehensive and searching. For example, has your patient with a CVA

---

**CASE STUDY 3.7** Delayed treatment of pneumonia

A 17-year-old youth was admitted with severe chest pain and malaise. Three weeks before admission he had become acutely unwell with a cough, shivering and breathlessness. He treated himself with aspirin. On examination he was pyrexial, pale and unwell looking. He had a productive cough, severe right-sided chest pain on inspiration and signs of a right-sided pleural effusion. His chest film showed a solid right lower lobe and fluid in the pleural space.

A diagnosis of unresolved pneumonia with possible empyema was made. His effusion was aspirated to dryness and sent for examination. He was started on ampicillin and erythromycin.

developed pneumonia because he cannot swallow and has aspirated? Your most important immediate task is to grade the severity of the pneumonia. This is simple to do and is based on the combination of vital signs (notably respiratory rate and blood pressure) and basic laboratory investigations. As a general rule, the more 'multisystem' the symptoms appear (e.g. diarrhoea, muscle pains, headache), the worse the pneumonia. Some organisms attack several systems at once. Has your patient with pneumonia, a splitting headache and photophobia also got meningitis? If you are lucky, the history may help you establish the cause of the pneumonia (for example on our unit a failure to seek out appropriate risk factors led to a lengthy delay in recognising an AIDS-related pneumonia). The history is more likely, however, to highlight other relevant medical conditions that will influence the speed of recovery.

Patients with pneumonia will be in need of reassurance (→ Box 3.6).

---

**Box 3.6 – Reassurance for the patient with pneumonia**

- Pneumonia is a treatable infection in the lungs. We are trying to trace its source.
- It would be very unusual for other members of your family to be at risk.
- The drip is to give you fluid and antibiotics.
- For the first few days you will be helped by continuous oxygen through the mask.
- The chest pain is due to inflammation in the lining of the lung; it is not from your heart.
- Your fever and sweats will take several days to subside.
- Your breathlessness is due to temporary lung damage, which is starting to heal. Although you will feel better in a few days we would not expect your X-ray to clear completely for 3 or 4 weeks.
- It is quite normal to have no appetite at all and feel very weak at first.
- You will probably be able to cough up sputum more effectively as you start to improve.

---

## CRITICAL NURSING TASKS DURING THE ACUTE ATTACK

- Provide timely therapy
- Provide explanations
- Monitor the patient's progress
- Assess the need for analgesia
- Watch for complications

*Five critical nursing tasks during the acute attack*

**Provide timely therapy.** Once the diagnosis is suspected, your patient must receive their antibiotics. Hypotension needs urgent attention with fluids. Hypoxia is treated with high concentrations of oxygen.

**Explain.** Explain the importance of continuous oxygen. Reassure the patient that the i.v. antibiotics are given for the first few doses only.

**Monitor the patient's progress.** The hypotensive and ill patient will need a urinary catheter to ensure an adequate (20+ ml/h) urine output. Oxygen saturations should be maintained above 92%. The pulse and temperature should start to decrease within 24–48 h of the start of treatment. Persistent confusion in your patient is a worrying sign.

**Assess the need for analgesia.** Opiates are not advisable because of respiratory depression, but you must try and relieve any pleuritic pain. The pain of pleurisy prevents an adequate cough and impairs deep inspiration.

**Watch for complications**

- Persistent fever and anorexia: pus in the pleural cavity or an abscess
- Ankle oedema and extreme lethargy: either cardiac failure or a low albumin due to systemic illness (lung abscess?)
- Low urine output and nausea: renal failure complicating sepsis

## ANSWERING RELATIVES' QUESTIONS IN PNEUMONIA

Pneumonia has a bad reputation with the lay public, who still associate it with death, especially in the elderly. This reputation is not undeserved, particularly when the pneumonia complicates other serious diseases such as cancer, diabetes and stroke. Many patients with pneumonia will have passed through a flu-like stage at home and will have seen their family doctor on two or three occasions, with or without the prescription of antibiotics. Many of you will recognise the words, 'why wasn't something done *sooner*!', and you may have had to deal with combinations of resentment and anger. You must remember that it is easy to diagnose pneumonia in hindsight, particularly with the aid of on-site chest films. It is probably best to explain to the relatives how the disease can progress rather than to imply any criticism of their initial management. Common questions that you will have to deal with are listed below.

*Is this bronchopneumonia, lobar pneumonia or double pneumonia?* The term 'bronchopneumonia' is commonly used to describe the terminal respiratory distress in a frail and usually elderly patient. In practice it means infection, usually in the lung bases, as a result of retained secretions and an ineffective cough.

'Bronchopneumonia' is often stated on the death certificate to be the immediate cause of death in patients in whom it was simply the terminal event after, say, severe stroke, advanced malignant disease or dementia.

'Lobar pneumonia' is a more exact term, indicating the extent (a lobe) of the consolidation. 'Double pneumonia' is an entirely lay expression, presumably indicating involvement of both lungs.

*Can the rest of us catch it?* There can be a common source of infection (such as a faulty water-cooling system in an outbreak of Legionnaire's disease), but person-to-person spread is rare.

*Will the confusion clear?* Providing the oxygen mask is kept on and the antibiotics work, the confusion will clear. It is, however, an indication of how severe a case this is that you are dealing with.

*Will there be any permanent lung damage?* There should be a complete recovery, but this should be seen as an opportunity to ensure that the patient stops smoking.

*What if he gets worse?* If your patient has poor prognostic signs, introduce the relatives to the possibility of ITU care and possible ventilation. One way to discuss this is as 'a stop-gap measure to allow the lungs to rest while the antibiotics get to work'.

*Can you feed him up? He has not eaten for days.* To start with, the priority is fluid, antibiotics and oxygen. As he improves his appetite will return.

*Why don't you X-ray him again to see how he is progressing?* Unless we need to look for complications, the chest X-ray will not improve for at least 2 weeks. The best sign of recovery is when the patient starts to feel better. Special tests such as CT scan are only helpful to sort out any complications.

## SPONTANEOUS PNEUMOTHORAX

A spontaneous pneumothorax occurs when a defect on the surface of the lung 'pops', letting air out under positive pressure into the pleural space. This pressurised air prevents expansion of the lung and can push the mediastinal structures to the opposite side of the chest (a tension pneumothorax implies a large, high-pressure pneumothorax with a major effect on lung function). The symptoms are pain, breathlessness and, in severe cases, cardiorespiratory collapse. As you can see, a pneumothorax can be confused with three major medical conditions:

● pulmonary embolus
● myocardial infarction
● pleurisy

Small pneumothoraces (a rim of air less than 2 cm wide on the chest X-ray) produce few symptoms and improve without treatment. A rim of more than 2 cm is a 'large' pneumothorax; the patient is usually breathless and intervention is necessary. Active treatment of a pneumothorax involves removing the air from the pleural cavity by simple aspiration or, in more difficult cases, by placement of an intercostal drain. Tube drainage is best performed with a small-bore (9–14F) catheter inserted very easily using a Seldinger technique and attached to either an under-water seal or a flutter valve.

Whether a patient is admitted for observation and possible intervention depends primarily on:

- the degree of lung collapse
- the amount of breathlessness
- the presence of pre-existing lung disease (patients with emphysema and asthma are prone to pneumothoraces. Even a small pneumothorax in a patient with severe lung disease or occurring during an asthma attack can be the last straw)

A *primary* pneumothorax occurs in otherwise normal lungs; a *secondary* pneumothorax is caused by underlying lung disease (usually emphysema) or trauma.

Simple aspiration is preferable to tube drainage for any primary pneumothorax and should be tried first. Aspiration is successful in 60% of cases, with re-expansion of the lung. These patients can be discharged rapidly but, as with *all* cases of pneumothorax, they must be told to return to hospital if they suddenly become short of breath and they should be given an early (1–2 weeks) appointment for the chest clinic.

If aspiration does not lead to re-expansion of the lung, or if there is expansion followed by further collapse within 72 h, then an intercostal drain will be needed (→ Fig. 3.4). Except when very small and asymptomatic, all *secondary* pneumothoraces require tube drainage.

Once a drain is in place:

- It should be clamped only under exceptional circumstances (*not* because the patient is going for a chest film).
- Chest drains that are still bubbling should not be removed unless they are to be replaced.
- If the drain is in place for more than 24 h, the patient should be referred at that time to the respiratory team.

The management of a pneumothorax can be troublesome, particularly if there is also chronic lung disease present. A safe course of action is to refer all cases of pneumothorax to the respiratory team.

## NURSING THE PATIENT WITH A CHEST DRAIN

Air, fluid, blood or pus in the pleural space can result in an acutely ill patient who is severely breathless and requires an urgent chest drain. The small Seldinger drains are easy to use, generally well tolerated and are increasingly used in preference to large-bore tubes. There are still occasions, however, when a large (24–28F) tube may be required.

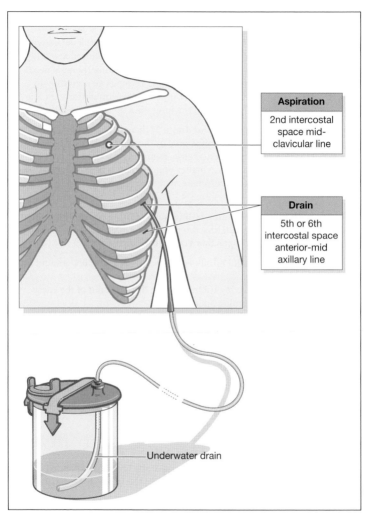

**Fig. 3.4**  Intercostal aspiration and drainage of a pneumothorax

Few procedures on the Acute Medical Unit cause as much fear and anxiety to the patient and the staff as the insertion of a large intercostal drain. Under stress they are put in and under darkness they fall out.

**Prepare your patient for the procedure.**  The patients are often young and distressed and will need a lot of reassurance, with an honest explanation of what to expect: 'There may be initial discomfort and a sensation of pushing, but the local anaesthetic will deaden any pain; if the pain is severe, tell us and we will put in more anaesthetic'. Explain that the breathlessness will go as soon as the tube is in place. It is wise to be non-committal about how long the tube will stay in. A sizeable proportion of pneumothoraces need prolonged drainage and surgical intervention: 'If things go according to plan, it will be removed in a few days, but if it is less straightforward, the tube will need to stay in longer until the lung goes up and stays up'.

**Alleviate the pain of the intercostal drain.** If there is no contraindication, a small dose of i.v. midazolam administered at the time of the skin incision may make the difference between a tense, panicking patient and one who is relaxed and cooperative. Check whether your patient is being given sufficient analgesia. Many doctors underestimate analgesic requirements in medical conditions.

**Problems with intercostal drains falling out or falling apart.** There should be a local protocol for a standardised technique for placing and securing a chest drain. Common problems that you will see include:

- sutures that are too small (3-0 silk is ideal) and are badly tied around the tube
- the weight of the connecting tubing pulling the drain out of the chest
- untaped connections coming apart
- failure to recognise, and act, on a displaced or disconnected tube (clamp an open-ended tube, seal over a sucking chest drain site)

Try and use transparent dressings, so that you can assess the state and site of the tube on at least a twice-daily basis. Simple follow-up measurements of how much tube is visible will warn of imminent displacement. Important nursing observations are of the amount of fluid drained (effusions), whether the tube is bubbling (pneumothorax) and whether it is swinging (confirming the tube is patent and remains in the pleural cavity).

**Three simple tube rules**

- bubbling tubes need to stay in
- swinging tubes can probably be removed if the lung has expanded
- non-swinging tubes are often blocked (hence the failure to re-expand?)

## FURTHER READING

### ASTHMA

Hart SR, Davidson AC 1999 Acute adult asthma – assessment of severity and management and comparison with British Thoracic Society guidelines. Respiratory Medicine 93 (1): 8–10

### COPD

Bardi G, Pierotello R, Desideri M, Valdisserri L, Bottai M, Palla A 2000 Nasal ventilation in COPD exacerbations: early and late results of a prospective, controlled study. European Respiratory Journal 15 (1): 98–104

### PNEUMONIA

Lim WS, Lewis S, Macfarlane JT 2000 Severity prediction rules in community acquired pneumonia: a validation study. Thorax 55: 219–223

### PNEUMOTHORAX

Hyde J, Sykes T, Graham T 1997 Reducing morbidity from chest drains. British Medical Journal 314: 914–915

Sahn SA, Heffner JE 2000 Spontaneous pneumothorax. New England Journal of Medicine 342 (12): 868–874

### WEBSITE

Access to all the British Thoracic Society Guidelines (Asthma, COPD, NIV, Pneumonia, Pneumothorax): http://www.Brit-Thoracic.Org.Uk/Public_Content.Asp?Pageid=7&Catid=36&Old

# ACUTE NEUROLOGICAL PROBLEMS

## INTRODUCTION

The major issue in the patient who presents as a neurological problem is to decide whether the patient needs supportive care or whether the patient needs active intervention. Many cases who present as neurological emergencies will recover fully, given time and good supportive treatment, because their underlying disorder is fully reversible. Examples include coma due to self-poisoning and the confusional states that follow an epileptic fit. Other cases require a much more active approach: typical examples are antibiotics for acute meningitis, glucose for hypoglycaemia and neurosurgery for subarachnoid haemorrhage. Therefore management decisions can only be made safely if the correct diagnosis has been established. Time is critical in neurological cases, as the nervous system has limited powers of recovery – the diagnostic path has to be followed with an appropriate degree of urgency. The Acute Medical Unit has a duty to ensure the safety of the patient during this time and the nursing staff have the key role in this process (→ Box 4.1).

---

**Box 4.1 – Role of the Acute Medical Unit in acute neurological problems**

1. Ensure the safety of the patient
2. Prioritise the initial management
3. Differentiate and manage 'medical' and 'neurological' coma
4. Identify and respond to neurological deterioration
5. Reach appropriate outcomes

---

# ROLE OF THE ACUTE MEDICAL UNIT IN ACUTE NEUROLOGICAL PROBLEMS

## ENSURING THE SAFETY OF THE PATIENT

There must be confidence in the ability to support the patient while the correct diagnosis is being reached. The role of the Acute Medical Unit at this stage is to prioritise the initial management. It may, for example, be necessary to stabilise the patient's condition before attempting to take a history.

There are four critical initial observations:

- Are the vital signs stable?
- Is the airway secure and is ventilation adequate?
- Is there a non-neurological condition that needs immediate attention?
- Is there anything neurological that needs urgent active intervention?

The most important examples in this latter category, and the ones we most fear missing, are:

- intracranial infection (most notably meningitis)
- subarachnoid haemorrhage
- expanding intracranial masses (bleeds in and around the brain, tumour, abscess)

It is critical that the patient reaches the appropriate service in the best possible condition, be it the acute neurosurgical unit, the stroke unit, the general medical wards or the ITU.

## PRIORITISING THE INITIAL MANAGEMENT

### GCS and ABCDE: Assessing and keeping the patient alive
Protection of the airway, ensuring adequate ventilation and maintaining the circulation are the immediate priorities in any patient. At the most basic level this means:

- ensuring the upper airway is patent
- giving sufficient oxygen
- securing i.v. access and maintaining the blood pressure

*Warning*: At this first stage, if meningococcal meningitis is suspected appropriate i.v. antibiotics must be given *straight away*.
   If there is any suspicion of a neck injury (an example would be a patient who had been found at the bottom of some steps, having had an apparent fall), the neck must be protected and immediately X-rayed. If there is a cervical spine fracture, manipulating an unsupported neck either to establish an airway or to move a patient around in bed can damage the spinal cord beyond repair. At least be aware of the risk, know how to apply a stiff collar and use sand bags to support the neck, and if there is any doubt protect the neck and log-roll the patient until the neck films have been cleared by a radiologist.

### Critical nursing observations
**Blood sugar.** Hypoglycaemia is the most important cause of a fully reversible neurological disorder. At blood sugars below 3 mmol/L the patient becomes comatose and may fit, but any neurological picture can be caused by hypoglycaemia. Providing the patient has not suffered irreversible damage from sustained hypoglycaemia, correction of the blood sugar will lead to a full and rapid recovery.

**Response of the pupils.** The size, symmetry and reactivity of the pupils are fundamental neurological observations. The most common cause of bilaterally fixed and dilated pupils is self-poisoning with tricyclic antidepressants, whereas poisoning with both opiates and diazepam-like drugs produces fixed constricted pupils.

**CRITICAL NURSING OBSERVATIONS**

- **Blood sugar**
- **Pupillary responses**
- **Temperature**
- **Pulse**
- **Blood pressure**
- **Respiratory rate**
- **Oxygen saturation**
- **GCS**
- **Top to toe examination**
- **A reliable history**

The major reason for following the change in the pupils is to identify 'uncal herniation': a shift of the brain because of cerebral oedema that results in the IIIrd cranial nerve being 'pinched' between the brain and part of the skull (→ Fig. 4.3). As the IIIrd nerve is responsible for pupillary constriction, an early warning of uncal herniation is pupillary dilatation followed by loss of the light reflex.

Any suspicion that a pupil is dilating and losing its light reflex must be reported to the medical staff for action to reassess the neurological status of the patients.

**Temperature.** In the right context, an increased temperature should be considered strong evidence of intracranial sepsis: meningitis, more rarely meningo-encephalitis, or even a collection of intracranial pus (intracerebral abscess).

Not every fever in a neurological emergency is due to intracranial sepsis, as there may be infection elsewhere such as aspiration pneumonia. High temperatures also characteristically occur in brain stem strokes. Nonetheless, intracranial infection should be the first consideration because of the need for immediate action.

**Pulse.** The rhythm and rate of the pulse are important. They may draw attention to non-neurological problems that need to be addressed. Extreme bradycardia, for example, may be the cause of an unexplained blackout. Atrial fibrillation is recognised by the irregularity of the pulse and its presence increases the likelihood that an acute stroke is due to a clot of blood finding its way from the left atrium (a fibrillating atrium encourages clot formation) to the brain: an embolic cerebral infarction. Changes in the pulse can be important: progressive slowing can indicate increasing ICP and is often accompanied by an increasing blood pressure.

**Blood pressure.** *Hypotension* must be evaluated in detail because it has several causes: heart problems, hypovolaemia due to dehydration, shock, sepsis and so forth. As a rule, in a patient with an impaired conscious level, hypotension suggests a metabolic cause such as sepsis, diabetes or hepatic encephalopathy. Postural hypotension (defined as a decrease in systolic pressure of more than 20 mmHg or a fall in the diastolic pressure of more than 10 mmHg 1 min after standing when accompanied by appropriate symptoms) is common especially in the elderly, is often drug-related and is a frequent cause of admissions with dizziness and unexplained falls.

*Hypertension* is commonly seen as an acute response to neurological events such as intracranial haemorrhage or large cerebral infarction. Severe hypertension can also complicate coma caused by self-poisoning with sympathomimetic recreational drugs such as ecstasy, amphetamines and cocaine, and may need urgent correction. However, in most neurological conditions, including stroke, lowering the blood pressure acutely to 'normalise' it is fraught with danger. The brain is usually fairly impervious to changes in blood pressure as the cerebral blood flow 'autoregulates': if the blood pressure drops, the vessels open up to allow greater flow through them. If there is a major neurological insult this autoregulation is lost, so if the blood pressure falls the blood supply also decreases, which may worsen the neurological deficit. Therefore in acute situations, especially in strokes, the temptation to 'treat' a high blood pressure should in most situations be resisted. The only exceptions are in special situations when very high levels, say around 230/140 mmHg, are considered dangerous. Nonetheless, any change in blood pressure must be gradual.

As already explained, the combination of a progressively falling pulse and an increasing blood pressure may, in the appropriate circumstances (such as the aftermath of a major intracranial bleed), be a sign of increased ICP.

**Respiratory rate.** The respiratory rate remains an essential observation in the patient who is critically ill, whatever the cause. It is particularly important to document any changes in respiratory rate. Thus in the neurological emergency a falling respiratory rate may reflect deepening coma. If the change in consciousness level is due to increasing ICP, the slowing respiration is accompanied by a falling pulse and rising blood pressure. It is instructive to contrast this with the signs that are seen in shock, in which a change in consciousness level is accompanied by an increase in the respiratory rate, an increase in the pulse and a decrease in the blood pressure.

**Oxygen saturation.** Hypoxia remains a common, yet easily correctable, cause of avoidable death on acute emergency wards. The normal oxygen saturation is around 97% and it must be appreciated that to decrease the saturation to 90% or less requires a major disturbance in ventilation that may be due to deepening coma and a worsening neurological state. A fall in oxygen saturation needs careful reassessment.

- Is the airway secure?
- Is the coma deepening?
- What about the lungs and the circulation?
- Should blood gases be checked?
- What is the respiratory rate?

It must be remembered that the oxygen saturation does not always reflect the level of ventilation. If the patient is on a high concentration of oxygen, the saturations can be more or less normal even when the patient is hardly breathing. The saturations must not be interpreted in isolation. There would be no reassurance from an oxygen saturation that had stayed constant for 4 h at 95% if, during that time, the GCS had dropped from 12 to 4 and the respiratory rate had fallen from 15 to 8 breaths/min. This patient should be on ITU with a view to immediate ventilation.

**Glasgow Coma Score.** The GCS was described in 1974 as a way to assess any patient with an altered level of consciousness. It is based on three categories of response: eye opening, the best motor response and the best verbal response (→ Table 4.1; Fig. 4.1). The GCS is the universal measurement of the depth of coma. It is simple to carry out and score and, provided it is performed properly, the result should be the same whoever makes the measurement.

| Table 4.1   Glasgow Coma Score | |
|---|---|
| *Response* | *Score* |
| Eye opening (E) | |
| Spontaneously | E4 |
| To verbal command | E3 |
| To pain | E2 |
| No response | E1 |
| Best motor response (M) | |
| Obeys commands | M6 |
| Localises pain | M5 |
| Withdraws to pain | M4 |
| Abnormal flexion to pain | M3 |
| Extension to pain | M2 |
| No response | M1 |
| Best verbal response (V) | |
| Orientated and converses | V5 |
| Disorientated and converses | V4 |
| Inappropriate words | V3 |
| Incomprehensible sounds | V2 |
| No response | V1 |
| **Total score** (3 to 15) | |

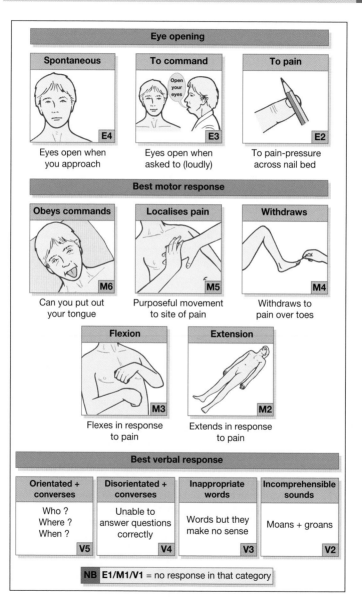

**Fig. 4.1** The Glasgow Coma Score

The GCS can be documented on a chart as the grand total from the three categories against time or as E4 M6 V5, etc. As a general rule the scores reflect the severity of the neurological status:

mild        13 to 15
moderate    9 to 12
severe      3 to 8

Coma is defined as a GCS of less than 9.

The initial GCS, often performed by the paramedics outside hospital, acts as a baseline. A low initial GCS score (less than 9) will mean the airway is vulnerable and the patient is at risk from aspiration.

*A change in the GCS is the single most important observation in the acute neurological patient.* A fall in GCS needs immediate attention. Deepening coma may need increased supportive measures, perhaps involving a move to ITU with a view to ventilation. More critically, a fall in GCS is often the first sign of increasing ICP, which occurs in active intracranial bleeding, intracranial sepsis and during the development of brain oedema following a cerebral infarct.

Some triage systems use an abbreviated assessment of the consciousness level based on the acronym AVPU:

A    Alert
V    Responds to voice
P    Responds to pain
U    Unresponsive

This is quick to perform and easy to recall. It is useful as part of a rapid primary assessment, but it is not detailed enough to use for serial observations.

**Top to toe examination.** Those closely involved with the care of acute neurological disorders should be aware of the importance of quite subtle physical signs in giving clues, particularly of head injury and infection. A head injury can result in local bogginess or scalp bruising, perhaps a palpable depressed skull and bleeding or loss of CSF from the ears and nose. Fractures to the base of the skull characteristically produce bruising around the eyes ('raccoon eyes') and behind the ears (Battle's sign). All these can and will be missed by clerking doctors, particularly if a 'stroke' label has been attached to the patient and the examination is less than thorough because of the pressures of time. Be particularly careful to look at any sites that appear to be the source of pain. Severe sinus sepsis is tender to the touch and very painful; falls from whatever cause lead to fractured hips; and grand mal fits can produce shoulder dislocation. A widespread haemorrhagic skin rash will clinch the diagnosis in meningococcal septicaemia, but it can appear with alarming speed, sometimes even after the patient has been clerked in.

**A reliable history.** One of the difficulties with neurology is the unreliability of the preadmission diagnosis. Unfortunately, diagnostic labels tend to stick and the consequences can sometimes be disastrous: the 'cerebrovascular accident' turns out to be a subdural bleed, 'off legs' a spinal cord compression, the 'well-known epileptic' a case of recurrent syncope due to intermittent heart block, and so forth. Every neurological patient who is admitted to hospital should be looked at afresh, particularly where there is a 'known' case of … Known by whom and with what degree of certainty? Are we sure that the original diagnosis still applies?

It is not advisable to make 'stroke' the initial diagnosis in a patient in coma, even if there is a past history of cerebrovascular disease. This is particularly the case in elderly patients. It is a dangerous tendency to attribute all changes in the consciousness level, all funny turns and all episodes of dizziness to a 'CVA' just because the patient is 80 years old.

Recent causes of coma initially labelled as stroke on our Acute Medical Unit included:

- post-ictal state
- respiratory failure
- overdose
- subarachnoid bleed

To make an accurate diagnosis, the history and eyewitness accounts are absolutely critical. By their nature, acute neurological problems are difficult to assess. The patients are often confused or uncooperative, making history taking and examination difficult. Nonetheless, these are the very patients in whom a correct diagnosis is paramount. Skills that are needed to assess patients with confusion or impaired consciousness levels must be perfected. Exact histories must be obtained from relatives and eyewitnesses, in particular to establish whether there is a possibility of trauma to the head or cervical spine. The typical sequence of events leading to a post-traumatic brain haemorrhage is of a head injury with transient loss of consciousness followed by amnesia for the event. The patient then becomes confused and aggressive and may fit. The GCS then starts to fall as a result of the haemorrhage. The patient may present at any of these stages. Intracranial infection is also easy to miss: here the critical questions are concerned with recent sinus or middle ear infections. Collections of pus in and around the brain present with stroke-like illnesses and are frequently missed because a proper history has not been taken and the conditions not even considered.

## MANAGING 'MEDICAL' AND 'NEUROLOGICAL' COMA

Coma is defined as a GCS of 8 or less. Broadly there are two types: 'medical' coma, which is coma due to conditions such as liver failure, respiratory failure and DKA, in which the management is primarily aimed at the underlying disease; and 'neurological' coma due to conditions such as stroke, subarachnoid haemorrhage and meningitis.

*The underlying mechanism in coma*

Consciousness is maintained by a constant stream of neurological traffic in the form of nerve impulses that are sent from the brain stem upwards into the two cerebral hemispheres. Loss of consciousness (coma) therefore has two general mechanisms that can form the basis of a practical classification of the causes of coma:

- Cerebral hemisphere malfunction
  — drug and alcohol intoxication
  — hypoxic brain damage (e.g. post-arrest)
  — stroke
  — metabolic disorders (DKA/hypoglycaemia, liver failure, respiratory failure)
  — infection (meningitis, encephalitis)
  — post-tonic–clonic convulsion
- Brain stem damage
  — direct damage
    - brain stem stroke
  — indirect damage (from downward shift of the cerebral hemispheres)
    - cerebral mass (clot, tumour, abscess)
    - cerebral oedema (due to stroke, anoxia, meningitis, etc.)

Coma that lasts more than 4 h is usually due to one of four groups of conditions (→ Box 4.2). By far the most common cause is self-poisoning (40%).

| Box 4.2 – The causes of coma that lasts 4 h or more | |
| --- | --- |
| • Self-poisoning with sedative drugs | 40% |
| • Post-hypoxic cerebral damage | 25% |
| • Stroke | 20% |
| • Metabolic disorders | 15% |

Several features of the patient's initial observations can be used to identify coma that is due to causes other than a stroke (→ Box 4.3). This has a practical purpose, because coma due to stroke has an extremely poor prognosis, whereas some of the other causes may be reversible.

| Box 4.3 – Features that suggest that a coma is not due to a stroke |
| --- |
| • Deep coma |
| • Reactive pupils |
| • Pyrexial |
| • No deviation of the eyes to one side |
| • Moves all four limbs |

> **Box 4.4 – The five 'S's: critical conditions that must not be missed**
>
> - Sugar (high or low)
> - Sepsis
> - Sub- (and extra-) dural haemorrhage
> - Special causes of coma (respiratory failure, renal failure and liver failure)
> - Secret overdoses (late presentation of paracetamol/tricyclic overdose)

There are five causes of coma that must not be missed as they are all treatable and relatively easy to diagnose, provided that they are considered at the time of the initial assessment ($\rightarrow$ Box 4.4).

### Practical management of coma

The systematic way to approach the patient with coma is to use the universal system of *primary assessment* based on the simple mnemonic ABCDE.

**A is the airway.** 'Are you all right?' If the patient responds appropriately, there is unlikely to be an airway problem. The airway can be maintained with a jaw thrust or chin lift. Placing the patient in the recovery position may be necessary (providing there is no sign or suspicion of spinal injury). Use a Guedel oral airway if it can be tolerated. Administer high-flow oxygen immediately. Look, listen and feel for expired air.

**B is the breathing**

- Count the respiratory rate (breaths/min):

    Less than 10      imminent respiratory arrest
    more than 20      ill
    more than 30      critically ill

- Listen for noise (wheeze, upper airway gurgling, 'croup')
- Assess the effort
- Perform oximetry
- Continue high-flow oxygen
- Keep the saturations greater than 90%

**C is the circulation**

- Assess pulse rate and strength
- Assess capillary refill (press finger pulp for 5 s and release; refill should be less than 2 s). This gives an idea of the peripheral circulation
- Measure the blood pressure

**D is the disability**

- GCS
- Assess pupil size, equality and reaction
- Measure blood sugar (give sugar for hypoglycaemia and, if there is a suspicion of alcohol abuse, thiamine)

**E is the exposure**

- Look for a rash and signs of trauma
- Check for hypothermia (core temperature)
- Look in the mouth (tongue biting)

*Importance of an eyewitness in coma*

Any relatives or eyewitnesses must be kept on the ward and interviewed (or if necessary telephoned). Their information may provide vital clues to the likely diagnosis. It is unacceptable for the doctor or the nurse ever to conclude that a history is either unobtainable or unavailable. Cerebral malaria is the classical example to emphasise this point: fatal if undiagnosed, curable with drugs, but too rare to remember to consider as a cause of coma. Only the patient's relatives will tell you of the safari holiday taken a week before the onset of headaches, fever and confusion. Patients who are most at risk are the least able to provide a good history for themselves. It is critical to ascertain whether there is a possibility of trauma. Patients with head injuries and trauma to the cervical spine are not usually admitted to the medical wards, but you should not lower your guard: in neurology the most challenging and difficult problems are those in which a history is unavailable and for which preadmission clinical details are scanty. Review all the details in the paramedics' record. Their information is often comprehensive and systematic and dates from soon after the event. A good paramedic assessment will give you important data on the circumstances in which the patient was found, the initial GCS and their clinical course in the critical early stages of the illness.

## RESPONDING TO NEUROLOGICAL DETERIORATION

It is not sufficient to document neurological observations. The reason for performing these time-consuming and exacting assessments is to act as soon as they change. The patient described below (→ Case Study 4.1) sustained

---

**CASE STUDY 4.1** A sudden change at 04.00

A 59-year-old man on warfarin for a valve replacement was taken to the AED having collapsed and fallen backwards, striking and bruising his head. He appeared well, but X-rays showed a basal skull fracture. In view of his 'medical' problems, he was admitted to the Acute Medical Unit, where he was described as 'drowsy and vague, complaining of headache'. He was moderately over-anticoagulated (INR 4.9). Half-hourly neurological observations recorded a systolic blood pressure increasing from 130 to 220 mmHg and a sluggishly reacting right pupil which, over $3\frac{1}{2}$ h, became more dilated. He was responsive to commands until 04.00 h, 6 h after admission, when he suddenly vomited copiously and became unresponsive (GCS 3). At this stage his right pupil was fixed and dilated. His anticoagulation was reversed with fresh frozen plasma. He was intubated, ventilated and sent urgently to the neurosurgeons.

traumatic intracerebral bleeding and was 'coning' (a shift of the brain as a result of raised ICP). The signs of increasing ICP were identified, but immediate action was not taken. A one-sided dilated pupil is often the earliest warning sign of elevated ICP which, if not corrected urgently, leads to a pressure cone.

*How the clinical state can change in the first hours of admission*
Case Studies 4.2–4.4 illustrate how the clinical state can change rapidly.

---

**CASE STUDY 4.2**   Confusion through delirium to coma

A 55-year-old man became acutely confused the day after returning from a Turkish holiday. Over the next 48 h his speech deteriorated and he became increasingly difficult to rouse. He then had a series of tonic–clonic convulsions. Investigations showed a severe viral encephalitis.

---

**CASE STUDY 4.3**   Fever to skin rash and meningitis

A 19-year-old student was admitted on Christmas Eve with an acute abdomen. In the recovery room after a negative laparotomy, the anaesthetist noticed a petechial rash. Lumbar puncture was normal, but treatment for meningococcal infection was started. Repeat lumbar puncture 8 h later yielded ginger-beer coloured CSF which grew meningococci. He recovered fully.

---

**CASE STUDY 4.4**   Aspiration pneumonia after a stroke

An 80-year-old man developed dizziness and a mild hemiparesis. On admission his GCS was 15 but he could not swallow at all. He would not tolerate an airway. Late the same night he vomited and dropped his GCS to 5. He became acutely short of breath and pyrexial. The cause of his deterioration was an aspiration pneumonia. In spite of physiotherapy and antibiotics, he deteriorated and died.

---

Other important examples include:
- deepening coma in an overdose
- deterioration due to missed infection elsewhere (blood, urine, chest, etc.)

## REACHING APPROPRIATE OUTCOMES

The combination of good nursing and medical care should aim to reach an appropriate outcome for every patient. Important outcomes and the principles by which they can be achieved are listed below.

**Making the correct diagnosis**

- Who needs a CT scan?
  - to decide the type of stroke (block or bleed?)
  - to exclude tumour, abscess, haematoma
  - to diagnose a subarachnoid haemorrhage
  - to evaluate suspected increased ICP
  - before a lumbar puncture if the patient is drowsy
- Who needs a lumbar puncture?
  - to diagnose meningitis
  - to diagnose a subarachnoid haemorrhage if the CT is normal

**Transfer to the stroke unit in an optimum condition**

- Coma management
- Swallowing assessment
- Early aspirin where indicated

**Avoiding major stroke after a transient ischaemic attack**

- Urgent investigation of suspected TIAs and minor strokes

**Surviving intracranial sepsis**

- Early treatment of meningitis
- Recognising and managing complications

**Reaching the neurosurgeons alive and on time**

- Recognising operable intracranial bleeds
- Diagnosing intracerebral masses
- Managing increased ICP

**Full recovery from self-harm**

- Responding to a changing GCS

**Recovery from reversible causes of neurological emergencies**

- Rapid and effective primary assessment
- Good coma management

## STROKE AND STROKE-LIKE EMERGENCIES

The World Health Organisation's definition of a stroke is a syndrome of rapidly developing clinical signs of focal (e.g. hemiplegia) or global (e.g. coma) disturbance of function, with symptoms lasting 24 h or longer (or leading to death) with no apparent cause other than of vascular origin.

The time frame of 24 h is to differentiate a stroke from a TIA, which recovers rapidly but is an important risk factor for developing a subsequent completed stroke. There are around 2.4 strokes per 1000 population per year. As 80% of these will be admitted as emergencies, most Acute Medical Units can expect to admit one to two strokes per day. It is important, however, not to overuse the stroke label on the Acute Medical Unit. Estimates suggest overdiagnosis, with up to a fifth of all 'strokes' turning out to be something else: post-epileptic states, toxic states due to infection, and metabolic problems such as respiratory failure.

Two factors have had a major impact on improving the outlook after a stroke: the introduction of Stroke Units, which have reduced mortality and long-term disability, and aspirin, which has reduced the risk of recurrence. Nonetheless, stroke remains the most frequent cause of major disability in adults.

There is increasing emphasis on other drugs that improve the outcome of stroke or prevent further damage. Recent studies have shown that, after a stroke, lowering the blood pressure (for example with the combination of the ACE inhibitor, perindopril, and the diuretic, indapamide) and lowering the cholesterol with a statin improve the outlook – and that this benefit is obtained even if the initial blood pressure and cholesterol level were normal. High blood sugars after a stroke may also be harmful and careful sugar control is likely to become a routine part of emergency stroke management.

## CAUSES

Most typical strokes are caused either by a cerebral infarction (an area of brain tissue death) or by an intracerebral haemorrhage (bleeding into and around the brain). Stroke-like illnesses are also caused by subarachnoid haemorrhage, subdural haemorrhage and extradural haemorrhage. Subarachnoid haemorrhage is an important cause of sudden severe headache and collapse and requires neurosurgical input. Subdural and extradural haemorrhages are rare but important causes of stroke-like illnesses that can be treated successfully if they are recognised in time.

### Cerebral infarction (approximately 80% of all strokes)

A cerebral infarction occurs when the blood supply to part of the brain is cut off, resulting in a focal area of brain-tissue death (an ischaemic stroke). There are two ways in which the blood supply can be interrupted: by a clot that travels through the arterial system and becomes lodged somewhere critical in the cerebral circulation (*cerebral embolus*), or by a clot that forms within the cerebral arteries themselves (*cerebral thrombosis*).

#### Cerebral embolus
Cerebral emboli can come from anywhere from the left atrium to the carotid arteries in the neck.

*Left atrial clot.* The most common cause of left atrial clot is atrial fibrillation. In atrial fibrillation, normal regular atrial contraction is replaced by irregular, uncoordinated atrial activity more akin to muscular shivering than proper contraction. As a result blood stagnates and can form a clot within the atrium. There is a particular risk of this happening if there is also heart disease in the form of heart muscle damage (which leads to further stagnation) or diseased valves (which can act as a focus for clot formation). Atrial fibrillation is a common age-related arrhythmia. It is found in around 10% of people older than 70 years and constitutes a major risk factor for stroke. However, the risk can be significantly reduced by anticoagulating patients who have atrial fibrillation so that there is less chance of clot formation, or by trying to restore a normal heart rhythm.

*Left ventricular clot.* It is quite common for a clot to form on the inside of the heart chamber over the scar of a recent myocardial infarction. In most cases the clot stays put, but there is always a risk of it breaking loose and travelling to the cerebral circulation. This is a particular problem in the first week or two after a myocardial infarction, when the clot is new.

*Carotid artery clot.* Atheromatous hardening of the carotid arteries has two relevant consequences for stroke formation. It may lead to critical narrowing (carotid artery stenosis) with a reduction in the blood supply to the brain. More importantly, blood clots form on the abnormally roughened arterial wall and can break off to lodge within the cerebral arterial tree. Small emboli produce minor stroke-like symptoms (TIAs), which are warning signs of a subsequent major stroke.

### Cerebral thrombosis
Hardening of the cerebral arteries (cerebral arteriosclerosis) leads to narrowing of the vessels and can progress to atheromatous plaque formation and localised thrombosis with blockage. As with atheroma elsewhere in the body, there are several causes; these include smoking, high cholesterol and a positive family history.

The two most important risk factors are:

- hypertension
- diabetes

Of the two, hypertension is the more significant: a diastolic blood pressure of 110 mmHg or more increases the stroke risk 15-fold. This compares with an increase of two to three times normal in diabetes.

The important point about these two risk factors is that they are both reversible. Controlling the blood pressure and controlling diabetes have a major impact in lowering the increased levels of risk.

### Clinical picture of a cerebral infarction
The clinical features depend on the site and extent of the infarct, and range from immediate coma and death to minor short-lived clumsiness of a limb. It is helpful to use clinical features to divide cerebral infarctions into two categories: those affecting the circulation to the front of the brain (*anterior*

| Type | Site on CT | Deficit | 1 year mortality % | 1 year dependency % |
|------|-----------|---------|--------------------|---------------------|
| TACI | 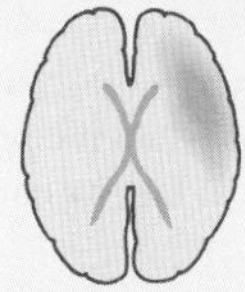 | One sided weakness/ sensory loss + Hemianopia + Cortical dysfunction | 60 | 35 |
| PACI | 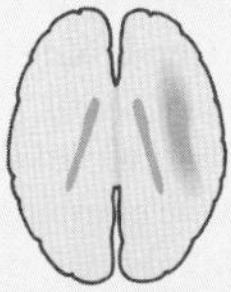 | Two of the following • One sided weakness or sensory loss • Cortical dysfunction • Hemianopia | 20 | 30 |
| LACI | 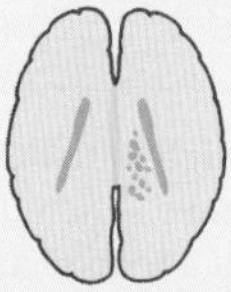 | One sided weakness/ sensory loss | 10 | 25 |
| POCI | 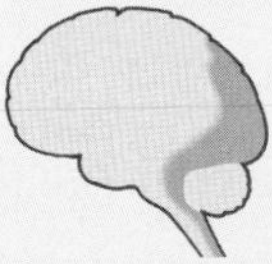 | Slurred speech Dysphagia Double vision Dizziness Unsteadiness | 20 | 20 |

**Fig. 4.2**   Types of cerebral infarct

*circulation infarcts*) and those affecting the back (*posterior circulation infarcts*) (→ Fig. 4.2).

**Anterior circulation infarcts.** Anterior circulation infarcts result in the picture of the 'classical' stroke with a variable combination of one-sided weakness (hemiparesis), one-sided sensory loss (hemianaesthesia), visual disturbance in the form of a gaze paralysis (the eyes are deviated away from the weak side) and partial loss of the visual field (the patient cannot see towards the weak side). In addition, there is a variable disturbance of higher functions (termed 'cortical function'): language disturbance (if the dominant side of the brain is damaged), neglect of the affected side and incontinence.

*'Total' anterior circulation infarct.* TACI is a combination of motor or sensory deficit, visual field loss and cortical dysfunction (e.g. language disturbance).

*'Partial' anterior circulation infarct.* PACI consists of any two of:

- unilateral weakness/sensory loss
- visual field defect (hemianopia)
- cortical dysfunction (language disorder or neglect)

*Lacunar infarct.* LACI consists of very small infarcts within the anterior circulation that pick off single pathways at critical points in the brain. They are particularly associated with a history of hypertension. The clinical picture is of a 'pure' one-sided motor or sensory loss.

**Posterior circulation infarcts.** POCI, also termed a 'brain stem CVA', result in symptoms that often affect both sides of the body (the brain stem transmits information to and from *both* sides of the brain) and characteristically affect coordination in four vital functions: talking, swallowing, looking and balancing. These patients have combinations of dysarthria (slurred speech), dysphagia (difficulty swallowing), double vision and dizziness.

### Site of the cerebral infarction and the outlook

Patients who suffer a TACI have a poor outcome: a high initial mortality and high levels of long-term dependence. Patients who have suffered a PACI have a much better outlook, with a low mortality but a high recurrence rate. A LACI is associated with a good outcome, low mortality and a low recurrence rate.

Posterior circulation strokes have the best overall outlook, although the swallowing difficulties need to be managed carefully to prevent the development of aspiration pneumonia. There is also a high recurrence rate.

### Transient ischaemic attacks

Transient ischaemic attacks are minor strokes caused by the passage of small emboli that negotiate the cerebral circulation without producing any permanent damage. The clinical picture depends on the route the emboli take and varies from a paralysed or clumsy limb (→ Case Study 4.5) to an isolated speech or visual disturbance. By definition the symptoms and signs of TIA

---

**CASE STUDY 4.5**  A 70-year-old man with episodic numbness

A man was admitted with episodic weakness of the right arm and leg lasting 5 min and associated with difficulties finding the right words. He returned to normal between attacks. During the previous week there had been four or five episodes. He had treated hypertension and a heart murmur. He was otherwise well. Subsequent urgent investigations showed a near total blockage of the right common carotid artery. His hypertension was controlled, and he was started on aspirin and referred for consideration of surgery to the blocked carotid.

last no longer than 24 h, but in practice the clinical picture is of an immediate onset with resolution within 5–20 min. It is unusual for any deficit to last longer than 1 h. Clearly, such short-lived symptoms can be confused with several other conditions, including epilepsy, migraine, hypoglycaemia, syncope and acute vertigo (giddiness).

The areas of narrowing and roughening within the carotid arteries from which the emboli usually arise can, in time, give rise to a major stroke. Someone who suffers a TIA is at more than 10 times the normal risk of having a major stroke and the risk is highest immediately after the event. As an approximate guide, the chances of a major stroke after a TIA or minor stroke are 8–12% at 7 days and 11–15% at 1 month. Treatment can significantly reduce these chances, but the situation is urgent and systems should be in place for those with TIAs and minor strokes to have specialist assessment within 24–48 h.

There are two ways to reduce the risk of both recurrent TIAs and a major stroke: long-term low-dose aspirin, and surgical intervention on the carotid artery. The benefits of surgery only outweigh the dangers of surgery in the first 3 months after a TIA when the risk for a stroke is at its peak. Furthermore, surgery only benefits patients with anterior circulation-type symptoms, in whom the carotid narrowing is very severe.

### Intracerebral haemorrhage (approximately 10% of all strokes)

Intracerebral haemorrhage occurs when the wall of an abnormally weak cerebral artery suddenly bursts and releases blood into the brain tissue with the formation of a clot (intracerebral haematoma) ($\rightarrow$ Fig. 4.3). The weakened areas consist of small outpouchings of the vessels, termed microaneurysms, which are the result of damage from chronic hypertension. As with cerebral thrombosis, controlling hypertension has a major role in primary prevention by reducing arterial damage.

#### Clinical features

A severe intracerebral haemorrhage presents as a dramatic collapse with headache and vomiting, leading rapidly to coma and then death. This is by no means the rule, however, and in many cases there are no clinical features that reliably differentiate a stroke caused by haemorrhage from that due to a cerebral infarct.

The distinction is critical because aspirin and, increasingly, thrombolytic drugs are being used to treat cerebral infarction and they would be absolutely contraindicated in cerebral haemorrhage. For this reason, early CT scanning has become an important part of acute stroke management, as it will show a haemorrhage within minutes of it happening. The longer the CT scan is delayed, the more difficult it is to distinguish a haemorrhage from an infarct. Ideally, patients with acute stroke should have access to a CT scan within hours of admission.

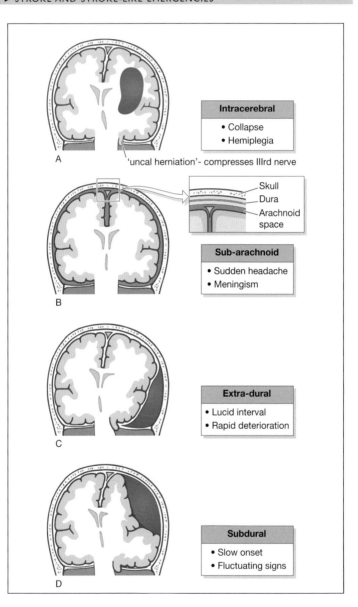

**Fig. 4.3** Types of brain haemorrhage

## Subarachnoid haemorrhage (approximately 5% of all strokes)

The arachnoid is a double-layered membrane that coats the surfaces of the brain and forms the subarachnoid space through which the cerebral arteries pass. Due to a genetic predisposition, some patients develop berry-like aneurysms on these vessels. The aneurysms are prone to rupture, particularly during periods of physical exertion. If an aneurysm bursts, there is acute haemorrhage that spreads throughout the subarachnoid space, typically causing intense meningeal irritation with severe sudden headache and vomiting (→ Fig. 4.3).

The major complications are:

- increased ICP
- spasm of the cerebral arteries, leading to further damage
- re-bleeding

The aneurysms are often multiple, so management is based on supporting the patient through the first episode and taking urgent neurosurgical advice on whether surgery to clip the aneurysms or embolisation to clot them off is needed to prevent any further bleeds. The drug nimodipine – 60 mg 4 hourly given either orally or by nasogastric tube – is used to lessen the risk of cerebral arterial spasm.

### Subdural haemorrhage

This is a low-pressure venous 'ooze' that slowly enlarges within the confines of the subdural space. The slowly forming haematoma presses on the brain and causes a progressive or fluctuating neurological deficit. Subdurals are usually caused by minor and frequently forgotten trauma, particularly in patients with other risk factors, most notably anticoagulant therapy or frequent falling (→ Case Studies 4.6). The classical presentation is with fluctuating drowsiness and rather vague one-sided weakness. The diagnosis is confirmed by CT scan.

### Extradural haemorrhage

This is a high-pressure arterial bleed virtually always associated with a fractured skull (→ Fig. 4.3). The rapid development of a large extradural clot compresses and shifts the cerebral hemisphere, producing coma and pupillary changes. Characteristically, but not always, there is a lucid interval after the head injury before the patient suddenly starts to deteriorate. It is the fear of a delayed extradural that keeps patients in hospital after head injuries.

In theory, extradural haemorrhages should not be seen on the medical wards, but an occasional patient may be admitted with an unrecognised head injury who suddenly deteriorates as a result of an extradural bleed. These patients survive only if the condition is recognised and they are sent for urgent neurosurgery.

**CASE STUDIES 4.6** Subdural haemorrhage

**CASE 1**
An 84-year-old woman was admitted from a nursing home where she was normally mobile, conversant and continent. Four days previously, she had fallen out of bed and banged her head. She was discharged from AED with a GCS of 14. The following day she became drowsy and incoherent. Her GP diagnosed a urinary infection. She deteriorated and was admitted. Her GCS was 8. There was bruising around the left eye. Her CT scan showed a large subdural haematoma. She was referred to neurosurgery to aspirate the haematoma.

**CASE 2**
A 75-year-old man was knocked down by a slowly moving bus and sustained a glancing blow to the side of his head, with transient loss of consciousness. On admission to the surgical ward his GCS was 13. He remained 'mildly' confused, but was discharged after 3 days. The relatives rang the surgical ward to say his mobility and confusion were worsening, but no action was taken. A week after discharge he was re-admitted to the medical ward. He was difficult to rouse: he had a GCS of 8 and was still confused. A CT scan showed a large subdural haemorrhage, with shift of the brain to the opposite side. Despite neurosurgical intervention, he made very poor progress.

The patients themselves may simply appear confused and aggressive after a head injury of which they have no recollection. The key, as with many of these neurological disorders, is to remember the possibility of the diagnosis, particularly where there is a dramatic change in the level of consciousness. It is, of course, critical to take a full history from the patient and witnesses with regards to possible head injury. It is also helpful to remember that vomiting after a head injury is a warning symptom of a skull fracture and these are the patients who are at risk of an extradural haemorrhage.

## NURSING THE PATIENT WITH A STROKE: THE FIRST 24 H

The nature of the emergency initial assessment of a patient with a stroke is determined by his condition. When there is impairment of the conscious level, the immediate assessment and management is that of any patient in coma, with the focus naturally being on securing the airway and performing resuscitation (ABCDE). When there appears to be a less severe disability such as a weak arm or speech disturbance in an alert and stable patient, the assessment may concentrate on the functional capacity of the patient, in particular vision, communication, balance and swallowing.

*Critical nursing observations and immediate management*
The immediate management of the stroke is that of coma and has already been described. The primary aim is to maintain oxygen delivery to the brain.

The initial examination should concentrate on the vital signs, the consciousness level (GCS) and the swallowing:

- assess security of the airway (recovery position ensures the safety of the airway)
- maintain an oxygen saturation > 95%
- pulse (atrial fibrillation?)
- temperature (aspiration pneumonia? hypothermia?)
- blood pressure

**Avoiding aspiration pneumonia and assessing the swallow.** About one in three stroke patients will have at least temporary swallowing problems after a stroke and will be at risk from aspiration; if they are also kept 'nil by mouth', there is the added problem of avoiding dehydration and even malnutrition. The fact that the conscious level is normal does not reliably predict that the swallow is safe (→ Case Study 4.7). There must be a formal swallowing assessment in every patient with acute stroke before oral fluids are allowed. The initial assessment will identify some of the features that are seen in patients who are at risk from aspiration:

- low GCS (less than 8)
- the voice sounds wet and rough and the gag reflex is reduced
- the cough is weak
- the larynx (Adam's apple) does not move upwards on swallowing
- the patient is elderly and frail
- previous stroke
- patients who are unable to sit upright and who have loss of balance

A simple water test must be carried out to identify disordered swallowing:

- support the patient in the sitting position
- give 5 ml of water and look for choking, coughing, dribbling, wet voice
- if swallowing is satisfactory, repeat the test with 50 ml of water
- if the test fails, keep the patient nil by mouth, start i.v. fluids and refer for advice

---

**CASE STUDY 4.7** Loss of swallowing

A 74-year-old man was admitted to hospital because he awoke and found that he could not swallow. He tried to get to the phone, but was unable to stand because of unsteadiness. On admission he had slurring of his speech and was unable to sit unsupported without toppling over. His arm movements were very uncoordinated; when he tried to touch his nose he was in danger of damaging his eyes. His blood pressure was 180/120 mmHg and he had loud bruits over both carotid arteries, suggesting arterial disease. He insisted he was well enough to go home but could not stand. On testing his swallow there was immediate choking and coughing. Investigations confirmed a POCI.

| Box 4.5 – Barthel ADL functional assessment scale | |
|---|---|
| Bowels | Mobility |
| Bladder | Transfer |
| Grooming | Dressing |
| Toilet use | Stairs |
| Feeding | Bathing |

If the swallow is unsafe, maintain the fluid intake with i.v. fluids. Refer the patient to the specialist team (either the dietician or the speech therapist) and consider re-testing in 24 h. As there is a risk of inhalation of oropharyngeal contaminants, particular care should be taken to ensure good oral hygiene.

**History.** The basis for making the correct diagnosis is the history from the patient and their relatives. It is important to evaluate pre-existing dependency using measures such as the Barthel ADL index (→ Box 4.5) and to find out the home situation in terms of carers, independent housing, warden control, residential care or nursing home.

If there has been a previous stroke, it will have to be established how much of the present problem is due to residual disability and how much is new. Risk factors for stroke can be identified from the history: hypertension, atrial fibrillation, diabetes and heart disease.

**Managing urinary incontinence.** Urinary incontinence suggests disordered higher (cortical) function and is common in anterior circulation strokes. Catheterisation causes infection and leads to a reduction in the bladder capacity; it should therefore be avoided, as it reduces the chance of the spontaneous recovery in bladder function that usually occurs after a stroke. Urge incontinence is a common early problem and is not helped by problems with communication and mobility. The focus for the nursing staff should be on the use of simple communication aids and in trying to anticipate or respond as rapidly as possible to the patient's toileting needs. The return of independent mobility is often associated with improved continence.

**Communication.** During the initial assessment, it will be apparent if there is a communication problem other than that due to an impaired conscious level. The three basic aspects to communication *must* be evaluated and documented at an early stage: this must be interpreted in the light of the relatives' description of the patient's pre-existing cognitive function.

*Vision.* The more extensive strokes are often complicated by visual disturbance. The pattern of visual loss that is usually seen is termed a hemianopia. This is a loss of the left or right visual field and involves both eyes. As a rule the visual loss is towards the paralysed side so, for example, a patient with a left hemiplegia would not be able to see towards the left. A person standing and talking from the patient's left-hand side will therefore not be seen and will often be ignored by the patient. Similarly, food and fluid placed to the left of the patient will not be seen. A hemianopia has to be specifically looked for, because many stroke patients will be unaware of its presence. It is also important to note if the patient is unable to move his eyes to one or other side (gaze palsy).

*Hearing.* Perhaps surprisingly, the most common cause of poor communication on the acute medical ward is a failure to appreciate simple deafness in an elderly patient. Hearing loss itself is not usually caused by stroke.

*Speech and language.* Slurring of the speech may be a problem, particularly after a POCI, but it is usually not a major barrier to communication. Much more importantly, stroke may be complicated by a problem with language: finding, using and understanding words, known as dysphasia (*dy*sphasia is *d*ifficulty with speech; *a*phasia is *a*bsence of speech). There are two types of dysphasia:

1. **Motor dysphasia.** There is a block in getting the words out, despite the patient understanding everything and knowing what he wants to say. This is most frustrating for the patient. Motor dysphasia is often accompanied by a hemiplegia.
2. **Sensory dysphasia**. The patient has difficulty finding the right words and in understanding what is being said. The patient's speech is jumbled and senseless, although the patient may not appear distressed by it. Sensory dysphasia is often accompanied by a hemianopia.

### Interventions in the first 24 h
**Acute drug intervention.** The only immediate active intervention that is universally acknowledged to reduce the recurrence rate and decrease mortality after a stroke is long-term aspirin treatment for proven cerebral infarcts. Long-term aspirin reduces the risk of further major vascular events in stroke patients by about 25%. The correct dose of aspirin remains controversial, but between 75 and 300 mg per day is usually given. Anticoagulation with warfarin reduces the recurrence of stroke in patients with atrial fibrillation. However, because of the risk of bleeding into the softened and damaged area affected by the stroke, most clinicians prefer to wait several days at least before starting warfarin therapy after a thrombotic stroke and, as with aspirin, only after cerebral haemorrhage has been excluded with a CT.

The role of thrombolytic ('clot-busting') therapy such as rt-PA (alteplase) in cerebral infarction remains controversial but its use is likely to increase, particularly once 'fast tracking' of strokes is introduced, much as has been the case for thrombolytic drugs in myocardial infarction (→ Box 4.6).

**Blood pressure.** The blood pressure often increases acutely after a stroke, only to settle without treatment over a matter of days. Reducing blood pressure with intervention may reduce the blood supply to an area of the

---

**Box 4.6 – Current status of rt-PA in cerebral infarction**

In patients with a large stroke and a normal CT scan, rt-PA given within 3 h of the onset gives a 12% chance of an improved neurological outcome at 3 months but with a 3% chance of an rt-PA-associated death from an acute intracerebral haemorrhage.

Estimates suggest that only 2–3% of stroke patients would at present be eligible for this form of treatment.

---

brain already threatened by ischaemia. Unless extreme hypertension (e.g. diastolic blood pressure of 140 mmHg) is encountered, it is safest to monitor the level and allow the blood pressure to settle. It is safe to discontinue usual antihypertensives for a week or so after an acute stroke, provided that the blood pressure is monitored.

**Temperature.** Pyrexia during the first 72 h of hospital admission is associated with early worsening of the neurological status. Apart from excluding infection, paracetamol can be used to bring the temperature down to normal.

**Cerebral oedema.** Cerebral oedema may develop after a severe stroke and produce a deterioration in the consciousness level within the first day or so. Provided that alternative causes of deterioration such as aspiration pneumonia or urinary infection have been excluded and the CT scan does not indicate a surgically treatable lesion, the management is supportive, as there is little evidence that measures to reduce ICP such as mannitol and steroids are helpful in this situation after a stroke.

**Avoiding pressure sores.** Many elderly patients who suffer a stroke do so alone and they may have been lying in one position for a number of hours, putting pressure on the skin and setting the scene for skin breakdown. This can be alleviated with appropriate physical measures such as the correct pressure-relieving mattress, combined with attention to nutrition and hydration.

The philosophy in the Acute Medical Unit should be based on initiating preventative measures and on starting to address nutritional issues as soon as the patient is admitted. In the past, hydration, nutrition and their effects on the risk of complications have been neglected. Not uncommonly, patients were admitted and eventually found their way to a rehabilitation unit only to find that 2 weeks or so had elapsed before the patient had received any proper food! The patients had lost weight and were at a major risk of pressure sores. As a rule, although fluids are appropriate for 24 h while the swallowing is assessed, after that nutrition is required. This often means passing a fine-bore nasogastric tube.

**Resuscitation status.** A judgement must be made and explicitly stated on the resuscitation status of the patient. This is based on a number of important factors that include:

- the wishes of the patient (in practice, these will seldom be known, and in the patients in whom the decision is most relevant – those who are critically ill – it is unlikely to be ascertainable)
- the chances of survival (as an example, patients who are comatose 24 h after a stroke have only a 20% chance of survival)
- the pre-existing dependency of the patient (the Barthel score will give an accurate picture of the patient's level of independence)
- the perceptions of close relatives and carers (due weight is given to their views, although ultimately the decision rests with the clinical staff in the absence of the patient's own views)
- coexisting diseases, e.g. advanced malignant disease
- the opinion of the relevant medical and nursing staff

Any resuscitation decision must be reviewed at predetermined intervals and on an Acute Medical Unit it would be appropriate to re-visit the question of resuscitation at least 12-hourly during the first 2–3 days.

## ANSWERING RELATIVES' QUESTIONS ON STROKE

*Will he recover?*  The answer to this depends on the severity of the stroke. Patients who are comatose on admission or who persistently ignore or neglect their paralysed side do badly. Stroke patients who start to recover within hours, particularly in terms of sitting balance, will do well. A 'cover-all' answer for all cases soon after admission would be to say that two out of every three stroke victims regain more or less full independence after a stroke. The patients who do badly are those with severe motor and sensory impairment, especially combined with hemianopias and urinary incontinence.

*Why cannot we simply dissolve the clot as in a heart attack?*  The evidence that clot busters work in acute stroke is controversial, and in any case, if they are given more than 3 h after the onset, they probably do more harm than good. At present they are not part of our usual care.

*Why have you not done MRI?*  We need to tell whether the stroke is a bleed or a blockage. The CT is the easiest test to do this. The MRI is reserved for particular types of stroke, but it is much less easy to do and the patient can find it quite an unpleasant test.

*Why can't you operate?*  Surgery can only rarely help stroke patients (cerebellar stroke and occasional superficial cerebral bleeds). There is a big risk that an operation can make any disability worse.

*What has happened?*  Part of the brain has been damaged and the function of that area has been affected. This explains why there is paralysis/speech problems/confusion. The cause is a blockage to the blood supply or a sudden leak of blood into the brain tissue from a leaking artery.

*Is it a heart attack – is the heart affected?* Although sometimes a clot causing the stroke comes from the heart, the heart itself is not affected. Nonetheless, the risk factors for stroke and for heart attack are the same, so any preventative measures we recommend, such as smoking cessation, will have a dual benefit.

*When will we know the amount of damage?* The main recovery takes place over the first days or weeks after a stroke, but some further more limited recovery is possible over a much longer period.

*Why is he not in a specialist unit?* All patients who are acutely ill and unstable are admitted to the acute ward. However, we work closely with the stroke/rehabilitation unit and we will transfer the patient there at the first opportunity. Physiotherapy and other specific treatment has, however, started already.

*What physiotherapy will he need?* The immediate emphasis is on positioning the limbs and body correctly and on assessing balance, rather than on simply seeing if the patient can walk. If you wish, you can talk to the physiotherapists about it.

*What about feeding?* At present his swallowing is not particularly good, so we are using a drip and restricting any oral intake for a day or so to allow time for it to improve.

*Was it stress that caused the stroke?* No, there is no relationship between the two.

*What is in the drip?* This is dextrose, which provides fluid and some calories. If we cannot feed the patient orally within 24 h, we will need to consider a thin feeding tube, possibly as a short-term measure, to give some nutrition.

*How much can he understand?*

1. This is a motor aphasia, which means he can understand but cannot find the right words.
2. This is a sensory aphasia, so there is quite a problem at present with understanding as well as the use of words.
3. He is in a coma, so at present we are unclear how much he can take in, but he may be able to hear and understand you.

*Will it happen again?* There is a chance of a further stroke if he has suffered one already, but we will do whatever we can to lessen the risks of recurrence. This will involve aspirin/cessation of smoking/control of blood pressure, etc.

*Were there any warning signs we/the GP could have seen?* Unless there were mini-strokes, there are few if any warnings of this sort of thing.

*Will he always be disabled/handicapped?* The degree of disability cannot be accurately predicted at this early stage. (However, if the patient is recovering already or has retained good power in the legs and has a clear understanding of the situation, you can be reasonably encouraging, particularly if he was not previously dependent for his care.)

*Is there anything we can do?* Once we know the level of ability with feeding and personal needs, you can assist with meals and other care if you wish.

### ✔ EXCELLENT ACUTE STROKE CARE

Documentation of:
- Conscious level
- Eye movements
- Swallowing
- Communication
- Understanding
- Vision (field and gaze)
- Sensation
- Neglect of the affected side
- Classification of the type of stroke
- Pre-stroke function

Early:
- CT scan
- Physiotherapist assessment
- Speech therapy assessment

## MENINGOCOCCAL MENINGITIS

Meningococcal meningitis is one of the most feared neurological emergencies: it affects children and young adults, it carries a 5% mortality rate and, even with treatment, patients can be moribund within hours of its onset. Since 1995, the number of cases in the UK has continued to rise: in 1998/99, 2962 cases were notified in the UK, compared with 1555 cases in 1994/95. The Acute Medical Unit will admit one to two cases per month, but many more patients than this will be admitted for investigations, including lumbar puncture, to exclude the diagnosis.

There are several strains of meningococcal bacteria, but in the UK groups B and C cause virtually all meningococcal infections (→ Table 4.2). This is not the case world-wide; for example in the Middle East and in the tropics, group A has been responsible for major outbreaks of meningitis.

Group B, which causes 60–65% of the cases in the UK, affects babies and toddlers, while group C causes the remaining 35–40% and particularly affects

| Table 4.2 | Incidence of meningococcal meningitis | | | |
|-----------|-----------|-----------|-----------|-----------|
| *Strain* | *Frequency* | *Max. age group* | *Vaccination?* | *Case clusters* |
| GROUP B | 60–65% | 0.5–4 years | Ineffective | No |
| GROUP C | 35–40% | 15–19 years | Effective | Yes |

young adults around university age. In recent years, the proportion of cases caused by group C (specifically the C2a serotype) has increased, with more cases being seen in patients in their late teens, in whom the mortality is the highest.

There are important public health implications when a case of meningococcal infection is admitted. It is an infectious disease that can be spread to close contacts, particularly in semi-closed communities such as university halls of residence. Close contacts of isolated cases receive prophylactic antibiotics to kill any meningococcal bacteria colonising the oropharynx. In meningitis outbreaks, whole groups may require prophylaxis and, in the case of group C infections, vaccination.

## CLINICAL PICTURE

Meningococcal bacteria normally live quite naturally in the oropharynx of about 10% of the healthy population. This figure rises to 25% in those living in close proximity, particularly when they are of school and university age. In meningococcal disease, for some unexplained reason the bacteria become virulent and invade the bloodstream. The result is meningococcal septicaemia and, if the nervous system is also invaded, meningococcal meningitis (→ Fig. 4.4).

There are therefore two components to meningococcal infections, either of which may dominate the clinical picture:

- septicaemia alone (mortality 30%)           10% of cases
- meningitis alone (mortality 5%)              50% of cases
- mixed features of meningitis and septicaemia   40% of cases

The key features of meningococcal infection are (→ Box 4.7):

- fever
- haemorrhagic rash
- altered level of consciousness

However, the early symptoms can be non-specific ones of fever, lethargy, abdominal pain, vomiting, joint pains and diarrhoea. The rash is caused by meningeal infection within the skin and is the major feature of septicaemia, but it can be difficult to recognise at first. It may start off as a red discolouration that blanches on pressure and only later develops into the

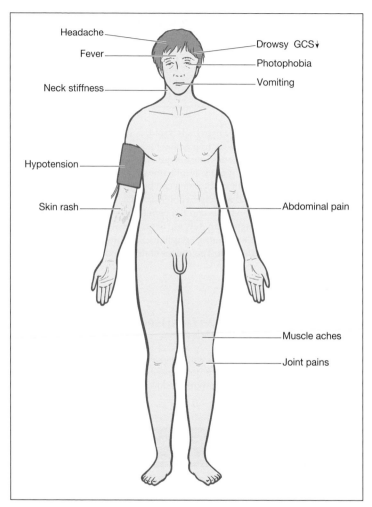

**Fig. 4.4** Clinical features of meningococcal septicaemia

non-blanching haemorrhagic spots that are so characteristic of meningococcal infection. Patients often have an extensive rash and an impaired conscious level during the septicaemic phase, with headache, photophobia and neck stiffness developing with the onset of meningitis. Patients with meningitis alone may not have a rash at all.

---

**Box 4.7 – Clinical features of meningococcal infection**

| Septicaemia | Meningitis |
|---|---|
| ● influenza | ● photophobia |
| ● vomiting | ● headache |
| ● muscle pain | ● neck stiffness |
| ● drowsiness | ● coma |

---

Clinical deterioration can be extremely rapid – of patients who die, almost a fifth die at home or on the way to hospital and, overall, 50% of the deaths occur in the first 48 h. Antibiotics must be given at the first suspicion of meningococcal infection – 2 g of i.v. cefotaxime or 2 g of i.v. ceftriaxone. Over a few hours, the patient with septicaemia can become confused, tachycardic, peripherally shut down and acutely hypotensive. The respiratory rate increases, the conscious level falls and the patient develops profound shock.

The patient with meningitis can develop acute elevation of the ICP, with deepening coma, fitting, hemiparesis, pupillary signs and the combination of a bradycardia and hypertension. The causes of death in meningitis are:

● septicaemic shock
● increased ICP

## NURSING THE PATIENT WITH SUSPECTED MENINGOCOCCAL MENINGITIS

If a patient is admitted to hospital with suspected meningococcal meningitis, there are a number of immediate critical nursing tasks that must be carried out. There are also a number of important nursing tasks.

### IMMEDIATE CRITICAL NURSING TASKS IN MENINGITIS

■ **Assessment of ABCDE**
■ **Give oxygen**
■ **Vital signs**
■ **Secure i.v. access**
■ **Administer *immediate* i.v. antibiotics (benzyl penicillin or cefotaxime)**
■ **Measurement of GCS: record serial data on a flow chart**
■ **Note any rash**

## IMMEDIATE IMPORTANT NURSING TASKS IN MENINGITIS

■ **Detain any relatives for further history and advice on contacts**
■ **Ensure there are no drug allergies**
■ **Ensure immediate specimens are taken for bacteriology**
   — **blood cultures**
   — **EDTA blood sample for urgent PCR (a special test to confirm infection)**
   — **clotted sample for meningococcal serology**
   — **oral or per nasal posterior pharyngeal wall swab (immediate culture)**
■ **Preparations should be made for a lumbar puncture, should it be needed to confirm a diagnosis of meningitis. There are several contraindications to a lumbar puncture, most notably progressive neurological deterioration such as fits or a GCS less than 13. Lumbar puncture is also not advisable if the patient is severely shocked or if increased ICP is suspected.**

*Nursing care*

The prime aims of nursing management are:

● to support the patient while the antibiotics take effect
● to be vigilant in recognising complications

The patient with meningococcal infection can be mildly unwell, extremely ill with classical features of meningitis, or in extremis with septicaemic shock. Most cases need intensive nursing input during the first few days of admission. Fortunately, most patients respond rapidly to i.v. antibiotics and supportive care – volume resuscitation and high flow oxygen – but in a minority the course will change rapidly with worsening septicaemia or a progressive increase in ICP.

Changes in the observations, particularly in the GCS, the pulse and the blood pressure, are vitally important. If the patient is doing badly, the GCS drops below 13, the pulse increases and the blood pressure falls (shock), or the pulse falls and the blood pressure increases (increased ICP; → Box 4.8). These patients need to be moved to an ITU.

Shock needs to be managed with inotropic support (dopamine or adrenaline), invasive monitoring and, probably, ventilation. Increased ICP caused by severe meningitis requires interventions to bring the pressure down, including raising the head of the bed by 30°, reducing external stimuli, i.v. mannitol, corticosteroids and ventilation (→ Box 4.8). The role of urgent

---

**Box 4.8 – Recognising and managing raised intracranial pressure**

**Clinical features**
- persistent vomiting
- falling GCS
- falling pulse
- rising blood pressure
- unilateral dilated pupil

**Management**
- raise the head 30°
- intravenous mannitol 20% solution 250–500 ml
- dexamethasone 4 mg i.v. qds
- reduce external stimuli, adequate pain relief
- ventilation to correct oxygen and blow off carbon dioxide
- CT scan and urgent neurosurgical opinion

---

use of steroids (dexamethasone 10 mg given i.v. with the first dose of antibiotics) remains controversial, but will be used in severe cases.

*Critical nursing observations in the first 24 h*
The frequency of observations should be modified according to the patient's condition.

---

 **CRITICAL NURSING OBSERVATIONS IN THE FIRST 24 H IN MENINGITIS**

- **Half-hourly GCS (fluctuation or deterioration are bad signs)**
- **Half-hourly pupillary responses (increased ICP)**
- **Half-hourly pulse, blood pressure, state of extremities (capillary filling) (shock/increased ICP)**
- **Half-hourly respiratory rate and saturations (shock/pulmonary oedema)**
- **Hourly urine volumes and strict fluid balance (shock/correcting hypotension)**
- **2-hourly temperature (response to antibiotics)**
- **ECG monitoring (arrhythmias due to septicaemic shock/heart muscle toxicity)**
- **Progression of any rash (worsening septicaemia)**

## Overview: The signs of worsening meningitis

- Rapidly progressing rash
- Poor peripheral circulation
  - capillary refill > 4 seconds
  - systolic blood pressure < 90 mmHg
  - falling urine output
- Respiratory rate < 8 or > 30 breaths/min
- Pulse < 40 or > 140 beats/min
- Falling (less than 12) or fluctuating (by more than 2) GCS
- Development of a focal limb weakness
- Fitting
- Falling pulse and climbing blood pressure

*Nursing management apart from the critical tasks and observations*

- Managing a confused, restless or aggressive patient
- Comforting and reassuring a critically ill young patient
- Antiemetic treatment
- Antipyrexia measures: tepid sponging, fan, adequate fluids
- Explaining the various observations and interventions
- Assessing headache, joint pains, neck stiffness, muscle pain
- Ensuring adequate analgesia is prescribed and given (dihydrocodeine by choice)
- Using appropriate handling manoeuvres to minimise patient's discomfort (e.g. log rolling)
- Minimising external stimuli: light, noise, visitors
- Ensuring a fully informed nursing handover, including a shared GCS assessment
- Ensure the consultant for CCDC knows about the case; he or she will be responsible for dealing with contacts
- Appropriate management plan for anticipated complications (e.g. fitting)

### ANSWERING RELATIVES' QUESTIONS IN MENINGITIS

The relatives of a young patient with meningococcal infection are understandably among the most distraught that will be encountered on the Acute Medical Unit. The lay perception is of young people struck down *en masse* at the threshold of their adult life by a 'killer infection' (there are currently around 260 deaths per year from meningococcal meningitis in the UK). The first task will be to reassure the family that 90% of all cases of meningococcal infection make a complete recovery.

*Should we have acted any sooner?* The early symptoms of meningitis are notoriously difficult to spot, and can be confused with flu or gastroenteritis, even by experienced doctors.

*When will we know whether he will pull through?* Complications, by which we mean shock and worsening of meningitis with increased pressure on the brain, usually occur within the first 48 h. We are aiming to head off complications by giving potent antibiotics to clear the infection before it spreads.

*What are the signs of improvement we should expect?* The patient will become less drowsy and the observations will stabilise, with a return to normal of the pulse, breathing rate and blood pressure.

*What are the signs that things are not going so well?* Drowsiness will increase and the patient may become more restless and confused. We may have to move the patient to ITU if we think ventilation (life support machine) and other forms of intensive support may be needed to get the patient through the next few days while the antibiotics get to work.

*Could there be any permanent brain damage?* Permanent damage is unusual but not unknown. The most common damage is hearing disturbance, but this is seen more commonly in children. Most adults make a full recovery. We can do further assessments if necessary, with special tests such as a CT scan at a later stage if we suspect complications.

*Are we all at risk now?* Yes, there is a substantial risk that close contacts, those who live with the patient and who may perhaps have been kissing their mouth, may develop symptoms of meningitis. The risk is greatest over the next week, but it remains high for several weeks. We will arrange for you to have urgent antibiotic treatment (usually rifampicin 600 mg 12-hourly for 2 days) to kill any bacteria that may be living at the back of your throat and reduce the risk of your getting meningitis. If you are worried about your own symptoms, you must see your doctor urgently.

*What about his friends?* Household contacts and 'kissing contacts' will be given preventative antibiotics and vaccination. We will need their details.

*Should we all be vaccinated?* Vaccinations against meningitis are now effective in preventing meningococcal infections and close domestic contacts (of group C cases) will be offered a vaccine.

*What vaccination is available?* Vaccination is available for groups A, C and two strains that cause occasional infections in travellers: W135 and Y. The original C vaccination is not suitable for children under 18 months and its protective effect is short lived. The recent introduction of a new group C conjugate vaccine (MenC), which gives long-term protection and is suitable for babies and toddlers, heralds the start of a routine vaccination programme against meningitis in the general population, in contrast to previous vaccinations that were used to protect household contacts and to control outbreaks when there were clusters of group C cases. As yet there is still no established vaccination for group B infections, the most common cause of meningitis in the UK, although in some countries, Cuba for example, a group B vaccination is given routinely to every child. Trials in the UK are under way, however, and it is likely that a group B vaccination will be available here soon.

*What about the university/school?* If this is a single case, preventative antibiotics are only recommended for close contacts (flat-mates, girlfriends/boyfriends, etc.). If the case proves to be part of a cluster (more than one case from the same group or class within 4 weeks), then preventative treatment may have to be given to a wider population. This is a matter for the public health specialists.

*Are the nurses and doctors at risk?* Nurses and doctors are only at risk if they have performed prolonged mouth-to-mouth resuscitation or have inhaled oral secretions during, say, attempts at intubation.

# ACUTE SEVERE HEADACHE

Patients are admitted to the Acute Medical Unit with headache because of two primary concerns:

- Is this meningitis?
- Is this a subarachnoid haemorrhage?

The three most common 'benign' causes of acute severe headache are:

- migraine
- tonsillitis/pharyngitis with meningism
- stress headache

However, the stakes are high, and most of us remember at least one case of 'missed subarachnoid' and 'missed meningitis' in our clinical practice. As with most neurological problems, the history is all important.

Bacterial meningitis has already been described in detail. Viral meningitis has a similar, though less severe, picture and the patients are not usually critically ill unless the inflammation has spread to the brain tissue (encephalitis).

## SUBARACHNOID HAEMORRHAGE

Subarachnoid haemorrhage occurs with the speed of a lightning strike: 'like a brick', 'like a sudden blow', 'like an explosion inside my skull'. It does not build up over an hour or so – it drops the patient in seconds. The headache is extremely severe and often spreads to the neck. There may be immediate loss of consciousness followed by immediate recovery or prolonged coma. The patient does not wake up with pain, struggles to work and has to come home to lie in the dark: that is migraine.

There are catches and exceptions: occasionally, patients with a subarachnoid haemorrhage have little warning bleeds in the days leading up to the major event, whereas some patients without a subarachnoid suffer so-called 'thunderclap headaches' that can be as severe as a subarachnoid but are entirely harmless. As a rule, however, a description of the exact onset will be the main way in which a provisional diagnosis is reached, to be confirmed or refuted by CT scan and lumbar puncture. Of the true explosive headaches, around one in eight patients will have had a subarachnoid haemorrhage. Interestingly, up to a fifth of all cases of meningitis are initially thought to be a subarachnoid haemorrhage.

### The CT and lumbar puncture in subarachnoid haemorrhage
It is critical not to miss a subarachnoid haemorrhage. The 30-day mortality is 45%, and most of this is due to re-bleeding. In view of the uncertainty of making a firm clinical diagnosis, a CT scan is always required to confirm a subarachnoid bleed. If the scan is done within 12 h, around 98% of the bleeds will be found and in 2% the scan will look normal. If the CT is delayed by 72 h, only 75% of the bleeds will be found and in 25% the scan will look normal, even though the patient has bled. Thus, if there is a suggestive history but a negative scan, the patient will need a lumbar puncture to look for blood and xanthochromia in the CSF.

### Nursing the patient with subarachnoid haemorrhage
The aim of the management is to keep the patient in the best possible condition until he can be transferred for neurosurgical assessment. The nursing principles are the same as those for a conventional stroke or a patient with coma, in terms of primary assessment with ABCDE and subsequent nursing care with attention to fluid balance, pressure areas and adequate pain relief.

**Headache and neck stiffness.** These symptoms are severe in patients with a subarachnoid and need powerful regular analgesia, conventionally using intramuscular dihydrocodeine and an antiemetic such as cyclizine. Opiates tend to be avoided because of their effects on the pupils, but may be required occasionally. Patients will be severely photophobic and will be most comfortable in a quiet, darkened room with a minimum of visitors.

**Neurological observations.** After a subarachnoid haemorrhage, the main complications and their warning signs are:

- Bleeding into the brain tissue (intracerebral haematoma)
  — falling GCS
  — development of stroke-like features (unilateral weakness, etc.)
  — seizures
- Spasm of the cerebral arteries
  — falling GCS

- Re-bleeding
  - further headache
  - falling GCS
- Increased ICP
  - falling pulse, rising blood pressure
  - falling GCS
  - pupillary changes

**Sequential neurological assessment.** GCS and pupillary responses, pulse and blood pressure and general nursing observations will identify the warning signs of complications. Any change in these parameters should be reported so that the overall clinical state can be reassessed with a view to repeat CT scanning and perhaps accelerated transfer to the neurosurgeons.

## ANSWERING RELATIVES' QUESTIONS IN SUBARACHNOID HAEMORRHAGE

*Where is the bleeding?* The blood has escaped from a ruptured artery on the surface of the brain. It has spread around the brain and into the spinal fluid.

*Why is he unconscious?* The bleeding can cause the brain to go into 'shock', which we are hoping will be temporary. We are supporting the breathing at present, but we are hoping there will be signs of recovery within the next 24–48 h.

*Will he recover?* The prospects of recovery depend on the extent of the bleeding and also on two other factors: whether there is spasm of the cerebral arteries and whether there is a second bleed.

*Why him?* The usual cause is an unexplained weakness in the artery wall that suddenly ruptures.

*Could the doctor not have seen the warning signs?* Occasionally there is a warning bleed, but these are often like migraine attacks. In most patients there is no warning at all.

*Was it all stress?* There is no relationship to stress.

*What about the well-man clinic visits, blood pressure, etc.?* There are no warning signs of a subarachnoid and it is not directly related to high blood pressure.

*Will there be brain damage?* That depends on whether there is bleeding into the brain substance itself and also whether the treatment we are using (nimodipine) is successful in preventing spasm of the leaking artery.

*Can you operate?* If the situation stabilises, we will transfer the patient to the neurosurgeons, who will assess whether surgery is needed to prevent a further bleed. The surgery is preventative and is unlikely to improve the patient's present condition.

*Will it happen again?* Sometimes there is more than one area of weakness or the weakened spot can itself leak again. About 10% of patients with aneurysms re-bleed within hours and, if untreated, up to 30% re-bleed within a few weeks.

*Can he drive again?* Non-vocational driving can be resumed in due course, providing recovery is complete. There will, however, need to be a certain period before driving can resume. You may need to inform the DVLC, and check with your insurance company if you are in any doubts.

*Can't you just send him to a specialist unit straight away and they can operate?* The best time to operate is when the patient is in the best possible medical condition, but before the peak time for re-bleeding. We are working in conjunction with the specialist unit and have taken their advice on the best time for a transfer.

## LUMBAR PUNCTURE

The lumbar puncture has a justified reputation as an unpleasant and potentially dangerous procedure. The main danger is from inadvertently doing a lumbar puncture when there is acute increase in the ICP, so that CSF is forced out of the breach in the subarachnoid space. The sudden release of increased CSF pressure sucks the brain in a downwards direction and can cause a dramatic deterioration in the neurological state (termed a 'pressure cone').

### Contraindications to a lumbar puncture

- Suspected increased ICP
- Patients in coma who have not had a CT scan
- Suspected cord compression
- Local sepsis over the proposed lumbar puncture site

### Indications on the Acute Medical Unit

- Suspected meningitis and encephalitis
- Suspected subarachnoid haemorrhage (after a negative CT)
- Suspected Guillain–Barré syndrome

*Suspected meningitis and encephalitis.* Although the lumbar puncture is important in the diagnosis and management of meningitis, it should not lead to a delay in giving antibiotics. In patients who are drowsy or with clinical signs of increased ICP or a possible cerebral abscess, the lumbar puncture is *only* performed once a normal CT scan has been obtained.

*Suspected subarachnoid haemorrhage.* The lumbar puncture is done to find the few cases of subarachnoid bleeding that the CT has missed. In a suspected subarachnoid bleed with a normal scan, fewer than 1 in 20 lumbar punctures will be positive.

*Suspected Guillain–Barré.* The CSF is examined to look for the characteristic changes seen in the Guillain–Barré syndrome (a high protein and few or no cells).

## Procedure

A full explanation of the reason for doing the lumbar puncture and a description of what to expect in terms of discomfort will help to allay the anxiety of most patients. The very restless and agitated patient may need cautious sedation with i.v. diazepam (i.v. flumazenil, which will reverse diazepam immediately, must be on hand in case of oversedation).

The patient should be warned of the following:

- the position
- the cold skin-preparation
- the poking around to find the correct entry spot over the back
- the burning of the local anaesthetic
- the pushing sensation in their back
- the possibility of an acute shooting pain in either leg
- the possibility of post-lumbar-puncture headache due to a low-pressure CSF leak

**The position.** It cannot be overstated that the correct positioning of the patient makes the difference between success and failure in performing a lumbar puncture.

The patient must be lying right on the edge of the bed curled up (comfortably, not forcibly) in the fetal position with the back and both shoulders perpendicular to the mattress. This position is easiest to achieve with a pillow under the head and two pillows between the knees and pushed into the abdomen, across which the patient can rest his upper arm (→ Fig. 4.5).

The two common mistakes are for the top shoulder to roll over rather than remain vertical, and for the spine to be curved rather than straight.

**The equipment.** The advice is to use a small (22G) lumbar puncture needle to reduce the risk of post-lumbar-puncture CSF leak and headache. The manometer is used to record the CSF pressure (normally 6–20 cmH$_2$O; if it is above 30 cmH$_2$O there is significantly increased ICP).

In suspected subarachnoid haemorrhage, three sequential bottles are needed (labelled 1, 2, 3) to identify the progressive decrease in blood staining of a traumatic tap. In addition, one specimen is sent for microbiology, one for biochemistry, one for cytology, and a fluoride oxalate (yellow label) tube is used for sugar. Blood is also drawn for determination of sugar level. In cases in which subarachnoid bleeding is not an issue, the three sequential bottles may not be used but should always be on hand.

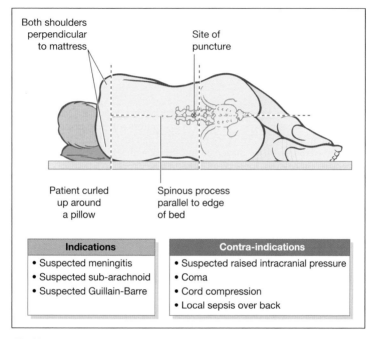

**Fig. 4.5** Positioning for a lumbar puncture

Normally, approximately five drops (1 ml) is sufficient in each bottle. Analysis of the results is summarised in Table 4.3.

**Aftercare.** Patients should stay flat on one pillow for 3–4 h after a lumbar puncture. Any post-lumbar-puncture headache should be recorded, analgesia

**Table 4.3   Diagnosis from analysis of LP results**

| Condition | CSF | Cell count (cells/ml) | Protein (g/l) | CSF sugar/ blood sugar |
|-----------|-----|-----------------------|---------------|------------------------|
| Normal | Clear | Less than 3 cells | 0.2–0.5 | >50% |
| Bacterial meningitis | Cloudy | Neutrophils up to 10 000 | 0.5–2.0 | <50% |
| Viral meningitis | Clearish | Lymphocytes up to 500 | <0.8 | >50% |
| Subarachnoid | Bloody | More than 100 red cells | >0.2 | >50% |
| Guillain–Barré | Clear | Fewer than 3 cells | 0.5–3.5 | >50% |

will be needed, and the patient should be reassured but kept flat until the headache improves.

If the CSF pressure is found to be very high, urgent neurosurgical transfer may be required. In these circumstances, frequent neurological observations (pupils, GCS, pulse and blood pressure) should be started as soon as the lumbar puncture has been completed. Measures to lower the pressure may be instituted before transfer. In the meantime, any changes in the neurological status must be recorded and reported.

*Xanthochromia: a practical guide to interpreting the CSF result in subarachnoid haemorrhage*

- Blood in the CSF from a recent subarachnoid haemorrhage can only be distinguished from a traumatic tap caused by the lumbar puncture needle by the finding of red/yellow pigmentation in the CSF specimen, due to breakdown of old blood. It appears as a yellow tinge (xanthochromia) after the CSF has been spun down in the laboratory. Xanthochromia can be seen with the naked eye or, in more subtle cases, by spectrophotometry. In traumatic bleeding caused by the lumbar puncture itself, this breakdown does not have time to occur and xanthochromia is absent.
- To allow breakdown to occur, 12 h should elapse between the subarachnoid haemorrhage and the lumbar puncture. Before then, especially within 4 h of a subarachnoid, it may be difficult to differentiate between a bleed and a traumatic tap. If there is no xanthochromia, three sequential CSF specimens from the lumbar puncture will show a progressive fall off in the amount of blood if the tap was traumatic. However, this is not as reliable as finding xanthochromia.
- The CSF (at least 1 ml of it) must be spun immediately, otherwise blood will start to break down in the tube, giving a false positive result; this means that the specimen must be dealt with urgently, day or night. Lumbar punctures are a major intervention and handling of the specimens cannot be left to chance. Careful liaison is needed with the porters and the laboratory staff.
- If the CSF is 'gin-clear' but the history was very suspicious, the specimen should be stored in darkness until it can be checked by the laboratory for xanthochromia using a spectrophotometer.
- Xanthochromia will be found in the CSF at lumbar puncture, even if it is performed 2 weeks or more after a subarachnoid haemorrhage.

## SUDDEN LOSS OF CONSCIOUSNESS: FAINTS AND FITS

Sudden loss of consciousness followed by a recovery is usually due to a faint (syncope) or a fit (tonic–clonic convulsion). These patients are frequently admitted to the Acute Medical Unit with a variety of labels (→ Case Study 4.8).

> **CASE STUDY 4.8** Sudden collapse: was this a fit or a faint?
>
> A 50-year-old woman was admitted with a 'fit'. She had awoken with severe abdominal colic and while being comforted by her husband turned ashen grey, started to sweat profusely and collapsed on the bed 'as though she had died'. She stopped breathing for a few seconds and then slowly came round over 2–3 min. On close questioning of the husband, there had been no convulsive movements, no confusion after the event, no incontinence and no tongue biting. A similar episode had occurred during a severe attack of calf cramp some years before. The diagnosis was of a vasovagal attack triggered by pain (a simple faint).

Provided that the underlying mechanisms and clinical features of epilepsy and syncope are understood, a correct diagnosis can usually be made without too many investigations, once a good eyewitness account has been obtained.

The history will differentiate fits and faints in 80% of cases. A witnessed account is vital and may have to be obtained by a phone call from the ward if necessary.

*Triggers.* Syncope will often be triggered by standing upright, by pain, strong emotion and by heat, particularly in crowded places. Fits do not have specific triggers – they occur anywhere, at any time.

*Onset.* Fits have an aura: often a feeling of anxiety or fear building up in the pit of the stomach. Faints start gradually and share a number of typical warning features: nausea; dimming of the vision; roaring in the ears; sweating and a feeling of heat; a sense of slipping away.

*The attack.* Generalised tonic–clonic attacks are accompanied by rapid, grunting respirations, foaming at the mouth and self-injury. In syncope the patient is cold, grey and clammy. There may be isolated convulsive jerkings, but not as the main feature of the attack.

*Recovery.* Recovery is slow after a convulsion, with drowsiness and confusion lasting at least 30 min. This is followed by a headache and generalised limb pains. Syncope recovers in a few minutes with no confusion, but often accompanied by a bout of vomiting. Self-harm is rare in syncope, in contrast to the tongue biting seen with many convulsions.

## THE BASIC MECHANISMS: SYNCOPE

Syncope (fainting) is due to a sudden reduction in the blood supply to the brain. In most cases, provided that the patient is allowed to stay horizontal, there is a full and rapid recovery. Sometimes the blood supply does not return rapidly – typically this is seen if the patient is wedged upright during a faint. As a result, the syncope may progress to an anoxic convulsion (termed *convulsive syncope*).

The reduction in cerebral blood supply has two possible causes:

- A sudden change in heart rate, e.g.
  — heart block
  — ventricular tachycardia
- A sudden change in blood pressure, e.g.
  — reflex syncope
  — acute gastrointestinal haemorrhage
  — acute pulmonary embolus
  — drug side-effect (postural hypotension)

### Reflex syncope

This is increasingly recognised as a cause for both sudden faints and misdiagnosed epilepsy. There are two forms of reflex syncope: *vasovagal syncope* and the *carotid sinus syndrome*. Vasovagal syncope includes the 'classical' faint commonly triggered by the sight of blood, intense pain and emotion and the less common form of vasovagal syncope in which the pulse or blood pressure drops acutely in an upright individual. The carotid sinus syndrome is syncope due to pulse or blood pressure changes in response to stimulation of the carotid sinus (an area of the carotid artery) resulting from sudden head movements or pressure from a tightly fitting collar.

Tilt-table testing, which examines the effect of posture on the pulse and blood pressure, has revolutionised the diagnosis of these various forms of syncope and is an important part of the follow-up of unexplained blackouts and 'drug-resistant' epilepsy (→ Case Study 4.9).

---

**CASE STUDY 4.9** Blackouts

A man of 75 years was admitted to hospital with blackouts. He had suffered a number of fainting attacks in recent months. His ears would start buzzing and he would black out 'for a few seconds'. In the past he had suffered two mild heart attacks and a small stroke. He had had negative tilt-table studies when the blackouts had been investigated previously.

On admission he had fully recovered but his pulse was 34 beats/min. His ECG showed that the atria and ventricles were beating independently (complete heart block). After settling into bed, he called the nurses suddenly and said he was 'going'. His ECG monitor showed ventricular standstill.

An urgent temporary pacemaker was inserted before his referral for a permanent device.

## THE BASIC MECHANISMS: EPILEPTIC SEIZURES

Two broad types of epilepsy are seen in adults: partial seizures and generalised tonic–clonic convulsions.

*Partial seizures*
Partial seizures arise from a single electrical focus in the brain and produce a localised focal fit during which the patient is usually conscious (→ Case Study 4.10). There is usually a 'march' of localised twitching, starting from a single area and spreading up a limb or from the face onto the same side of the body. At times the fit can become generalised into a classic tonic–clonic attack.

The clinical picture can be very similar to, and must be distinguished from, those seen in TIAs and in the initial stage of a migraine attack.

---

**CASE STUDY 4.10** Partial seizure in a diabetic (not hypoglycaemia)

A 45-year-old woman was admitted following two transient episodes of numbness and tingling of the right side of her face and right arm. There was slight slurring of her speech. Each episode lasted 15 min and cleared completely. She was an insulin-dependent diabetic with good control and had normal blood sugars on admission. A CT scan showed a focal abnormality in the left cerebral hemisphere in the area concerned with movement to the face and arm. At surgery, a large meningioma was found and successfully removed.

---

*Generalised convulsions (tonic–clonic fitting)*
In adults over 25 years, first-time generalised fits usually have an underlying cause – either a structural abnormality such as vascular disease or a brain tumour, or a metabolic cause such as alcoholism or hypoglycaemia (→ Case Studies 4.11).

## NURSING THE PATIENT WHO HAS SUDDEN LOSS OF CONSCIOUSNESS

*Nursing tasks*
**Patients who have regained consciousness**
- Primary assessment ABCDE
- Blood sugar measurement
- Measure the blood pressure lying and either sitting or standing
- 12-lead ECG and cardiac monitor/telemetry for arrhythmias
- Look for injuries, painful areas, bruising and swelling (document on a chart)
  — wrists (commonly fractured by falls in the elderly)
  — ankles

**CASE STUDIES 4.11** Generalised convulsions

## CASE 1: Epilepsy due to old cerebrovascular disease

A man aged 55 with a known previous stroke was admitted to hospital having
collapsed at home. The assumption was that this was another stroke. On
admission, his GCS was 6. He had bitten his tongue and both plantars were
up-going (suggesting some disturbance to both sides of the brain). He made a
full recovery after a period of confusion over the next 24 h, but had a
witnessed grand mal fit 3 days after admission. The diagnosis was epilepsy
triggered off by the scar of an old stroke.

## CASE 2: Post-traumatic epilepsy

A man with learning disability was admitted after his first generalised
convulsion. Three years previously he had suffered a single fit a few days after a
blunt head injury with a depressed skull fracture. On admission to hospital, he
had a GCS of 13 and had bitten his tongue. A diagnosis of post-traumatic
epilepsy was made. He had a further three fits after admission and was started
on carbamazepine.

## CASE 3: The importance of a drug history

A 60-year-old woman with a residual hemiplegia from a past cerebral
haemorrhage was admitted with confusion. Several hours after admission she
had a generalised convulsion followed by a series of rapidly recurring
convulsions, with no period of recovery between them. She was intubated and
ventilated, but continued to fit on weaning despite diazepam, chlormethiazole
and phenytoin. Five days after admission, her GP informed us that she had
recently discontinued long-term phenobarbitone. A diagnosis of barbiturate
withdrawal-induced fits was made and she was commenced on
phenobarbitone.

## CASE 4: Unexplained convulsion

A 45-year-old man collapsed at the wheel of his car while driving to the local
shops, and collided with a roundabout. He had no memory of the event and
was still confused when he was seen in AED. When he was admitted, it was
noted he had a fine petechial rash over his upper torso and had bitten his
tongue. These changes were consistent with the effects of a major convulsion.
There was a past history of ischaemic heart disease and mild angina.

A diagnosis of epilepsy was made. He was also investigated to exclude a
cardiac cause, in particular an abnormal heart rhythm, for the collapse.

## CASE 5: Epilepsy due to alcohol?

A 68-year-old woman was admitted with a 4-day history of rigors and
confusion. There had been a single convulsion immediately before admission.
On examination, she had a GCS of 14 and a fever. The suspicion was of heavy
alcohol consumption, with fitting precipitated by abrupt alcohol withdrawal.
Twenty-four hours after admission, she remained pyrexial and mildly confused.
She then had a series of tonic–clonic convulsions. The patient was sedated and

**CASE STUDY 4.11** (continued)

investigated by urgent CT scan and LP. The scan was normal and the CSF showed a protein of 0.8/L. Urgent tests on the CSF showed a positive result for the herpes simplex virus, confirming a viral encephalitis. She was treated successfully with acyclovir.

— hips
— shoulders (can be dislocated during convulsions)
- Look for signs of upper gastrointestinal blood loss
  — coffee-ground vomit around mouth
  — melaena (inspect first bowel movement after syncope)
- Look for signs of DVT (pulmonary embolism as a cause of syncope)
- Detain the relatives, telephone witnesses, contact nursing home/GP, etc.
- Obtain a drug history (postural hypotension due to drugs, hypoglycaemics, etc.)

**Patients who are fitting (→ Fig. 4.6)**

- Primary assessment: ABCDE
  — with the emphasis on the airway and good venous access (wide bore)
  — do not insert anything in the mouth
- Ensure the patient cannot injure himself; stay with him, summon help
- Give high-flow oxygen
- Place the patient in the recovery position, cushion the head, do not restrain
- Carry out blood sugar measurement, bloods for drug levels, biochemistry, clotting, etc.
- Initiate anticonvulsant drugs: i.v. diazepam 10 mg
- If there is a history of alcohol abuse, consider i.v. thiamine as Pabrinex
- Take a full history, especially concerning drugs and alcohol, from a relative

**Patients with status epilepticus.** Status epilepticus is defined as fits that continue for 30 min or more without intervening periods of recovery *and is a medical emergency.* Without treatment there is a risk of brain damage, hypoxia, shock, other major complications and death. Two groups of patients with pre-existing epilepsy are at particular risk of status: those with severe learning disability (who often have structural brain damage and are on complex therapeutic regimens) and those undergoing anticonvulsant withdrawal.

However, a third of patients with status epilepticus have no previous history of fitting. Occurring *de novo* status can be triggered by stroke, intracranial infection, brain tumour, head injury and metabolic disturbances such as electrolyte abnormalities and alcohol abuse.

The management is the same as for a single fit in terms of resuscitation and preventing harm to the patient. However, because more intensive drug

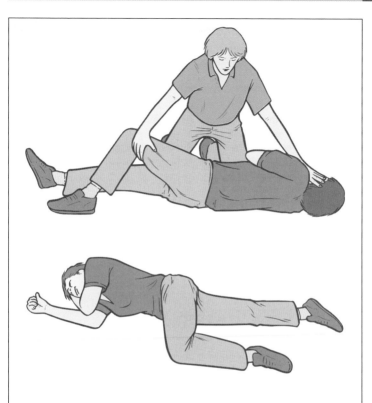

**Do** cushion the head with hands/forearms if nothing else available

**Do** administer oxygen via a face mask

**Do** turn them over into the above position once it is over – it will help them breathe

**Do** have suction available

**<u>Do not</u>** move them during the seizure unless in danger

**<u>Do not</u>** put anything between the teeth

**<u>Do not</u>** restrict their movement

**<u>Do not</u>** leave them until fully recovered

**Fig. 4.6** First aid for seizures

therapy is required, there is a risk of drug-induced respiratory depression. Close monitoring is therefore needed, particularly of the respiratory rate. If the patient's convulsions cannot be stopped within an hour, the patient needs ITU care with a view to ventilation.

### Drugs commonly used in status epilepticus

*Lorazepam*

- This is now the drug of choice for status epilepticus
- 4 mg i.v. to be repeated after 10 min
- If there is no response, load with phenobarbitone or phenytoin with diazepam

*Diazepam*

- 10 mg i.v. bolus, repeat 5–15 min later
- Immediate effect
- Repeated dosing can result in unpredictable response (respiratory depression)
- Can be given rectally if no i.v. access (not active intramuscularly)

*Phenytoin*

- Slow onset, so give with a bolus of diazepam
- 1000 mg intravenously (18 mg/kg) over 20 min is a typical dose for an adult
- Must be given with ECG monitoring

*Chlormethiazole (Heminevrin)*

- Rapid onset, therefore the infusion rate can be tailored to the patient's needs
- 0.8% solution: 5–15 ml/min for 100 ml as the loading dose
- 0.5–4 ml/min as maintenance infusion for 12 h

*Phenobarbitone*

- Effective, but slow onset
- 700 mg (10 mg/kg) over 7 min i.v. is a typical dose for an adult

*Paraldehyde*

- Safe but smelly
- A single dose can be effective for hours
- Can be administered intramuscularly but only by *deep intramuscular injection*
- 10–20 ml of paraldehyde diluted with an equal volume of 0.9% saline
- Glass syringes unnecessary for injections drawn up and given immediately

### Common reasons why management is unsuccessful

- Prescribed drug doses are inadequate
- Initial i.v. drugs not followed up by maintenance therapy

- Uncorrected hypoxia, acidosis, hypotension
- Missed underlying cause, e.g. encephalitis, drug withdrawal
- Complications of status, e.g. DIC, hyperpyrexia
- Pseudoseizures rather than true convulsions

## SUDDEN UNEXPLAINED DEATH IN EPILEPSY

Unexplained sudden death in epilepsy is of increasing concern, because it reflects an overall picture of suboptimal epilepsy care and may therefore be avoidable. SUDEP is particularly associated with long-standing, early-onset epilepsy in patients with multiple handicaps who are not under epilepsy specialists and whose drug regimen is disorganised, out-dated, or both.

## PSEUDOSEIZURES (NON-EPILEPTIC SEIZURES)

Pseudoseizures are similar to, and can be confused with, true tonic–clonic fits. The attacks represent conscious or unconscious manipulative behaviour, simple malingering or are a manifestation of an underlying psychiatric disorder. Pseudoseizures are commonly misdiagnosed, particularly by inexperienced staff in the emergency situation. The diagnosis can be particularly difficult in patients who have a combination of true and pseudo-fits. However, there are several characteristics that help to identify pseudoseizures:

- the movements are semi-purposeful and include kicking out
- the head thrashes from side to side; there are often pelvic thrusts
- the posture is often a hyperextended back with the patient lying on his side
- examination is resisted and the eyes remain tightly screwed up
- incontinence and tongue biting can occur in pseudoseizures
- some patients with pseudoseizures just collapse limply to the ground
- cyanosis occurs only in true tonic–clonic convulsions
- true convulsions last between 50 and 90 s
- pseudoseizures last between a few seconds and many minutes

*Management*
Once pseudoseizures are suspected, anticonvulsant medication should be cautiously tailed down and the patient referred to a neurologist with a special interest in epilepsy. It is not helpful to confront the patient at this stage. A simple explanation that further tests are needed is sufficient, particularly as the diagnosis may not be straightforward.

# ACUTE PARALYSIS OF THE LOWER LIMBS ◀

Patients who are admitted to hospital with sudden weakness of both legs are a rare but important group, as misdiagnosis can leave the patient paraplegic.

For practical purposes, there are two basic conditions that need to be considered:

- spinal cord disorders
- Guillain–Barré syndrome (ascending polyneuropathy)

*Spinal cord compression*

Acute diseases of the spinal cord are compressive (e.g. spinal secondaries or spinal abscess) and need urgent surgery; inflammatory (e.g. multiple sclerosis; → Case Study 4.12) and may need specific drug therapy; or vascular (spinal cord stroke; → Case Study 4.13). Urgent MRI will differentiate between the three groups.

---

**CASE STUDY 4.12** Cord compression or multiple sclerosis

A 30-year-old woman awoke with non-specific lumbar pain that progressed over a few hours to involve numbness of both legs and difficulty passing urine. Within 48 h of the onset, she had painless retention and weakness of both legs.

On examination, the legs were weak and she could not stand. Her bladder was palpable and there was loss of sensation from her upper abdomen down to her feet. An emergency MRI was normal, so the provisional diagnosis was not cord compression but an inflammatory lesion, probably multiple sclerosis.

---

**CASE STUDY 4.13** Diabetic lady 'off her legs' with a vascular cord lesion

A 65-year-old obese Type II diabetic was admitted with acute 'left-sided stroke'. On the Consultant's round, it became clear that the weakness involved the extensor muscles of both arms as well as the left leg. She could not stand, and the pattern of the change in her reflexes suggested a high cord lesion. An urgent MRI scan showed a vascular lesion (acute spinal cord ischaemia) in the mid cervical cord. She remained immobile, and was referred for rehabilitation.

---

The key for the Acute Medical Unit is to recognise that a patient who comes in 'off his legs' could well have a progressive neurological problem in both lower limbs. The nursing staff are well placed to assess lower limb movement, power and sensation when they first expose the patient during the primary assessment. Patients who have acutely weak legs, bladder dysfunction and escalating back pain (characteristically worse on lying flat) need to be taken particularly seriously, for they are the ones with probable cord compression. The site of the problem can often be identified from the site of the back pain and any points of maximum tenderness over the spine. It is important to look at bladder function in such cases, as painless urinary retention may be one of the early warning signs and always needs urgent investigation.

### Guillain–Barré syndrome

The Guillain–Barré syndrome is an ascending paralysis that starts in the feet and moves progressively up the body, to an extent that the respiratory muscles are often involved. The disease can progress rapidly over a matter of hours and put the patient's breathing at risk.

Respiratory monitoring is particularly important in the Guillain–Barré syndrome. Impending critical respiratory muscle involvement is suggested by breathlessness and an inability to cough and perhaps swallow effectively. The best way to monitor for deterioration is to take serial FVC measurements with a spirometer (the peak flow rate is not a useful test in this particular situation). As a general rule, once the FVC decreases to 1 L the patient needs ventilation, although a downward trend on hourly readings should prompt a transfer to an HDU or ITU.

## FURTHER READING

### COMA

Addison C, Crawford B 1999 Not bad, just misunderstood – Glasgow Coma Scale. Nursing Times 95 (43): 52–53
Shah S 1999 Neurological assessment. Nursing Standard 13 (22): 49–56

### STROKE

Bath PMW, Lees KR 2000 Acute stroke. British Medical Journal 320: 920–923
Gubitz G, Sandercock P 2000 Acute ischaemic stroke. British Medical Journal 320: 692–696
National clinical guidelines for stroke. March 2000. Royal College of Physicians, London

### MENINGITIS

Cohen J 2003 Management of bacterial meningitis in adults. British Medical Journal 326: 996–997

### EPILEPSY

Heafield MTE 2000 Managing status epilepticus. British Medical Journal 320: 953–954

### WEBSITES

Guidelines for acute stroke management:
http://www.rcplondon.ac.uk/pubs/books/stroke/stroke_guidelines_2ed.pdf
Guidelines for managing meningitis in adults:
http://www.britishinfectionsociety.org/meningitis.html

# GASTROENTEROLOGY

## INTRODUCTION

It is common for patients on the Acute Medical Unit to have gastrointestinal symptoms either as their presenting complaint or complicating another medical condition. The common medical gastroenterological emergencies are upper gastrointestinal bleeding – haematemesis and melaena – and acute infective diarrhoea. The issues in gastrointestinal bleeding are those of adequate resuscitation and the problems caused by re-bleeding; those in acute diarrhoea are of distinguishing simple viral gastroenteritis from bacterial diarrhoea and its associated complications. Unfortunately, both groups of emergencies are still mismanaged and associated with an unacceptable mortality rate. Due to the overwhelming influence of alcohol abuse on the pattern of acute medical admissions, there will also be a significant number of emergencies in which liver disease is the dominant problem. These admissions pose a major nursing and medical challenge, with issues concerned with fluid balance and transfusion in the sick, bleeding patient who may be confused, septic and in impending liver failure.

Other medical conditions also present with gastrointestinal symptoms: on our unit, we have recently seen two young patients presenting with acute abdominal pain, one with diabetic ketoacidosis and the other with meningococcal meningitis. Acute myocardial infarction, basal pneumonia and pulmonary embolus are all known to masquerade as an acute abdomen from time to time. More commonplace is the problem of nausea and vomiting – common diagnostic dilemmas in themselves, but also occurring as accompanying symptoms in diseases as diverse as cerebral haemorrhage and septicaemia.

The Acute Medical Unit nurse must be familiar with the causes and clinical course of the common acute gastrointestinal emergencies, in particular with the complications that can occur in the first 24 h and which often determine whether the patient will recover. Nurses must also have a working knowledge of the common gastrointestinal symptoms that they will encounter – what will be the likely cause and what will be the best form of management.

## NAUSEA AND VOMITING

Nausea is one of the most distressing acute symptoms, but it is easy to relieve, provided that:

- the underlying mechanism is understood
- the cause is identified and corrected
- the appropriate drugs are used

Vomiting is a common but potentially serious problem:

- it can occur in response to a minor illness, but it can indicate serious disease
- it can itself lead to metabolic problems

## THE PATIENT WHO IS VOMITING: THE GENERAL APPROACH

*Consider the underlying mechanisms and potential causes (→ Fig. 5.1)*
Severe pain, particularly when associated with anxiety, causes nausea through a direct effect on the cerebral cortex. Chemical toxins, notably opiate drugs, ketones and urea, act through chemoreceptors in the brain stem, the area of the brain that can also be affected by increased intracranial pressure and posterior circulation stroke, both of which can present with nausea and vomiting.

Local gastrointestinal causes include acute gastritis and gastroenteritis (especially staphylococcal food poisoning), liver inflammation and cholecystitis.

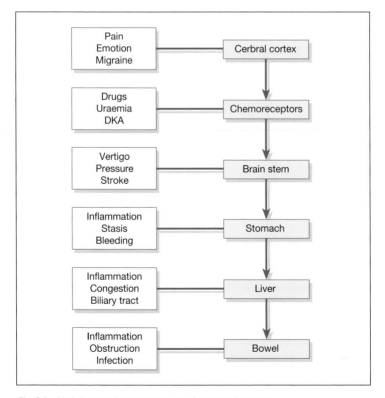

**Fig. 5.1** Underlying mechanisms and causes of nausea and vomiting

*Establish the history*

- When and how did it start?
- Did it occur in the setting of another illness?
- Is there pain anywhere?
- What other symptoms are present (e.g. headache, giddiness, abdominal pain)?
- Has it happened before?
- Has anyone else got the same symptoms?

*Is this gastrointestinal disease?*

- Is there any diarrhoea?
- Is there or has there been any abdominal pain? (Try to identify abdominal pain other than that due to the mechanical effects of retching.) Vomiting is a common feature of cholecystitis and pancreatitis
- Are there any features of obstruction (absolute constipation, cramps, abdominal distension, a tender lump in the groin may be a strangulated hernia)?
- Is the cause acute liver damage (hepatitis or paracetamol overdose)?
- Is there alcohol abuse?

*Is this drug-related?*

- What drugs have been started or increased in recent days?
- Is this digoxin toxicity/opiate side-effect?

*Could this be raised intracranial pressure?*

- What is the accompanying clinical setting?
  — headache (meningitis/subarachnoid haemorrhage)?
  — malignant disease (cerebral secondaries)?
  — altered conscious level (cerebral mass/encephalitis, etc.)?

*Could this be metabolic?*

- Is there renal failure?
- Are the sodium and calcium levels normal?
- Could this be ketoacidosis (the patient may be diabetic)?

## NAUSEA AND VOMITING IN ACUTE MEDICAL CONDITIONS

*Migraine*

Migraine is commonly accompanied by vomiting. Other more worrying causes of headache – meningitis, increased intracranial pressure and subarachnoid haemorrhage – are also associated with vomiting, so the symptom itself is of little diagnostic help in this setting. In these situations, other features such as a skin rash or stroke-like symptoms help to clarify the underlying diagnosis.

### Myocardial infarction

Vomiting is an important feature that distinguishes the pain of a myocardial infarction from that of angina and is often accompanied by nausea and sweating. In the elderly patient, vomiting may be the only symptom of a myocardial infarction.

### Sepsis

Vomiting can be the only symptom of hidden infection, even of frank septicaemia, particularly in the elderly or immunocompromised patient. This is particularly the case in infections in the kidneys and lower urinary tract.

### Acute gastric dilatation

Acute gastric dilatation is important because it is an easily preventable cause of sudden death. In this condition, gross gastric distension leads to upper abdominal swelling associated with nausea, often accompanied by hiccups and belching. These patients are often already unwell and a common outcome is sudden vomiting, aspiration and cardiorespiratory arrest. Factors that can trigger acute gastric dilatation include electrolyte disturbance, bacterial toxins and, most commonly, DKA. Treatment is simple – anticipate the possibility (in DKA, in severe infection and in any critically ill patient), recognise the condition, and prevent aspiration by decompressing the stomach with a nasogastric tube.

## ACUTE UPPER GASTROINTESTINAL HAEMORRHAGE

Acute upper gastrointestinal bleeding is a common cause for acute admission. In a catchment population of 200 000, around 300 acute gastrointestinal bleeds will be admitted per year. Some will be trivial (a young man who has light blood streaking after repeated vomiting the 'morning after') and can be discharged home very quickly. The majority will be of moderate severity, can undergo endoscopy on the next available list and will stop bleeding of their own accord. A minority, however, will be life-threatening and complex: a truly multidisciplinary approach will be needed, involving gastroenterologists, radiologists, surgeons and several junior doctors.

At the centre, in the severe cases, is the nurse. It is the nurse who will be the first to assess the initial blood loss, who will personally witness any re-bleeding and who will be on the ward at critical times – when the patient returns from endoscopy, when the consultant surgeon arrives seeking an urgent update and in the early hours when the observations deteriorate. Also caught up in the frenetic activity will be a critically ill patient who, possibly in a confused and agitated state, may be frightened and uncertain about what is going on. The nurse's role is:

- to ensure the immediate safety of the patient
- to assess the degree of initial blood loss
- to collect information for assessing the risk to the patient of the bleed
- to identify the earliest signs of re-bleeding
- to coordinate the management of fluid replacement, transfusions and fluid balance
- to reassure the patient and ensure that there is appropriate symptomatic relief

The are some critical issues in the presentation and management of gastrointestinal bleeding on the Acute Medical Unit:

- early diagnosis and adequate resuscitation are the keys to successful management
- patients with significant haemodynamic disturbance or who need transfusion will need urgent endoscopy
- patients who do badly are older, lose a larger quantity of blood and either continue to bleed or stop and then bleed again
- there is an overall mortality of 8–10%, which has not improved in recent years
- the mortality is almost entirely confined to patients over 60 years and with significant co-morbidity

## CAUSES OF ACUTE BLEEDING

The success of the management of acute gastrointestinal bleeding lies in making an early diagnosis of its likely source. Unfortunately, there are several potential bleeding sites: from the oesophagus to the duodenum in patients with haematemesis and from the oesophagus to the beginning of the colon in patients with melaena. The cause of the bleeding determines the outlook: some types (e.g. gastric erosions) will always stop bleeding on their own; some will often need intervention (e.g. varices) (→ Fig. 5.2). Once the

| Box 5.1 – Age and the common causes of upper gastrointestinal bleeding | |
|---|---|
| **Young** | **Old** |
| Mallory–Weiss – – – – Varices – – – – | Gastric/oesophageal cancer |
| Duodenal ulcer | Gastric ulcer |
| Acute gastritis | Oesophageal ulcer |
| Acute duodenitis | Oesophagitis |

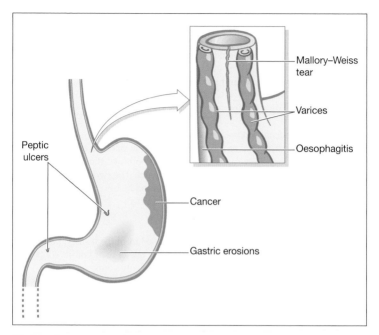

**Fig. 5.2**   Common causes of upper gastrointestinal bleeding

initial bleed has settled, some lesions will have resolved completely (e.g. Mallory–Weiss tears), whereas others have a high risk of re-bleeding (e.g. arterial bleeds from a peptic ulcer). Diagnosis rests on knowing the likely source, bearing in mind the patient's age (Box 5.1) and history and, most importantly, the findings at early endoscopy – which ideally means within the first 24 h of admission.

*Peptic ulcer disease*
Duodenal and gastric ulcers are the cause in half of all cases of acute upper gastrointestinal bleeding. Most ulcers (eight out of ten) stop bleeding of their own accord; the remainder need intervention at endoscopy (injection/heat probe/laser), in the radiology department (embolisation), or possibly by surgery.

Helicobacter pylori *infection and bleeding peptic ulcers*
About 60–70% of all gastric ulcers and 80% or more of all duodenal ulcers are caused by *H. pylori* infection within the stomach (most of the remainder are associated with use of NSAIDs). Eradication of the infection speeds ulcer

healing and, of importance to the Acute Medical Unit, if the ulcer has bled, eradication lessens the risk of re-bleeding. Eradication therapy is simple – a week of ampicillin, omeprazole and clarithromycin – and should, arguably, be given to all bleeding duodenal ulcers after the patient is stable. This aspect of management is frequently neglected. The situation with bleeding gastric ulcers is more controversial and in most cases re-endoscopy is advisable 6 weeks after the initial bleed, at which time tests for *H. pylori* can be performed and eradication therapy given if necessary.

### Acute gastritis, duodenitis and acute erosions ('stress ulcers')

Acute gastric and duodenal erosions are common in patients taking NSAIDs and aspirin. Although they can cause massive blood loss, the bleeding will stop provided the patient survives the initial event. The two major issues are adequate resuscitation and ensuring that the blood loss is not arising from a more serious source such as a chronic ulcer or varices.

### Mallory–Weiss tear

Acute oesophageal mucosal tears can be diagnosed from the history: patients retch and vomit several times before noticing that one of their vomits contains a varying amount of fresh blood. The patients are usually young, and acute alcohol intake is often involved. The bleeding can be heavy and the patients can be very alarmed. The outlook is almost universally excellent, with the bleeding stopping of its own accord and the tear healing completely within 24 h.

### Oesophageal varices

Less common, but more frightening for everyone concerned, oesophageal varices account for around 10% of acute bleeds. Blood loss can be massive and can itself result in death, but more commonly it triggers acute liver failure – in patients whose livers are already performing badly. Varices need active intervention to stop them bleeding and to reduce the risk of a re-bleed. Overall death rates are high, up to 30%. Fortunately, there have been important improvements in the field using endoscopic (injection sclerotherapy and banding) and radiological (transjugular intrahepatic portosystemic anastomosis) techniques. It is to the general relief of many that the Sengstaken tube is now making progressively fewer appearances on the medical ward.

### Gastric and oesophageal cancer

Gastric and oesophageal cancer occur in the older patients, and the bleeding is often preceded by a history of weight loss, anorexia and, in the case of oesophageal cancer, swallowing difficulty.

### Dieulafoy's erosion

This rare cause of massive bleeding is due to erosion of a congenitally abnormal artery in the lining of the stomach. Emergency surgery is often required.

## MANAGEMENT OF UPPER GASTROINTESTINAL HAEMORRHAGE

*Ensuring the safety of the patient: ABCDE*
Patients with major gastrointestinal bleeding need instant assessment and urgent resuscitation.

The conscious level may be impaired, either as part of shock (poor cerebral blood supply) or because the bleeding has occurred in a patient with liver disease and has triggered liver failure. However, unless the bleeding has taken place, say, as a stress reaction to an acute stroke, the airway is unlikely to be at risk.

Administer high-flow oxygen immediately if the patient is hypotensive or has a pulse over 100 beats/min – on the assumption there has been a major bleed. Monitor the oxygen saturations to assess the response.

Check the patient for any pain: severe abdominal pain is unusual in upper gastrointestinal bleeding and needs urgent medical assessment. In the elderly, blood loss can readily trigger an anginal attack or even cause myocardial infarction.

Anticipate that large-bore i.v. cannulae (e.g. grey Venflons) will be inserted into both arms and that either immediate saline or polygeline (Haemaccel) may be needed. If there is haemodynamic disturbance (say: pulse 110 beats/min, systolic blood pressure 100 mmHg, respiratory rate 30 breaths/min), it would be appropriate to give 2 L of isotonic saline rapidly and then, if there is no improvement, consider polygeline (Haemaccel), as at least 20% of the blood volume will have been lost.

*Who needs urgent endoscopy?*
Young patients with minor gastrointestinal bleeding in whom there is no change in pulse or blood pressure can be safely discharged and do not require endoscopy. Most other patients with gastrointestinal bleeding can safely be endoscoped on the next available endoscopy list. Indeed, the risks of emergency endoscopy in an inadequately resuscitated patient in the middle of the night can outweigh the potential advantage. However, urgent endoscopy to establish the site of blood loss, assess the risk of re-bleeding and attempt endoscopic haemostasis is required:

- when oesophageal varices are suspected
- after massive bleeding
- in the high-risk elderly
- when the problem is a re-bleed

*Assessing the degree of bleeding*
The history is invaluable in assessing blood loss:

- haematemesis with melaena indicates greater bleeding than either alone
- clots in the vomit and recognisable blood in the stool both indicate heavy bleeding

- bleeding accompanied by syncope is an ominous sign
- postural dizziness and overwhelming thirst suggest a major bleed

The examination adds supporting evidence to the history. However, the patient's age will influence the signs – a young person can lose 500 ml or more of blood before any of the observations change, but a similar loss in an elderly person would have a major impact. The patient with major bleeding characteristically:

- is pale and clammy
- has a tachycardia of more than 100 beats/min
- has a systolic blood pressure of less than 100 mmHg
- shows postural hypotension, with a 20+ mmHg fall in the systolic pressure on sitting

### Assessing the risk to the patient from the bleed (→ Case Study 5.1)

*Age – is the patient over 60 years of age?* The mortality rate in upper gastrointestinal bleeding is 20 times higher in the elderly than in the young:

- the underlying causes are more serious (e.g. gastric ulcers and gastric cancer)

---

**CASE STUDY 5.1** Death due to re-bleeding in a high-risk patient

An 84-year-old independent man presented with two syncopal episodes followed by a large vomit of recognisable blood. He had a 1-week history of upper abdominal pain and was taking regular low-dose aspirin. There was a past history of chronic angina and Type II diabetes.

On admission the patient was pale, alert and orientated with blood visible around the mouth. The pulse was 80 beats/min and the blood pressure 135/65 mmHg lying and 80/35 mmHg sitting. There was mild epigastric tenderness and rectal examination revealed soft brown stool.

The initial assessment was of an acute upper gastrointestinal bleed in a high-risk elderly man with ischaemic heart disease. Haemaccel, 2 units, was given while awaiting the first of 6 units of blood that were ordered. The surgeons were contacted and agreed to visit 'if there was a second bleed'. A central line was inserted.

Three hours after admission the patient vomited 500 ml of fresh blood. Emergency endoscopy showed a 1.5-cm deep gastric ulcer. This ulcer was not actively bleeding and was injected with adrenaline. Twenty-four hours later the patient appeared to be stable, having had a total of 5 units of blood. A second endoscopy was ordered by the surgeons and showed a 'spurting vessel'; this was re-injected. After this the patient's condition remained stable. Surgery was planned in the event of further bleeding.

Six days after admission the patient had a sudden massive bleed and suffered a cardiac arrest. The patient aspirated blood into the lungs. Resuscitation was unsuccessful and the patient died.

- ageing arteries do not stop bleeding so readily
- pre-existing heart disease may complicate the effects of acute blood loss

*Amount – small, moderate or large?* The initial assessment of pulse, blood pressure and direct observation should be interpreted in combination with the results from the endoscopy. Clearly, the finding of 'a spurting arterial bleed from the base of a chronic gastric ulcer' is much more significant than 'no visible blood in the stomach or duodenum'.

*Is there another complicating condition present?* The three most important diseases that will influence the chances of recovery are:

- liver failure (abnormal clotting, varices, encephalopathy)
- kidney failure (worsened by acute blood loss and reduced renal blood flow)
- heart failure (impairs the corrective responses to blood loss, increases the risks of transfusion)

*Is there an underlying malignancy?* This may be the direct source of the bleeding, or the bleeding may be from stress ulceration caused indirectly by a malignancy elsewhere. Upper gastrointestinal bleeding is quite a common problem in terminal malignant disease.

### Looking for evidence of re-bleeding

Patients who stop bleeding initially and then re-bleed are at special risk.
There are several endoscopic features that predict a high risk of re-bleeding:

- active arterial bleeding (90% risk)
- a vessel visible at the base of an ulcer (50% risk)
- an adherent clot over an ulcer crater (30% risk)

Features that indicate re-bleeding are fresh haematemesis or melaena associated with disturbed haemodynamics – a pulse rate over 100 beats/min, a systolic pressure less than 100 mmHg, a fall in CVP more than 5 cmH$_2$O or a fall in haemoglobin of more than 2 g in 24 h. Depending on the underlying diagnosis, patients who re-bleed will need further endoscopic procedures and, if these are unsuccessful, a second re-bleed will almost certainly lead to emergency surgery. Reliable, well-charted observations are critical in the close monitoring of these patients during the first 48 h of their admission. The pulse rate is the single most useful measurement, as it is the first to change if the patient re-bleeds (or remains high if bleeding does not stop in the first place). The drop in blood pressure lags behind the increase in pulse rate, although a postural decrease also provides a useful early warning. Half-hourly observations are needed in the first 4 h after an acute bleed.

In major bleeds, the CVP provides the most reliable guide to re-bleeding, because it falls before there is any increase in the pulse rate. It is invaluable in the elderly in whom the risks are high and other factors such as beta-blocker therapy and cardiac arrhythmias render the pulse rate unreliable as a sign of blood loss ($\rightarrow$ Case Study 5.2).

---

**CASE STUDY 5.2**   Re-bleeding in the early hours?

An 87-year-old woman was admitted with haematemesis and melaena. Endoscopy showed oesophagitis, pyloric stenosis and a bleeding duodenal ulcer, which was injected, with apparent success. At 01.00 h her pulse suddenly increased from 100 to 140 beats/min and her blood pressure fell acutely (Fig. 5.3). There were no external signs of further bleeding. Her ECG showed rapid atrial fibrillation at 140 beats/min. She remained hypotensive for half an hour before she reverted spontaneously to normal rhythm, when her pulse and blood pressure also normalised. She did not re-bleed after admission and made a good recovery. Any acute illness in the elderly can trigger rapid atrial fibrillation, which in itself can lead to a sudden, but reversible, deterioration in the patient's condition.

---

The patient described in Case Study 5.1 is typical of the type of patient who is commonly admitted to the acute medical wards. He was at high risk in terms of:

- age
- existing health
- the degree of blood loss
- the source of the bleeding
- early re-bleeding

Many personnel were involved, and the patient needed extremely close monitoring. Characteristically, there was uncertainty over the indications and timing of surgery – in circumstances in which a clear management plan from the outset is a fundamental requirement. An early, combined and well-documented consultation between the physicians, surgeons and nursing staff is invaluable in cases such as this, in which the risks of major complications can be anticipated from the moment the patient is first seen.

While difficult management decisions are being considered, it is also critical that the nurse is focused on the immediate condition of the patient:

- Quarter-hourly observations may be necessary during the first few hours after a massive bleed to determine whether the bleeding has stopped. These can be reinstated at the first sign of re-bleeding (e.g. a fall in a previously stable CVP or a large fresh melaena stool).
- Reassuring signs are a decrease in the pulse rate and reduction in any postural hypotension.
- The respiratory rate is raised in shock, but will also increase if the patient develops pulmonary oedema due to over-transfusion – this is a particular risk in an elderly patient with pre-existing heart disease who has needed vigorous resuscitation with fluids and blood.

Intensive monitoring and urgent investigative procedures are likely to lead to disorientation and distress in these elderly patients. Constant reassurance is

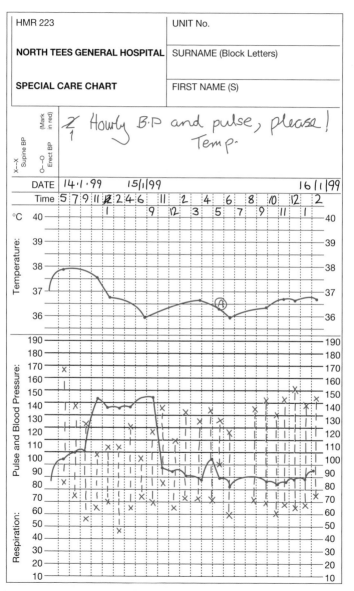

**Fig. 5.3** The importance of careful nursing observations: sudden deterioration after a gastrointestinal bleed

needed, combined with careful explanations of the various interventions and staff that the patient is suddenly encountering. It will be a great comfort to the patient to be able to identify at least one familiar face among the frenetic activity of the first 12–24 h. Patients with significant blood loss are extremely weak and debilitated. If there is frequent melaena, the effort of calling for, and using, a commode at short notice will be exhausting (and often extremely embarrassing) for the patient. Nursing staff have to be readily available to assist the patient and to deal with the distress of melaena or haematemesis with sensitivity and professionalism.

*Role of the nurse in facilitating communication*
Case Study 5.3 illustrates how poor communication can affect a patient's treatment. This was a very high-risk case in terms of the bleeding source, the age of the patient and the pre-existing health of the patient. There was good early liaison with the surgeons, but the problems arose because of the quality of the communication. An issue as simple as the orientation of an endoscope photograph had serious consequences and underlines the enormous value of effective communication. In this case, it would have been invaluable to have had a senior member of the surgical team present at the endoscopy.

The nurse is in an ideal position to facilitate the liaison between surgeons and physicians.

● Are the observations and transfusion charts clearly documented and displayed so that the surgeons can judge whether the patient is still bleeding or is re-bleeding?

---

**CASE STUDY 5.3** Unusual cause of bleeding not helped by problems with communication

A 71-year-old woman was admitted with major upper gastrointestinal bleeding: there were large fresh clots in her vomit bowl and dark red blood mixed in with melaena. A week before admission an exercise test had been aborted because of early ischaemic changes on her ECG. She had also suffered a myocardial infarction 6 months previously. Emergency endoscopy revealed a typical Dieulafoy anomaly with a visible arterial bleed, high in the lesser curve.

After unsuccessful attempts at endoscopic injection and embolisation she was taken as an emergency to theatre. There was no direct communication between the senior surgeon and the endoscopist; much of the information transfer was either through a third party or from the endoscopy form, which itself was filled out ambiguously. Furthermore the first operation, a partial gastrectomy, was done under adverse conditions with the patient actively bleeding and hypotensive. The lesion was not included in the resected gastric tissue. She continued to bleed after surgery and so further surgery with a total gastrectomy was done. She made an uneventful recovery after this.

- Is the most recent bowel action/vomit available to be seen and documented in the nursing notes?
- Are the most up-to-date blood results available (especially the blood count and clotting studies)? Ideally, they should be displayed on a flow chart.
- Is there an informed member of the medical team (e.g. the endoscopist or the registrar) available on the ward?
- Are the case-notes available and, most importantly, is the endoscopy record available?
- Does the patient understand why a surgeon has been involved?
- Has an ECG been performed and seen by the medical team?

## ANSWERING RELATIVES' QUESTIONS IN ACUTE UPPER GASTROINTESTINAL BLEEDING

*How serious is the bleeding?* The answer depends on the patient. Although the average mortality from upper gastrointestinal bleeding is 10%, it varies by a factor of 20 between the young and the elderly, and from extremely low rates in acute gastritis to perhaps 20–30% in acute bleeding varices.

*Will the ulcer stop bleeding of its own accord?* Eight out of ten ulcers stop bleeding on their own; the rest are treated at endoscopy with injection or coagulation. In these cases nine out of ten will stop bleeding, but a very small number will need to go on to urgent surgery, either because the procedure does not work or because it is only temporarily successful.

### EXCELLENT CARE FOR ACUTE UPPER GASTROINTESTINAL BLEEDING

- Following an established management protocol based on national guidelines
- Intensive nursing input during the initial period of instability
- Clear guidelines for the changes in observations to be reported to medical staff
- Combined medical and surgical input in high-risk patients
- Use of central venous lines in high-risk patients
- Good liaison with the gastroenterology team
- Access to early endoscopy and endoscopic haemostatic techniques
- Appropriate monitoring, including clotting studies in all high-risk patients
- Patients for emergency surgery to see the senior surgeon preoperatively

*How will the telescope examination help?* It will tell us the cause of the bleeding and will give some idea if it will stop. Heavy bleeding from an artery, for example, is more likely to come to surgery than a superficial area of inflammation in the gullet. It may be necessary to try and seal off the bleeding at the time of the examination, using locally applied heat or an injection into the bleeding point.

*What is the outlook in bleeding from oesophageal varices?* Although treatments have improved greatly in recent years, this remains a very serious condition. Much will depend on whether the bleeding can be stopped and, if it can, whether there is further bleeding in the first 2–3 days. About a fifth of all patients who bleed from varices re-bleed in the first few days, and for them the outlook is not particularly good.

*Can the patient eat and drink?* The patient will need to remain nil-by-mouth in preparation for urgent endoscopy. Depending on the findings and the subsequent progress, they may then be able to start fluids and a light diet.

## IMPORTANT QUESTIONS TO ASK THE PATIENT OR RELATIVES

- What is the patient's alcohol intake?
- Is the patient on NSAIDs, low-dose aspirin, steroid tablets or warfarin?
- Is there a history of abnormal bruising or bleeding?
- Has there been previous surgery, and if so what was it?
- Has there been a problem with blood transfusions?

## REASSESSING THE PATIENT ON RETURN FROM ENDOSCOPY

Patients will have been away from the ward for an hour or more undergoing endoscopy. Systematic nursing observations may have been curtailed during

## CRITICAL NURSING TASKS IN UPPER GASTROINTESTINAL BLEEDING

- Ensure the safety of the patient
- Correct the oxygen saturation
- Secure the venous access
- Measure the pulse, blood pressure and respiratory rate
- Identify the signs of shock – pallor, sweating, restlessness, confusion
- Ask about liver disease and clotting disorders

## IMPORTANT NURSING TASKS IN UPPER GASTROINTESTINAL BLEEDING

- ■ Assess the likely severity of the initial blood loss and chart further loss
- ■ Take an appropriate history
- ■ Complete baseline observations
- ■ Reassure the patient and attend to the patient's basic comforts
- ■ Follow the vital signs at appropriate intervals
- ■ Ensure accurate fluid balance charts
- ■ Report signs of re-bleeding/changes in the vital signs
- ■ Save any important evidence (vomited blood, fresh melaena)
- ■ Warn the patient about the likely need for an endoscopy
- ■ Report any abdominal pain
- ■ Initiate careful oral hygiene measures

and after the procedure. Fluid balance charts and transfusion needs may not be correctly documented and the patient, who is already sick, has the after-effects of the procedure and sedation to overcome. It is vital to reassess the patient on return to the ward.

- Is the airway secure (most patients will have been sedated for the endoscopy)?
- Is the patient in the recovery position while the sedation wears off?
- Is the patient oxygenated?
- Has resuscitation been adequate (pulse, blood pressure, CVP, capillary filling)?
- Are the management plans clear?
  - What did endoscopy show (spurting/oozing arterial bleed, varices)?
  - Are there prescriptions for fluids and blood?
- Are there any special requirements (octreotide, omeprazole infusion, platelets, FFP)?
- Can the patient eat and drink? Patients who remain stable 4 h after endoscopy can usually drink and start a light diet
- Is the fluid balance chart accurate and is adequate blood available?
- Has there been liaison with the relatives?

At this point, the intensity of nursing input depends on whether the patient is in a high-risk category. A sick patient with heavy blood loss (more than 4 units of blood transfused in the first 12 h) and with a high chance of re-bleeding will require continuous and close observation; a young patient with superficial gastritis and little evidence of bleeding will need much less intensive input.

## PORTAL HYPERTENSION AND THE MANAGEMENT OF OESOPHAGEAL VARICES

Nutrients, drugs and potential toxins are carried in the *portal vein* from their main site of absorption, the stomach and small intestine, to be processed and detoxified within the liver. To enable these substances to reach the liver cells, the portal vein divides into small capillaries (venules), which form a delicate network throughout the substance of the liver. The branches of the portal vein are vulnerable to any disease process such as cirrhosis or severe hepatitis that causes structural damage within the liver – the venules become obliterated and the portal venous blood flow is obstructed. If the venous drainage from the upper intestine to the liver is obstructed, pressure builds up behind the blockage (*portal hypertension;* → Fig. 5.4) and the blood is forced into finding an alternative route. In this situation, veins at the lower end of the oesophagus, which drain into the inferior vena cava (part of the systemic venous system) and normally only carry small amounts of blood, find themselves the main route of venous traffic from the upper gastrointestinal tract (*portosystemic shunting*). These veins have to enlarge and in doing so form *oesophageal varices* (Fig. 5.4).

There are two consequences of portosystemic shunting for the patient:

● substances absorbed from the gut bypass the liver and pour straight into the vena cava. The resulting accumulation of toxic dietary components, in particular ammonia, can lead to increasing confusion, drowsiness and ultimately coma – *hepatic encephalopathy*
● the varices enlarge progressively, and may rupture and bleed

The logical way to stop bleeding from oesophageal varices is either physically to obliterate the varices themselves or to reduce the pressure in the portal vein. Varices can be obliterated by injection sclerotherapy using an irritant inserted directly into the bleeding varices through an endoscope. A newer technique, oesophageal banding, uses an endoscopic device to lasso the varices with small elastic bands. These techniques have largely replaced the use of direct oesophageal compression with an inflated balloon (the Sengstaken tube).

Several drugs will stop variceal bleeding by lowering the portal pressure and reducing the flow of blood through the varices. Octreotide (a relative of the hormone somatostatin) and Glypressin, given by i.v. infusion, are the most commonly used, and when combined with injection sclerotherapy will stop variceal bleeding in eight out of ten patients. In patients with known liver disease, octreotide is often given at the first sign of significant upper gastrointestinal bleeding, to be discontinued later if endoscopy does not confirm that the blood is coming from varices.

Transjugular intrahepatic portosystemic shunting (TIPS) is a new radiological technique for reducing the portal pressure when other methods to stop the bleeding fail. The procedure, performed through a cannula

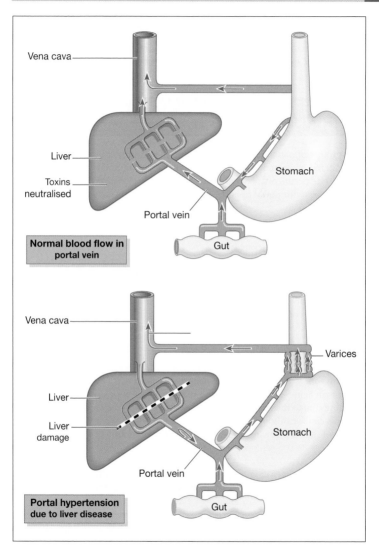

**Fig. 5.4**  Portal hypertension and oesophageal varices in liver disease

inserted into the jugular vein, involves making a channel within the substance of the liver between the portal vein and the systemic veins – an artificial portosystemic shunt – which reduces the pressure in the portal vein (although the extra shunting may trigger or worsen hepatic encephalopathy).

# ACUTE LIVER FAILURE AND HEPATIC ENCEPHALOPATHY

Two groups of patients present with acute liver failure: those in whom it is precipitated by an acute event such as viral hepatitis, and those in whom the episode occurs on a background of chronic (most commonly alcoholic) liver disease with portal hypertension. Acute liver failure has a number of components that make it a particularly challenging nursing problem (→ Fig. 5.5).

*Impairment of the conscious level*
The combination of poor liver function and portosystemic shunting means that toxic substances from the gut, in particular ammonia, are either dealt with ineffectively by the liver or bypass it altogether. The result is a toxic encephalopathy with impairment of the conscious level that can progress rapidly from confusion and agitation to deep coma. When it does, the patient has usually developed cerebral oedema and requires intensive care, preferably in a specialist liver unit. It is useful to assess and follow changes in the hepatic encephalopathy using a standard scoring system (→ Box 5.2).

*Bleeding varices and clotting abnormalities*
Patients in acute liver failure are at great risk from upper gastrointestinal bleeding due to the combination of varices and impaired clotting. Not only will this cause cardiovascular instability, but blood in the gut provides a source of toxins that can worsen hepatic encephalopathy.

*Sepsis*
Infection can trigger or complicate acute liver failure and can be difficult to recognise. Blood and ascitic fluid are routinely cultured and broad-spectrum

| Box 5.2 – Hepatic encephalopathy scoring system | |
|---|---|
| 0 | normal |
| 1 | mood change |
| 2 | drowsy |
| 3 | confused/disorientated |
| 4 | coma/unrousable |

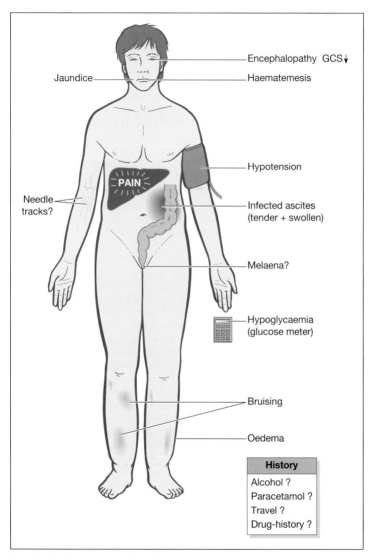

**Fig. 5.5** The features of acute liver failure

antibiotics are often prescribed as a precaution. It is also important routinely to culture urine and sputum in these patients.

*Metabolic abnormalities*
The main problems are hypoglycaemia and renal failure. Hypoglycaemia is important because it will contribute to confusion and can be readily corrected. Patients in liver failure who develop renal failure do particularly badly. At presentation, these patients are often hypovolaemic; careful early fluid replacement (monitored with a CVP line) can improve their renal function.

## MANAGEMENT OF ACUTE LIVER FAILURE IN THE FIRST 24 H

Patients with acute liver failure need supportive care until there is either spontaneous improvement or they are transferred to a specialist unit with a view to more intensive treatment; this may include, as a last resort, transplantation.

*Hepatic encephalopathy*
Hepatic encephalopathy is managed according to its severity and its mode of onset. Acute liver failure with grade 3 or grade 4 encephalopathy (confusion or coma) is usually associated with cerebral oedema. The patient needs to be sedated, paralysed and ventilated, as agitation and restlessness increase intracranial pressure. Intravenous mannitol (0.5 mg/kg) can be used in the emergency situation to reduce cerebral oedema. Acute on chronic liver failure with encephalopathy (such as may occur in decompensating alcoholic liver disease) can be treated less aggressively: the intake of protein, the main source of ammonia, is reduced and the bowel is cleared using lactulose, which reduces production of ammonia in the bowel and also empties it through its action as a laxative. The dose of lactulose is adjusted until there are between two and four soft stools per day. Oral neomycin, which sterilises the bowel of all ammonia-producing gut bacteria, can also be used.

*Bleeding*
Bleeding can be minimised by correction of any clotting abnormality. The safest way to monitor bleeding and fluid replacement in the unstable phase is to use a central venous pressure line. There is a fine line between under- and over-transfusion in these patients, with the constant risk of pulmonary oedema (particularly when saline is infused) to be balanced against the deleterious effects of under-transfusion on kidney function.

*Sepsis*
Bloodstream infection and peritonitis are common in patients with acute or chronic liver disease, particularly after acute gastrointestinal bleeding, and

can precipitate encephalopathy. Gut bacteria are usually to blame, so most regimens for liver failure include aggressive blind antibiotic therapy aimed at these organisms. Alcoholics with liver disease are often heavy smokers and are prone to respiratory infection, particularly pneumonia.

*Metabolic problems*
Hypoglycaemia must be avoided by hourly checks on the BM stix and the appropriate use of i.v. 10% or 20% dextrose. Patients with acute on chronic liver disease have often been on diuretics for ascites and may have acutely low potassium levels that need to be corrected.

*Critical nursing tasks in acute liver failure*
**Ensure the safety of the patient: ABCDE.** The airway is at risk in grade 4 encephalopathy, although most patients with acute liver failure will be confused and restless rather than comatose. Oxygen is administered and oxygen saturations are monitored. A baseline respiratory rate is required, because hypoxia and an increase in respiratory rate are early signs of pulmonary oedema, but could also indicate aspiration pneumonia. The pulse and blood pressure are critical for assessing blood loss and septicaemic shock – septicaemia from gut organisms often gives a picture of hypotension, fever and warm vasodilated extremities. Measure the BM stix urgently; hypoglycaemia is the one important cause of reversible neurological disturbance. The patient should be rapidly assessed for signs of gastrointestinal bleeding (nature of the stool, evidence of haematemesis).

**Gaining venous access.** Large peripheral venous cannulae will be inserted using a careful aseptic technique (these patients are, in effect, immunosuppressed). Most patients with complex liver failure will need central venous pressure monitoring.

**CRITICAL NURSING TASKS IN ACUTE LIVER FAILURE**

- Ensure the safety of the patient: ABCDE
- Gain venous access
- Carry out top-to-toe examination
- Liaise with the patient's family
- Ascertain the possible causes of liver failure
- Explain the likely interventions in the first 48 h
- Obtain a drug history

**Carry out top-to-toe examination.** Examine for signs of sepsis, infected needle tracks (hepatitis) and tender abdominal distension (infected ascites?).

**Liaise with the patient's family.** It may not be possible to obtain the necessary details from the patient. It is critical to try and obtain some form of psychosocial history. If emergency transplantation becomes an issue, a major determinant of likely success is the patient's pre-existing psychological status.

**Ascertain the possible cause of acute liver failure.** The most common causes of acute liver failure are paracetamol poisoning and acute hepatitis. It is critical to exclude the possibility of a paracetamol overdose; by the time the patient presents with liver failure the drug may be undetectable in the blood; and yet specific intervention with the antidote, N-acetylcysteine (Parvolex), can be life-saving even at this late stage. The various forms of hepatitis can be suspected from the history: recent travel, i.v. drug abuse, transfusions. Acute on chronic liver failure is most commonly seen in alcoholic liver disease; but other causes include various forms of non-alcohol-related cirrhosis such as primary biliary cirrhosis and autoimmune liver disease.

### Explain the likely interventions in the first 48 h

- **Endoscopy** – this will be done urgently if there is active bleeding
- **Radiology** – possible interventions to control bleeding
- **Transfusions** – blood products and clotting factors may be necessary
- **Multiple infusion lines** – central and peripheral infusions, urinary catheter to monitor output
- **Transfer** – some patients with acute severe liver disease may need intensive care, either locally or at a regional liver unit. The patient will need to be stabilised before transfer can be considered or safely undertaken

**Obtain a drug history.** It is vital to obtain an accurate drug history. Some drugs are directly toxic to the liver or may have important side-effects – hypokalaemia associated with diuretic use is a common problem in liver disease. Non-steroidal drugs increase the risk of gastrointestinal bleeding and also increase the likelihood of problems with kidney function. Intravenous drug abuse increases the risk of both acute and chronic hepatitis.

### Important nursing tasks in acute liver failure

**Determine accurate fluid balance.** Fluid balance in acute liver failure is complex, but its management is made easier if there are accurate input and output charts. Several infusions can be running simultaneously: dextrose, N-acetylcysteine (Parvolex), clotting factors and central lines. Vomit and any bowel action must be strictly documented. Hourly urine output measurements are critical to the assessment of kidney function; an output of less than 30 ml/h is a cause for concern.

---

**IMPORTANT NURSING TASKS IN ACUTE LIVER FAILURE**

- Determine accurate fluid balance
- Identify sepsis
- Reassure the patient and manage confusion and disorientation
- Carry out general nursing measures

---

**Identify sepsis.** Primary bacterial peritonitis – infection of the patient's ascitic fluid – is a common problem in liver failure and can be difficult to diagnose. Patients with peritonitis may complain of generalised abdominal pain, associated with tenderness and discomfort when they are moved around the bed. There may be a fever. Chronic liver disease, especially in malnourished alcoholic patients, is often associated with skin sepsis, as infected abrasions, skin abscesses or infected pressure sores. The mouth is also an important focus of infection.

**Reassure the patient and manage confusion and disorientation.** Patients with acute liver disease are often distressed and agitated. There may be hepatic encephalopathy and some may be suffering from alcohol withdrawal. Sedation has a limited role to play, unless the patient is a danger to himself, as it can worsen liver failure. In the less confused patient, simple measures such as nursing the patient in a well-lit room, constant reassurance and explanation and bringing in close relatives are often sufficient. In severe encephalopathy, however, sedation and ventilation may be the only option in the face of worsening cerebral oedema. It is important to exclude a reversible cause for the restlessness, such as hypoxia, hypoglycaemia, pyrexia or acute urinary retention. Venous access is often difficult, so infusion sites should be well protected.

**Carry out general nursing measures.** The safety of these acutely ill patients is at risk. Pressure areas and the skin in general are often poorly nourished and in poor condition. Oral hygiene is usually poor and needs careful attention. Restless patients will need close observation, which may have to incorporate safety measures such as cot sides.

---

**EXAMPLE CASES IN ACUTE LIVER FAILURE AND HEPATIC ENCEPHALOPATHY**

Case Studies 5.4 and 5.5 give examples of management of cases of acute liver failure.

**CASE STUDY 5.4** A 34-year-old woman with jaundice and abdominal swelling

A 34-year-old woman was admitted to hospital with a 4-week history of abdominal swelling and a 3-day history of increasing jaundice. There had been a general deterioration in her health, with lethargy and anorexia. For the past 2 weeks she had been taking regular paracetamol for a constant headache, but she denied taking an overdose.

She had been a heavy drinker since the age of 16 years, predominantly cider – between six and ten cans every day. She had been tremulous in the morning for some time and was spending all her money on alcohol. She was unable to remember a day when she had not had a drink. She was married, with a 4-year-old son and smoked 25 cigarettes per day.

On admission the patient was jaundiced and smelt of alcohol. The patient was agitated but not confused or drowsy and there was a fine tremor. The BM stix reading was 6 mmol/L. Temperature was normal, pulse 110 beats/min and blood pressure 130/70 mmHg, with no postural drop. Her abdomen was distended but not tender but both her liver and spleen were enlarged. There was no melaena on rectal examination.

The working diagnosis was acute alcohol-induced liver damage, possibly associated with an additional insult from excess paracetamol ingestion.

Bloods were taken for:

- liver function tests
- clotting studies
- haemoglobin (to exclude bleeding), WCC (to exclude infection) and platelets (low in alcoholics)
- blood sugar
- kidney function (the kidneys are very vulnerable in liver disease)
- alcohol level
- paracetamol level (to exclude acute paracetamol toxicity)
- culture (infection can trigger off liver failure if there is pre-existing liver disease)

Ascitic fluid was tapped and cultured.

### Important initial questions

- Why is she agitated?
  — hypoglycaemia?
  — alcohol intoxication?
  — alcohol withdrawal?
  — early hepatic failure (encephalopathy)?
- sepsis?
- *Is there any gastrointestinal bleeding (i.e. bleeding varices)?*

### Initial and subsequent investigations

The results of the investigations are shown in Table 5.1. Paracetamol levels were negative and alcohol levels were three times the legal driving limit.

*(continued overleaf)*

**CASE STUDY 5.4** (continued)

## Progress

The patient was started on i.v. cefuroxime and metronidazole. Intravenous N-acetylcysteine (Parvolex) was given but discontinued once the paracetamol levels were available. She was prescribed intravenous thiamine–vitamin C combination (Pabrinex) and oral lactulose.

| Table 5.1 Results of investigation | | | |
|---|---|---|---|
| | Day 1 | Day 2 | Day 3 |
| Bilirubin (μmol/L) | 313 | 393 | 396 |
| AST (I.U./L) | 623 | 1477 | 1282 |
| Albumin (g/L) | 33 | 28 | 26 |
| Sodium (mmol/L) | 132 | 121 | 124 |
| Urea (mmol/L) | 3.8 | 6.7 | 12.3 |
| Creatinine (μmol/L) | 45 | 87 | 148 |
| Prothrombin time (s) | 17 | 24 | 20 |

Half-hourly observations including BM stix were started. Four hours after admission, she became more drowsy and her BM stix fell to 4.5 mmol/L. Intravenous glucose 20% was started. After some discussion, she was given 10 mg vitamin K i.v.

The patient was observed overnight and by the next day she was confused and increasingly restless in spite of normal blood sugars. Her liver function had deteriorated and she had developed a flapping tremor.

At this stage the differential diagnosis was between alcohol withdrawal and hepatic failure with encephalopathy. The liver function tests had deteriorated and the high liver enzyme results suggested acute alcohol-induced liver damage: alcoholic hepatitis. There was no evidence of acute infection and no evidence of active upper gastrointestinal bleeding, both of which could have triggered liver failure in a patient with underlying liver disease.

Over the next 48 h, the patient's increasing confusion became difficult to manage and so she was cautiously given oral Heminevrin®. Her renal function was noted to be deteriorating and her urine output had fallen to less than 20 ml/h. After discussion with the Liver Unit she was started on oral prednisolone (a treatment for alcoholic hepatitis). Twenty-four hours later, as her confusion had increased, she was transferred with a view to assessment and possible liver transplantation.

**CASE STUDY 5.5** A heavy-drinking 55-year-old man with melaena

A retired 55-year-old man was admitted to hospital, having collapsed at home after passing a large amount of black stool. According to his wife, he had been unwell for 3 weeks since returning from a holiday in Spain: a graze on his leg had become infected, he had developed swelling of both ankles and his motions had been very dark for a week. He had been drinking heavily for around 10 years to cope with business worries, and on the recent holiday had consumed between five and ten pints of beer daily. He had previously been told that he was suffering from alcoholic cirrhosis.

On admission, he was drowsy but rousable and responding appropriately: GCS = 14 (E3 M6 V5). His BM stix result was 8.5 mmol/L. His pulse was 120 beats/min and his blood pressure was 105/80 mmHg lying and 90/60 mmHg sitting up. He was apyrexial. Oxygen saturations were 94%. Capillary filling was normal. He was obviously jaundiced and had gross abdominal distension, with tense oedema of both ankles. There was an infected skin abrasion on his right calf and scattered bruising. While being admitted, he used a bedpan and passed 400 ml of black stool containing fresh clots.

This man had the features of advanced (decompensated) liver disease. These are:

- **failure of the liver to manufacture enough albumin** – *ascites and oedema*, and low serum albumin
- **failure of the liver to excrete bilirubin** – *jaundice* and a high bilirubin level
- **failure of the liver to manufacture enough clotting products** – *bruising or bleeding*. The liver is the main source of several important clotting factors and if, as a result of liver damage, these fall to a third or less of their normal levels, the patient will be at risk from bleeding. This results in spontaneous bruising and, more importantly, an impaired clotting response to any gastrointestinal bleeding. Vitamin K, which is needed to activate these factors, may also be in short supply because, as one of the fat-soluble vitamins, it needs normally functioning bile for it to be absorbed from the diet. The prothrombin time tests these vital aspects of liver function: it should not normally exceed 11–13 s
- **failure of the liver to destroy toxic products** – a major function of the liver is to break down the body's toxic products. In liver failure the accumulation of toxins, in particular ammonia, leads to increasing drowsiness, confusion and ultimately coma – so-called *hepatic encephalopathy*
- **upper gastrointestinal bleeding** – the main worry in this man is that he is bleeding from oesophageal varices, a common and potentially fatal complication of severe liver disease. Because of their lifestyle, patients with alcoholic liver disease are also prone to peptic ulcer disease: the management of a bleeding ulcer is so fundamentally different from that of bleeding varices that the exact source of the haemorrhage has to be identified as soon as possible

### Ensuring the safety of the patient: ABCDE

The consciousness level of the patient was impaired, but with a GCS above 8 the airway is not at risk. However, an abnormal GCS must always be

*(continued overleaf)*

**CASE STUDY 5.5** (continued)

monitored. In acute liver failure, for example, the GCS can fall abruptly due to complications: worsening encephalopathy and, in particular, the sudden development of cerebral oedema. The BM stix result of 8.5 mmol/L excluded hypoglycaemia (a complication of liver failure) as the cause for the altered conscious level.

The circulatory changes suggest significant blood loss: tachycardia and postural hypotension supported by the appearance of fresh melaena. Recognisable fresh blood in a melaena stool is a sign of massive upper gastrointestinal bleeding. The patient will need initial resuscitation with i.v. fluids and blood, close serial observation of the pulse, blood pressure and urine output will be critical, blood loss will have to be documented and central venous cannulation will be required.

Exposing the patient revealed the infected skin abrasion on the lower limb. Any infection in this critically ill man is potentially important; the wound should be carefully documented and swabbed.

### Reassurance and explanation

The initial assessment indicates that the patient should be forewarned and reassured about the intense activity that will take place in the next day or so. Losing blood from internal bleeding is a frightening experience, and initially the patient will be very distressed and will feel out of control. Although pain is not usually a problem, there is likely to be intense thirst (blood loss), nausea and perhaps vomiting.

### The patient's subsequent progress

The patient was given oxygen via a high-flow mask. Large-bore cannulae were sited in both arms and i.v. (Haemaccel) was given – 1 unit over 30 min – while awaiting blood for transfusion. The transfusion technician, the laboratory and the endoscopy unit were alerted to the potential severity of the problem.

The initial blood tests confirmed marked anaemia (haemoglobin 6.0 g/dl), moderately deranged clotting and grossly abnormal liver function tests.

Within the first hour, the following procedures were completed:

- cardiac monitor
- central line (internal jugular approach)
- urinary catheter (to monitor the exact urine output)
- ascitic tap (to exclude infection in the ascitic fluid as the cause of the deterioration)

The initial phase of treatment involved:

- **careful transfusion aiming to maintain a CVP of +5 cmH$_2$O** – patients with liver failure handle excess fluid, particularly saline, badly. However, there is a risk of kidney failure if adequate fluids are not given at an early stage. Despite a careful approach, a subsequent chest film on the patient showed pulmonary oedema

(continued overleaf)

**CASE STUDY 5.5** (continued)

- **i.v. vitamin K 10 mg** – this will help, but not totally correct, the abnormal clotting. Specific clotting factors provided as fresh frozen plasma (FFP) will also be needed
- **i.v. antibiotics: cefuroxime and metronidazole** – these are administered on the basis of an assumption that infection is already present, or very likely to occur, as a complication. This combination was chosen as most effective against gut organisms that may infect the ascitic fluid or biliary tree

One hour after admission, the patient had received 2 units of blood, 3 units of FFP and a unit of Haemaccel. His CVP had risen to +19 cmH$_2$O and his chest film (to show the central line) showed pulmonary oedema.

Emergency endoscopy, after treatment of the pulmonary oedema, showed confluent oesophagitis and fresh bleeding from an oesophageal varix. The varix was injected with a sclerosant (ethanolamine oleate) and as this appeared to control the bleeding the patient was returned to the ward and started on an octreotide infusion at 50 µg/h.

His observations did not stabilise; his pulse remained high at 115–120 beats/min, his systolic blood pressure stayed below 95 mmHg and 6 h after admission his CVP dropped to +2 cmH$_2$O and he had a large fresh haematemesis. Repeat endoscopy confirmed further active variceal bleeding and the injections were repeated.

He returned to the ward and overnight his pulse, blood pressure and CVP stabilised with further blood transfusions and FFP. Hourly urine outputs however had dwindled to 10–20 ml/h and the patient was difficult to rouse.

His blood results showed worsening kidney function. At mid-morning he had a further very large haematemesis associated with worsening confusion. A Sengstaken balloon was passed as an emergency procedure and he was transferred to the ITU.

At this stage the problems were:

- uncontrolled variceal bleeding
- worsening hepatic failure
- pulmonary oedema
- hepatorenal syndrome (kidney and liver failure in a critically ill patient)

The outlook in this situation is extremely poor.

## ACUTE JAUNDICE

Jaundice is caused by a build-up of the yellow pigment, bilirubin, a breakdown product of haemoglobin and related proteins, which is normally produced and excreted by the liver. Virtually all cases of jaundice on the acute medical unit will be due either to acute liver damage from viral hepatitis (→ Case Study 5.6) and toxins (usually alcohol) or to obstruction of the bile ducts by gallstones or, less commonly, tumour.

**CASE STUDY 5.6** Acute jaundice and malaise in a 60-year-old man

This man was admitted with a 2-week history of vomiting after meals and a 1-week history of increasing jaundice, dark urine and pale stools. There was no history of pain, gallstones or risk factors for hepatitis (transfusions, travel or at-risk behaviour). He was on no medication and was a light social drinker.

On examination he was fully alert, markedly jaundiced and had a slightly enlarged and tender liver. There were no signs of chronic liver disease.

Blood tests were available from 4 days before and from the day of admission. His bilirubin level had doubled over 4 days but his liver enzymes were falling from markedly high levels (AST from 2800 to 590 IU/L). The albumin and clotting tests (which are the two most important tests of how well the liver cells are working) were normal.

A liver scan showed no abnormality in the liver, no signs of obstruction to the biliary tree and a normal pancreas. A day after admission the tests for glandular fever came back positive. A diagnosis of viral hepatitis due to glandular fever was made.

Acute hepatitis presents with flu-like symptoms, joint pains, nausea and discomfort in the right upper abdomen. Most of the symptoms improve with the sudden appearance of jaundice, although the nausea and vomiting may increase. Occasional cases progress to acute liver failure, but for the majority treatment with rest, a light, low-fat diet and alcohol avoidance will lead to a full recovery. Half of the cases of infective hepatitis are due to hepatitis A. This is transmitted by the orofaecal route, but spread to close domestic contacts can be prevented by vaccination. Hepatitis B is less common and tends to be associated with transmission through bodily fluids: transfusion, infected needles and other high-risk behaviour. Close contacts such as sexual partners also require protective vaccination.

*Gallstones, acute cholecystitis and ascending cholangitis*
Gallstones usually present with biliary colic – severe upper abdominal pain going through into the back. If they become wedged in the bile ducts there is a risk of infection, either confined to the gall bladder (acute cholecystitis), or spreading up the bile ducts to the liver (ascending cholangitis; → Case Study 5.7). In these situations there is pain, but also signs of sepsis (fever, high white cell count) and, with spreading infection, abnormal liver function tests. Nursing management is focused on assessing the patient's progress and ensuring that while investigations are in progress there is adequate pain relief. An overall deterioration, continuing or worsening pain and fever that fails to respond to i.v. antibiotics indicate a need for intervention, either by endoscopic attempts to remove the impacted stones (ERCP with sphincterotomy) or a direct surgical approach.

**CASE STUDY 5.7** A man with chest pain and chills

A 75-year-old man was admitted with the sudden onset of prolonged shivering episodes lasting 15 min at a time. This was followed after about 4 h by an attack of retrosternal chest pain associated with nausea. There was a past history of peptic ulcer disease and chronic atrial fibrillation.

On examination he was mildly jaundiced and sweating profusely. His pulse was 85 beats/min in atrial fibrillation and blood pressure normal; the temperature was 38°C. His liver was mildly enlarged and he was tender over the gall bladder.

The liver function tests were abnormal, with a high bilirubin and moderate elevation of the AST (79 IU/L) and alkaline phosphatase (325 IU/L). An urgent ultrasound showed gallstones and a dilated biliary tree.

A diagnosis of infection in the biliary system spreading to the liver (ascending cholangitis) was made and the patient started on i.v. fluids, ampicillin and gentamicin.

# ACUTE ABDOMINAL PAIN

Abdominal pain is a common complaint on the acute medical ward. Although it is a feature of several medical conditions such as cardiac failure (liver congestion) and acute gastritis, it can also be due to a 'pure' surgical condition such as acute appendicitis or intestinal obstruction in a patient who has been admitted for medical reasons because the diagnosis was not immediately apparent (→ Fig. 5.6).

*Critical nursing tasks in acute abdominal pain*

**Establish the site and pattern of the pain.** Midline localised pain is likely to arise from the stomach, duodenum or bowel. Severe pain that radiates into the back suggests either acute pancreatitis (→ Case Study 5.8), a deep peptic ulcer or an abdominal aortic aneurysm. Right-sided pain may arise from the liver, gall bladder or appendix. Kidney pain starts in the loins and radiates to the front or into the groin. An intra-abdominal catastrophe such as a perforation or a sudden blockage of the blood supply to part of the gut causes severe acute generalized pain from the outset. Pain that waxes and wanes (colic) occurs in acute gastroenteritis but is also seen in obstruction, in which case the pain becomes progressively more severe. If obstruction is suspected, look for evidence of a strangulated hernia – a tender swelling in the groin.

**Assess the severity of the pain.** Patients with severe abdominal pain are often grey, restless and clammy, and may be either lying still not wanting to be moved (acute peritonitis) or doubled up by intestinal colic. Oesophageal and peptic ulcer pain are not usually severe unless there are complications

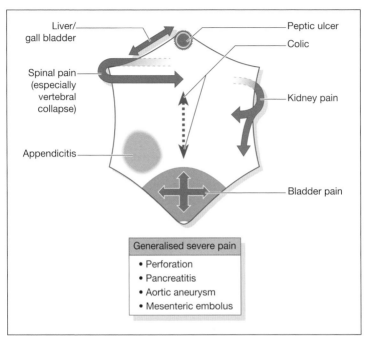

**Fig. 5.6** The common causes of acute abdominal pain

---

**CASE STUDY 5.8** Severe abdominal pain and jaundice in a 56-year-old woman

A 56-year-old woman was admitted with a 6-month history of intermittent abdominal pains and a 3-week history of jaundice with pale stools. The pain was situated below the rib cage on the right and would be constant for an hour or so before easing off. On the day of admission, the pain was much more severe and prolonged. It also radiated into the back and was associated with vomiting.

On examination she was in pain, mildly jaundiced and looked unwell. There was a low-grade fever, a pulse of 110 beats/min, respiratory rate of 20 breaths/min and a blood pressure of 110/60 mmHg, with no postural drop. Oxygen saturation was 92%.

She was tender over the gall bladder and there were only scanty bowel sounds. The abnormal blood tests were as follows:

WCC 16.5 × 10⁹/L, bilirubin 59 μmol/L, AST 182 IU/L, amylase 5727 IU/L

An urgent abdominal ultrasound showed gallstones and a dilated biliary system.

A diagnosis of gallstone-related pancreatitis was made. The patient was transferred to the surgeons for further management.

### CRITICAL NURSING TASKS IN ACUTE ABDOMINAL PAIN

- Establish the site and pattern of the pain
- Assess the severity of the pain
- Look for signs of shock
- Examine for abdominal rigidity and peritonitis
- Prepare for resuscitation

such as perforation (→ Case Study 5.9). Gall bladder pain is generally very severe (→ Case Study 5.10), as is the pain of acute pancreatitis.

### CASE STUDY 5.9  Peptic ulcer pain

A 28-year-old man was admitted with 6 h of epigastric pain. He gave a long story of similar, less severe pain occurring an hour or so after food or alcohol and relieved by indigestion tablets. He looked well, but had marked epigastric tenderness.

### CASE STUDY 5.10  Biliary colic

A 40-year-old woman was admitted with severe constant pain under the right rib margin that radiated into the back. She was restless and in pain, with marked tenderness over the gall bladder area. There was a trace of bile in her urine and she appeared mildly jaundiced. Over the next 24 h she developed nausea, vomiting and a fever and was started on i.v. antibiotics for a diagnosis of presumed acute cholecystitis.

**Look for signs of shock.** Severe abdominal pain with signs of shock – tachycardia, hypotension and increased respiratory rate – suggests a serious intra-abdominal catastrophe: perforation, acute bowel ischaemia, ruptured aneurysm or acute pancreatitis. A rising pulse rate, increasing pain, falling blood pressure and decreasing hourly urine output suggest an impending intra-abdominal disaster. These patients require urgent resuscitation and medical evaluation, including abdominal films and an immediate surgical opinion.

**Examine for abdominal rigidity and peritonitis.** The most obvious features of acute peritonitis are localised pain on coughing and board-like abdominal rigidity, accompanied by few, if any, bowel sounds. The patient does not want to move, appears shocked and is usually vomiting. If the condition has been developing over several days, the signs may be less dramatic: abdominal distension, vague tenderness, but a silent abdomen. Common causes of peritonitis are perforation of a peptic ulcer or acute appendicitis. Acute peritonitis may be accompanied by signs of sepsis – hypotension, rapid thready pulse and cold, mottled extremities.

**Prepare for resuscitation.** Patients with an acute abdomen, particularly peritonitis, need urgent resuscitation, often in preparation for surgery. The basic requirements are oxygen, i.v. fluids, nasogastric intubation and urinary catheterisation to ensure an adequate urine output. Once a provisional diagnosis and management plan is in place, the patient must be given adequate analgesia, which may require i.v. opiates.

*Important nursing tasks in acute abdominal pain*
**Look at associated clinical features.** A review of the reasons for the admission is helpful in evaluating the nature of the pain. Right upper abdominal pain in a patient with heart failure may be due to liver congestion. Pain with jaundice may be due to gallstones. Severe pain developing in a patient with a bleeding ulcer may be due to perforation. Acute pancreatitis is common in alcoholics, but can also complicate gallstones and DKA.

**Review the previous history.** Review any similar previous pain, particularly if it has been investigated already. Some drugs are commonly associated with upper gastrointestinal ulcers and erosions: NSAIDs, aspirin and steroids. Old notes are needed urgently, with a particular view to the previous surgical history (→ Case Study 5.11).

**Review the urine test results.** Urinary infection is one of the most common causes of abdominal symptoms, either suprapubic discomfort from bladder distension or loin pain from the kidneys. Inspect a urine sample – if it is cloudy and strong-smelling, infection is likely.

---

## IMPORTANT NURSING TASKS IN ACUTE ABDOMINAL PAIN

- Look at associated clinical features
- Review the previous history
- Review the test results
- Review the stool chart
- Prepare the patient for further investigations

---

**CASE STUDY 5.11** Renal pain

A 60-year-old man was admitted with a 4-day history of severe intermittent pain in the right loin, radiating around into his abdomen. For the past 12 h he had a number of sudden 'chills' and had mild urinary frequency. In the past, his left kidney had been removed because of 'infection'. An urgent ultrasound showed a large renal stone wedged in the right ureter and an enlarged and obstructed right kidney. Blood cultures were positive for *Escherichia coli*.

---

**Review the stool chart.** The nature of the patient's bowel actions is of fundamental importance in assessing the cause of abdominal pain. Obstruction is associated with absolute constipation: no motions and no flatus. Colic with diarrhoea suggests colitis, particularly if there is blood in the stool, or gastroenteritis.

It is important to document the exact type of stools that are passed. If the problem includes diarrhoea, the volume and quality of the stool is vital in assessing the fluid replacement needs of the patient. Bloody diarrhoea is a serious problem that has relatively few causes: severe colitis, campylobacter enteritis and, in the elderly, acute ischaemic colitis. Fresh stool specimens must be sent (*and processed by the laboratory*) urgently.

**Prepare the patient for further investigations.** Basic blood tests are done on admission to assess the degree of shock (renal function) and to look for

---

**CASE STUDIES 5.12** Acute abdominal catastrophe

## CASE 1

Two weeks after a myocardial infarction, an 80-year-old woman was admitted to hospital, severely ill with hypotension, tachycardia and acute generalised abdominal pain. Her abdomen was diffusely tender with very few bowel sounds. She remained critically ill despite fluids and antibiotics, and underwent emergency laparotomy. The findings were of a gangrenous intestine due to an embolus lodged in the mesenteric artery. The embolus had arisen from the scar at the site of her myocardial infarction.

## CASE 2

A 60-year-old woman awoke with constant midline upper abdominal pain. During the day, the pain persisted and became more severe. The general practitioner visited and diagnosed constipation. By the evening she was confined to bed with generalised, constant abdominal pain; she had started to shiver and was unable to get warm. On admission to hospital, she was in shock and had marked generalised abdominal tenderness. She was resuscitated with oxygen and i.v. fluids and transferred to the surgeons. At operation she had a ruptured diverticular abscess of the large bowel, with faecal peritonitis.

evidence of infection (white cell count and blood cultures). It is vital to obtain an up-to-date ECG to help identify the at-risk cardiac patient. Abdominal and chest films identify perforation; abdominal ultrasound and CT can look for other causes such as gallstones, pancreatitis, intra-abdominal abscesses (→ Case Studies 5.12) and abdominal aneurysm.

# ACUTE DIARRHOEA: SOURCES AND COURSES

## INFECTIVE DIARRHOEA

There are six common causes of infective diarrhoea:

- Campylobacter
- Salmonella
- Escherichia coli
- Clostridium difficile (due to antibiotics, particularly oral cephalosporins)
- SRSV
- rotavirus

The main features are listed in Table 5.2.

Patients are usually admitted to hospital with diarrhoea because of the worries about them maintaining their fluid intake against loss from both the upper and lower gastrointestinal tract. The secondary problem involves distinguishing between acute infective diarrhoea and the acute inflammatory bowel diseases – ulcerative colitis and Crohn's disease.

**Assessment**

- History of recent foreign travel
- Ask about other possible cases
- Have there been recent doubtful meals/mass catering, etc.?
- History of recent antibiotic therapy

**Table 5.2   Features of infective diarrhoea with different causes**

| Organism | Food | Incubation | Main clinical features | Complications |
|---|---|---|---|---|
| Campylobacter | + | 5 days | Bloody diarrhoea | Acute colitis |
| Salmonella | + | 2 days | Vomiting and diarrhoea | Shock |
| E. coli (0157:H7) | + | 2 days | Cramps and diarrhoea | HUS |
| Clostridium difficile | − | 10 days | Acute severe colitis | Acute colitis |
| SRSV | − | 1 day | Nausea and vomiting | Outbreak |
| Rotavirus | − | 1 day | Diarrhoea and vomiting | Outbreak |

**Is this patient at special risk?**

- Elderly
- Diabetic
- Immunosuppressed
- Cardiac disease
- Kidney disease

**Is there a history of recurrent diarrhoea?**  A background of recurrent diarrhoea, especially associated with blood and mucus, makes an acute episode of diarrhoea more likely to be due to inflammatory bowel disease than to infection.

*Nursing assessment in acute diarrhoea*
At all times the nurse should ensure the safety of the patient: ABCD.

**Assess fluid loss**

- How much is being passed and for how long?
- What has the fluid intake been?
- What have the urine volumes been (approximately)?

**Look for evidence of shock**

- Confusion/drowsiness
- Hypotension
- Oliguria (less than 30 ml/h)
- Evidence of sepsis/fever
- If antibiotic-induced, has the original infection resolved?

**Diagnosis.**  Infective diarrhoea is diagnosed from stool cultures, which must be obtained as soon as the patient is admitted to hospital. The organisms are easy to culture and in the case of *Clostridium difficile* the toxin can be identified in the stool.

*Nursing management in acute diarrhoea (Fig. 5.7)*
To protect staff and patients, infection control *must* always be instituted in cases of acute diarrhoea until stool cultures are available. Most cases are self-limiting, provided that attention is paid to correct fluid balance. This is particularly the case with the viral diarrhoeas: SRSV and rotavirus. Patients who are most at risk are the elderly and frail. The principle of treatment is to correct fluid deficit and keep up with the loss of fluid in the stool and vomit (→ Case Study 5.13). It follows therefore that the fluid balance and stool charts must be accurate. By its nature, diarrhoea will impair the accurate collection and measurement of urine, but the combined volume of stool and urine in a commode or bedpan can be estimated relatively easily. It is critical to keep a reliable stool chart.

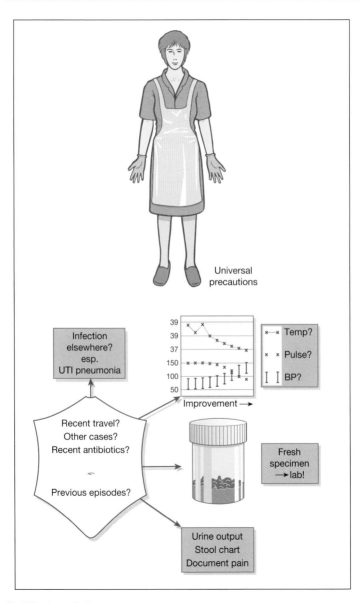

Universal precautions

Infection elsewhere? esp. UTI pneumonia

Temp?
Pulse?
BP?

39
39
37
150
100
50

Improvement →

Recent travel?
Other cases?
Recent antibiotics?

Previous episodes?

Fresh specimen → lab!

Urine output
Stool chart
Document pain

**Fig. 5.7**  Acute diarrhoea

**CASE STUDY 5.13** *Salmonella* gastroenteritis

Twenty-four hours after a family celebration, a 75-year-old woman developed nausea, short-lived vomiting and acute diarrhoea that persisted for 4 days, culminating in an emergency admission. By this time, she was too weak to stand and complained of persistent mid-abdominal cramps.

### Initial nursing assessment

**ABCDE.** The patient was conscious and orientated, complaining of severe thirst and generalised episodic abdominal pains. The respiratory rate was 25 breaths/min, oxygen saturation 90%, pulse rate 120 beats/min and a lying blood pressure of 90/70 mmHg, decreasing to 70/40 mmHg on sitting upright. The temperature was raised, at 38.5°C, and the BM stix was normal at 6.0 mmol/L in spite of 4 days of virtual starvation. There were early pressure sores over the buttocks, perianal faecal soiling and mild bilateral ankle oedema. The patient's abdomen seemed soft but generally tender, with very active bowel sounds.

**History.** There was no previous history of diarrhoea, recent antibiotic treatment or other significant illnesses. Several other guests at the function had also developed diarrhoea. There had been around eight bowel actions in the past 24 h, but only two or three small amounts of urine had been passed over the previous 4 days.

### Immediate management

- The assessment was of an elderly unwell woman with infective diarrhoea and dehydration, with a marked reduction in urine output, raising the possibility of renal failure. The elevated temperature suggested possible sepsis from the gut, or perhaps a urinary infection
- Oxygen was administered to bring the saturation to 95%
- Peripheral venous access was not possible and so a central cannula was immediately inserted
- A urinary catheter was passed to measure an accurate output
- Rehydration was started, with a combination of isotonic saline and potassium chloride supplements
- Bloods were taken for FBC, biochemistry and culture. An urgent stool specimen was sent directly to the on-call bacteriology technician. The consultant microbiologist was warned of the possibility of a food poisoning outbreak
- Abdominal X-rays were taken in view of the persistent pain, to exclude complications – severe colitis of any cause can lead to distension and, ultimately, perforation of the large bowel ('toxic dilatation')

### Progress

The initial tests confirmed dehydration and renal failure (urea 54.1 mmol/L, creatinine 504 μmol/L); the sodium and potassium levels were low due to loss of electrolyte in the stool. Oral rehydration was not possible because of

*(continued)*

**CASE STUDY 5.13** *(continued)*

nausea and vomiting. Correction of the CVP from −3 to +5 cmH$^2$O over the first 4 h with i.v. saline brought up the blood pressure. Urine outputs over the first 3 days of admission were 450 ml, 800 ml and 1500 ml, indicating a return of renal function (this was 'prerenal' rather than established renal failure, as it responded promptly to fluid replacement). After discussion with the consultant microbiologist, the antibiotic ciprofloxacin was administered.

*Salmonella enteriditis* were isolated from the initial stool specimen and, as usually happens with this infection, the abdominal pain and diarrhoea settled over the first 7–10 days of admission.

Antibiotics are rarely needed unless there are signs of complications:

- persistent fever with a failure to improve
- development of severe colitis
- development of shock
- signs of infection elsewhere, e.g. infected heart valve
- severe colitis with the risk of haemorrhage, toxic dilatation and perforation
- HUS

Ciprofloxacin is the drug of choice except for *C. difficile*, for which treatment is usually oral vancomycin or metronidazole.

## INFECTIVE DIARRHOEA VERSUS ACUTE ULCERATIVE COLITIS

Some cases of severe diarrhoea will be due to acute ulcerative colitis rather than to an infective cause such as *Salmonella* or *Campylobacter*. The history is usually longer, with evidence of previous bowel symptoms. The patients are often more acutely ill with systemic features of anaemia, weight loss and fever associated with copious watery diarrhoea, which is usually bloody, as opposed to the typical green and offensive stool of infection.

However, the emergency assessment is similar:

- Is there hypovolaemic shock?
- Are there signs of sepsis?
- Is the abdomen tender, silent, board-like or distended (toxic dilatation)?
- What has been the output of stool and urine over the immediate past few days?
- What is the nutritional state (ankle oedema often indicates a low-protein state)?

## IMPORTANT NURSING TASKS IN ACUTE ULCERATIVE COLITIS

- Reassure the patient and his relatives
- Examine the pressure areas and perineum for evidence of damage, initiate protection
- Explain the management plan
- Ensure the patient understands the significance of the stool and urine output charts
- Involve the dieticians at an early stage
- Avoid prescriptions for opiate analgesics or antidiarrhoeal drugs that can trigger toxic dilatation

## CRITICAL NURSING TASKS IN ACUTE ULCERATIVE COLITIS

- Look for evidence that the colitis is improving:
  - a falling pulse rate
  - a resolving fever
  - less frequent diarrhoea
- Look for signs of toxic dilatation of the colon:
  - persistent abdominal pain and tenderness
  - increasing pulse rate
  - increasing daily abdominal girth
  - sudden cessation of diarrhoea
- Look for signs that the colitis is not responding:
  - persistent fever and tachycardia
  - persistent severe diarrhoea
  - continuing or increasing lower gastrointestinal blood loss
  - no improvement in malaise or abdominal pain

# MEDICAL CONDITIONS PRESENTING WITH GASTROINTESTINAL SYMPTOMS

## CARDIOVASCULAR DISEASE

*Congestion*
Hepatic congestion with stretching of the capsule that surrounds the liver leads to right-sided abdominal pain below the ribs, anorexia and nausea. In extreme cardiac failure the liver can fail, with the development of jaundice and grossly abnormal liver function tests.

*Ischaemic bowel*
Acute shortage of the blood supply to the gut due to an embolism or to reduced cardiac output after, say, a myocardial infarction can cause acute lower abdominal symptoms: pain and diarrhoea that is often bloody.

*Abdominal aneurysm*
Rupture of an aortic aneurysm leads to acute severe abdominal pain and circulatory collapse. Immediate surgical intervention can be life-saving.

*Drug-induced side-effects*
Common gastrointestinal-related drug side-effects are warfarin-induced upper gastrointestinal bleeding and the clinical features of digoxin toxicity: nausea, vomiting and anorexia.

*Cardiac cachexia*
Extreme anorexia and weight loss are recognised features of advanced cardiac disease, particularly progressive congestive cardiac failure due to chronic valvular disease. This can be sufficient to mimic the development of a gastrointestinal malignancy, particularly when associated with other gastric symptoms such as abdominal distension (ascites) and the pain from liver congestion.

## RESPIRATORY DISEASE

*Diaphragmatic pleurisy*
The pain from diaphragmatic pleurisy can be referred to the upper abdomen and can be confused with biliary colic or peptic ulceration. The clue is that there are usually associated features of pneumonia (cough, breathlessness and fever), and the pain is much worse on inspiration.

*Congestion in cor pulmonale*
Right-sided heart failure in COPD can give rise to hepatic congestion and right upper quadrant pain. In patients with COPD, particularly those who

are acutely short of breath, there is often also upper abdominal discomfort, arising from the ribs and diaphragm, that appears to be associated with the extra respiratory effort that these patients have to make.

*Steroid-induced side-effects*
Patients on long-term oral steroids – chronic asthmatics and those with severe COPD – are prone to gastritis and peptic ulceration. More importantly, as they age these patients are also liable to osteoporotic collapse of their thoracic and lumbar vertebrae. This presents with pain spreading like a girdle from the back around to the front of the abdomen. The pain can be severe and can be confused with an acute abdominal crisis.

## DIABETES

Diabetic ketoacidosis can typically present with acute abdominal pain and vomiting. The picture can be very similar to that of acute pancreatitis, with similar biochemical changes in the blood. Interestingly, there is also an increased risk of true acute pancreatitis complicating severe ketoacidosis.

## FURTHER READING

### LIVER DISEASE
Campbell J 1999 Nursing care for jaundice. Nursing Times 95 (4): 53–55
McCarthy M, Wilkinson ML 1999 Clinical review: Recent advances in hepatology. British Medical Journal 318: 1256–1259

### DIARRHOEA
Ghosh S, Shand A, Ferguson A 2000 Clinical review: Ulcerative colitis. British Medical Journal 320: 1119–1123

### WEBSITE
Guidelines for the management of non-variceal gastrointestinal haemorrhage 2002: http://www.bsg.org.uk/clinical_prac/guidelines/nonvariceal.htm
Guidelines for the management of variceal gastrointestinal haemorrhage 2000: http://www.bsg.org.uk/clinical_prac/guidelines/man_variceal.htm

# CHAPTER 6

# DIABETIC COMPLICATIONS

# DIABETES ON THE ACUTE MEDICAL UNIT: THE GENERAL APPROACH

Diabetes is closely linked with a number of common acute medical conditions. It is a major cause of premature vascular disease involving the heart, brain and kidneys, and therefore diabetes will be encountered in a significant proportion of emergency patients with myocardial infarction, angina, heart failure, stroke and renal insufficiency.

The illnesses to which diabetic individuals are susceptible will, in turn, have an adverse effect on diabetes control. Insulin requirements are increased in most acute medical conditions and diabetes control can become disrupted. Diabetic patients already on insulin may need careful adjustments; those not usually requiring insulin may need to have it introduced. Severe illness such as pneumonia or meningitis can even precipitate DKA. The level of short-term diabetes control may alter the longer-term outcomes in an acute illness. Recent evidence in acute myocardial infarction, for example, has shown that careful initial management of the blood sugars using an intensive insulin regimen can reduce the 1-year mortality rate by almost a third. There is increasing evidence that the same may be true in acute stroke: high blood sugars in the acute situation appear to have an important adverse influence on long-term stroke outcome. Clearly, the acute medical patient who is also diabetic can present some of the most taxing problems in terms of nursing and medical management.

*The Acute Medical Unit nurse is presented with a dual challenge: to manage the primary acute medical problem and to ensure that the patient's diabetes control does not have an adverse effect on the eventual outcome.*

Diabetic emergencies, most notably ketoacidosis and hypoglycaemia, need immediate, expert management. Insulin-dependent diabetes can give rise to dramatic metabolic disturbances due to extreme changes in the blood sugar. The speed and accuracy of the initial assessment of the patient and the treatment in the first 2–3 h of admission will have an important bearing on the prognosis. Box 6.1 lists the key points that should be checked for in the acute admission of a diabetic patient.

Diabetic individuals are prone to infections: healing is often impaired and extensive soft tissue damage and loss can occur. The feet, in particular, are at risk from acute infection as a result of the combination of diabetic neurological and diabetic vascular damage. Such infections often present as emergencies with spreading infection, uncontrolled diabetes and, in many cases, a lower limb at risk of amputation.

Finally, it is important to take advantage of the opportunities that can arise on the Acute Medical Unit to influence long-term management. In particular, there is an important link between poor compliance and the risk of diabetic complications. A significant proportion of patients with diabetes only seek medical advice when major problems arise. For these patients, their acute

---

**Box 6.1 – Key points for an acute admission in a diabetic patient**

1. Is the patient hypoglycaemic?
2. Is this a diabetic emergency or an emergency in a patient with diabetes?
3. Confirm the timing of the last insulin/oral hypoglycaemic and the last meal
4. What is the usual regimen in this patient?
5. Critical nursing observations: GCS, pulse, blood pressure, temperature, respiratory rate, oxygen saturation, blood sugar, urinary ketones
6. Check vision
7. Skin: examine pressure points (heels, soles of the feet, ankles), *remove dressings*
8. Look for infection: cellulitis (legs and feet)/groins/vaginal discharge?
9. Examine the feet: numb/painful/infected/gangrenous?
10. Urgent venesection for biochemistry, etc.

---

admission provides an important chance to look for unrecognised complications and initiate a review of their overall diabetes management.

*Aims of this chapter*

- To provide an understanding of normal and abnormal blood sugar control
- To present an overview contrasting Type I and Type II diabetes
- To examine the acute medical conditions that are associated with diabetes
- To explain how to control the blood sugars in adverse medical situations
- To present the management of diabetic emergencies
- To look at the treatment of infection in the diabetic patient
- To identify opportunities on the Acute Medical Unit to influence longer-term management

# NORMAL BLOOD SUGAR CONTROL AND THE NATURE OF DIABETES

The normal blood sugar level is kept within the range 4 mmol/L to 8 mmol/L by a balance between:

- the rate at which glucose is removed from the blood to be used by the muscles
- the rate at which glucose is manufactured by the liver and released into the blood

Insulin is released from the pancreas and *reduces* the blood sugar by:

- increasing glucose uptake and utilisation by the muscles
- reducing glucose formation and release by the liver

Normally, the pancreas senses the increase in blood sugar that occurs after food is eaten and secretes a carefully controlled amount of insulin. The insulin lowers the blood sugar and drives metabolism by pushing glucose into the cells, where it is used for energy.

If there is no insulin present, the body behaves as though it is in a state of acute starvation:

- the liver compensates by producing and releasing excessive glucose
- the muscles stop taking in and using glucose
- as a result, there is an acute increase in the blood glucose level
- fat is burnt as the alternative source of energy to produce fatty acids. These, in turn, form ketones, which are acids. Ketones appear in the blood and the urine
- the patient becomes acidotic (the blood pH falls)

Diabetes occurs in two situations:

- there is a complete failure of insulin production. This is the situation in *Type I diabetes*
- there is a reduction in insulin production and the tissues themselves are resistant to the actions of insulin. This is the situation in *Type II diabetes*

## AN OVERVIEW OF TYPE I AND TYPE II DIABETES

Type I (or 'insulin-dependent', IDDM) diabetes mellitus occurs when there is a progressive failure of insulin production.

Type II (or 'non-insulin-dependent', NIDDM) diabetes mellitus occurs when there is a combination of two factors:

- the tissues fail to react to insulin
- the rate of insulin production is reduced

There are fundamental differences between the two types of diabetes ($\rightarrow$ Table 6.1).

- Type I diabetes
  — there is little or no naturally occurring insulin
  — unless supplied with regular carbohydrate and insulin, the patient will become ketotic
- Type II diabetes
  — there is a relative lack, but not a complete absence, of insulin
  — blood sugars are elevated, but the patient is not usually at risk from DKA

| Table 6.1 | A comparison of Type I and Type II diabetes | | | | |
|---|---|---|---|---|---|
| | *Clinical onset* | *Natural insulin* | *Risk of DKA* | *Obesity* | *Relative frequency* |
| Type I | Sudden | Nil | Yes | No | 20% |
| Type II | Slow | Low | Rare | 80% | 80% |

### Type I diabetes

Type I diabetes is an autoimmune disease. In order to develop it, the patient needs to have an inherited tendency that is activated in some way by a viral trigger to switch on a progressive destruction of the body's own ability to produce insulin. Antibodies are produced that are directed against both the insulin hormone and the pancreatic beta cells that produce and release insulin. Once 80% of the beta cells have been destroyed, insulin concentrations fall to such low levels that the patient develops diabetes.

### Type II diabetes

Type II diabetes is a partially inherited, age-related, 'Western' condition that has a strong association with obesity, a poor diet and physical inactivity. Insulin levels are moderately low (the number of pancreatic beta cells is reduced by around 20%). More importantly, the patient's tissues are resistant to the action of insulin.

## RECENT DEVELOPMENTS IN THE TREATMENT OF DIABETES

### Type I diabetes

There is increasing emphasis on tight blood sugar control to lessen the risks of long-term complications. In order to achieve this, there is a wide choice of insulin regimens and insulin injection devices. Many patients are now established on regimens with a basal background of single-dose, long-acting insulin that is fine-tuned by thrice-daily short-acting insulin regulated according to fingerprick blood sugar profiles. The importance of minimising postprandial increases in blood sugars has been realised and some patients use ultra-short-acting insulin (Lispro) with or even just after food to achieve this aim. New analogues such as insulin glargine and determir are replacing isophane, the traditional basal insulin. Designed to be slowly released from the injection site, these insulins give a more physiological blood sugar profile and represent an important improvement in the management of Type I diabetes. The dietary treatment of Type I diabetes remains based on an adequate calorie intake with complex carbohydrates, high fibre and a reduced fat intake.

### Type II diabetes

Traditionally, management is based on dietary control with or without oral hypoglycaemics. The aims of dietary treatment in Type II diabetes are to reduce the energy intake, correct the blood lipids and reduce the patient's weight. Drug treatment with oral hypoglycaemics acts by stimulating insulin secretion (e.g. glibenclamide and gliclazide), by re-sensitising the tissues to the action of insulin, or by directly reducing the release of glucose by the liver (metformin). In time, blood sugar control deteriorates – within 6 years of diagnosis, 25% of patients with Type II diabetes will require insulin. The effectiveness of combining once-daily insulin glargine with oral metformin has facilitated a much more active approach to blood sugar management, with the knowledge that this will improve the outlook.

There have been major changes in our approach to the prevention of complications in Type II diabetes. Complications, and in particular vascular complications, are common in Type II diabetics. Up to 20% of new cases will have evidence of complications at the time of diagnosis and there is overwhelming evidence that the traditional 'bad companions' of diabetes have a major impact on the frequency with which they occur. Predictably, these are:

- hypertension
- hyperglycaemia
- hyperlipidaemia
- smoking

Large studies at the end of the 1990s have altered the perception of the importance of addressing these factors in patients with Type II diabetes. The evidence indicates that we must take every opportunity to re-enforce the need for good diabetic control and the need to reduce the other risk factors, notably hypertension and smoking. For example:

- Good long-term blood sugar control:
  — reduces the risk of major diabetic eye disease by a quarter
  — reduces the risk of early kidney damage by a third
- Lowering abnormally high blood pressure in these patients:
  — reduces death from long-term complications by a third
  — reduces the risk of strokes by a third
  — reduces the risk of serious visual deterioration by a third

This represents a change of emphasis in management. The aim must be to keep the blood sugar and blood pressure in Type II diabetes as near normal as possible. The Acute Medical Unit often affords the first opportunity to address these issues, with both new and established diabetes.

## ACUTE MEDICAL CONDITIONS ASSOCIATED WITH DIABETES

The presence of widespread arterial damage in many diabetic patients makes them prone to a number of major acute medical problems. The cause of the damage is a combination of direct tissue toxicity from abnormally high sugar levels and the elevated blood lipids that are so common in diabetes. The effect of the damage depends on whether large (e.g. main coronary and cerebral arteries) or small (e.g. skin microcirculation and arteries within the kidney) vessels are predominantly affected (→ Box 6.2). Unfortunately, in many of the older Type II diabetics there is damage throughout the arterial

---

**Box 6.2 – Acute medical conditions resulting from large vessel and small vessel disease in diabetes**

| **Large vessel disease** | **Small vessel disease** |
|---|---|
| Stroke | Retinopathy (visual impairment) |
| Myocardial infarction | Renal failure (proteinuria/hypertension) |
| Cardiac failure (coronary arteries) | Cardiac failure (heart microcirculation) |
| Amputation | Foot problems |
| Sudden death (cardiac) | Sudden death (cardiac) |

---

system, and these people are at risk from ischaemia affecting the coronary, cerebral and renal circulation.

Although there are no fundamental differences between the management of medical conditions in those with and without diabetes, diabetics as a rule fare less well than non-diabetics with the same disease. Thus diabetics with ischaemic heart disease have more widespread and more severe coronary artery disease and if they suffer infarct they have twice the mortality compared with non-diabetics. Complications are common, and often remain unrecognised by the patient. Thus a middle-aged patient with Type II diabetes may have heart muscle damage that only becomes apparent during other severe illnesses. Similarly, silent diabetic renal disease may lead to hypertension and its complications. It is therefore important that, when a patient with diabetes is admitted with a seemingly unrelated problem such as a urinary infection, the opportunity is taken to make a general assessment: for ischaemic heart disease, for hypertension and for kidney damage.

Tissues become damaged more easily and heal more slowly in diabetes. Immune function is reduced and organ damage is likely, especially where the blood supply is already compromised by diabetic vascular disease. Thus pneumonia is more likely to be complicated by empyema, renal infections may end in abscess formation and pressure sores may progress to osteomyelitis. Opportunistic infections may occur: examples include *Candida* infection of the skin creases and mucous membranes, pseudomonal infections of the ear and an unusual form of meningitis caused by the organism *Listeria*.

*Diabetic renal disease*
One-third of Type I and between one-quarter and one-half of Type II diabetic patients develop diabetic kidney disease (diabetic nephropathy). Diabetic nephropathy is the main cause of end-stage renal failure in the UK. Urinary protein loss is often the first indication of renal disease. Normally, we lose less than 30 mg of albumin per 24 h in the urine. An early sign that diabetes is affecting the kidneys is the presence of 'micro' albuminuria – a loss of 30–300 mg per 24 h – which can be detected using a specialised screening

test. Once the protein loss exceeds 300 mg per 24 h, however, conventional testing of a random urine sample with Albustix will be positive for protein. It is important to appreciate the significance of finding proteinuria in a diabetic patient on the Acute Medical Unit. It does much more than simply alert us to the possibility of a urinary infection.

- Proteinuria indicates probable renal involvement. (What are the patient's urea and creatinine? Are there any previous records of kidney function in the notes?)
- Proteinuria goes hand-in-hand with cardiovascular complications and diabetic eye disease
- Proteinuria is strongly associated with hypertension
- Switching off the renin–angiotensin–aldosterone system ($\rightarrow$ p. 18) with ACE inhibitors (e.g. lisinopril) or angiotensin II receptor blockade (e.g. irbesartan) slows down the deterioration from microalbuminuria to advanced diabetic nephropathy.

If diabetic renal disease is discovered on the Acute Medical Unit for the first time, the patient must be referred on for specialist management so that the risk of further complications can be reduced by:

- careful blood pressure control
- treatment with ACE inhibitors and related drugs
- tight diabetic control
- correction of lipids
- advice on cessation of smoking

*Diabetic neuropathy*

Diabetic nerve damage is very common – it occurs in around one-third of patients with Type II diabetes. There are two types of diabetic neuropathy: peripheral neuropathy and autonomic neuropathy. Both are very relevant to the Acute Medical Unit nurse. Peripheral neuropathy gives problems in the feet: numbness, poor skin nutrition and impaired mobility. The patient has no warning of trauma to the feet, so minor abrasions can develop painlessly into infective ulceration. Nerve damage and muscle imbalance lead to foot deformity (claw toes) and pressure damage (calluses and ulcers) over abnormal bony prominences. Elsewhere in the body, nerve damage can lead to neuralgia with severe, recurrent and often undiagnosed pain in the thighs and abdomen.

Autonomic neuropathy leads to abnormal regulation of involuntary muscle activity, notably in the bladder, in the control of the blood pressure and in gastric emptying. Bladder involvement leads to painless retention, overflow and recurrent urinary infection. Abnormal blood pressure control can lead to severe postural hypotension (decreases in the systolic pressure of more than 20 mmHg) resulting in dizziness, poor balance and recurrent falls. Acute gastric distension can result in regurgitation and aspiration of the stomach contents – an important cause of death in severely ill diabetics and yet fully preventable by timely nasogastric intubation.

### Cardiovascular disease

Cardiovascular disease is a major problem in diabetes and shortens the life expectancy of the diabetic patient by between 5 and 10 years. Diabetics with ischaemic heart disease have more widespread and more severe coronary artery disease than the non-diabetic. The main manifestations of cardiovascular disease are angina, myocardial infarction and heart failure. Due to diabetic neuropathy and an increased pain threshold, angina can present late and myocardial infarcts can be painless. It is not unusual for an infarct to present as a sudden deterioration in diabetic control. The risk of a myocardial infarct is increased in diabetes – by a factor of two to three in Type II diabetes and by an order of a magnitude in Type I diabetes sufficient, for example, to cancel out the protective effect of their sex in a premenopausal diabetic female. There is also increased mortality both in hospital and during long-term follow-up. The heart muscle fares badly in these patients and the risk of re-infarction is high. The strong association between diabetes and hypertension also accelerates many of the cardiovascular complications.

### Cerebrovascular disease

The vascular damage in diabetes affects both the larger cerebral vessels and the cerebral microcirculation. Patients with diabetes are at two to three times the normal risk of having a stroke. Should they suffer one, the mortality is higher and the functional outcome is worse than the equivalent stroke in a non-diabetic. Diabetic cerebrovascular disease presents with typical stroke-like symptoms due to thrombosis or hypertension-related cerebral haemorrhage. It is critically important, however, *not* to misdiagnose a neurological presentation of hypoglycaemia as a stroke. It should be assumed that any change in the consciousness level of a diabetic patient has a metabolic cause until proved otherwise.

### Peripheral vascular disease

Diabetic peripheral vascular disease presents as an emergency with ischaemic problems in the limbs due either to acute arterial occlusion or to vascular complications in the feet: ulceration, infection and gangrene.

## BLOOD SUGAR CONTROL IN ADVERSE MEDICAL SITUATIONS

### How good should control be during acute severe illnesses?

Any severe illness will disrupt diabetic control and, in the case of an insulin-dependent patient, may put them at risk from DKA. In the non-insulin-dependent patient, uncontrolled hyperglycaemia can produce a diuresis sufficient to lead to dehydration and hypovolaemia. There is also increasing evidence that elevated blood sugars *per se* are damaging to some patients, even in the short term. Hyperglycaemia reduces the body's immune function: white cell function, for example, is markedly impaired with blood sugars above 20 mmol/L. This may be of critical importance when the body is trying to deal with acute infection. Similarly, as discussed earlier, hyperglycaemia has a damaging role in influencing recovery from myocardial infarction. There is increasing evidence that the same may be true in acute stroke. As a rule, therefore, it is prudent to optimise diabetic control during any acute medical illness, on the assumption that it will avoid the risk of ketoacidosis and may improve the overall outlook.

*Assessing control*

**What are 'osmotic symptoms'?** Heavy glycosuria draws water into the urine by osmosis. Osmotic symptoms are therefore polyuria and thirst, and are a sign either of the onset of diabetes or of diabetes that is out of control. The strength of the osmotic diuresis can lead to dehydration but also to electrolyte loss, most notably of potassium and sodium.

**Laboratory blood sugar versus fingerprick testing.** Although the fingerprick blood sugar tests give values that are around 15% less than the laboratory blood sugars, they are an invaluable way to assess diabetic control in the acute, unstable situation. The main problem is the unreliability of the glucose stix at low blood sugar levels. Normally, the BM stix is used as the initial test in suspected hypoglycaemia, so that immediate action can be taken. Ideally, blood should be drawn simultaneously for checking in the laboratory.

**Modern blood glucose meters.** Glucose meters and glucose test strips have improved considerably in recent years. At one time they were difficult to use and prone to user error: too little blood on the strip would lead to under-reading; timing had to be to the second; and the technique for wiping blood off the strip was critical. Fortunately, the manufacturers have removed many of the user-dependent problems that led to their unreliability. Ideally, the system in use should now have the following characteristics:

- the strips should function accurately, even with small drops of blood
- the strip's test pad should absorb the blood so that wiping or blotting is not required. With modern strips, the blood can be dropped or scraped on to the strip
- accuracy should not be affected if the pad is touched accidentally
- it should be possible to put the strip in the meter and then place the sample on the strip (no more critical time intervals or stop watches and little risk of blood contaminating the inside of the meter)
- there should be very easy manual, or preferably automatic, calibration of the meter

---

**Box 6.3 – Good practice in fingerprick testing**

- Have you re-read the instructions recently?
- Has your machine been calibrated?
- Is the finger warm, dry and clean? Are your hands dry and clean?
- Prick the side, not the pulp, of the finger tips
- Produce a large drop of blood by milking up from the finger base
- Don't let the skin touch the test strip
- Apply the drop to the strip so that it covers the test area – do not smear it on
- Follow the instructions
- If you have to, wipe or blot off the blood as instructed
- Use the meter as instructed
- Do you audit your practice?
- How do your results compare with the laboratory sugars?
- Is your ward's blood glucose monitoring subject to a Quality Control Programme?

---

- the new, 'virtually' pain-free, adjustable finger-pricking devices should be in use
- the lancet should be enclosed in the removable platform of the device, making both sharps injuries and inadvertent re-use impossibilities

Good practice in fingerprick testing is outlined in Box 6.3.

**What about urine testing?** Urine testing for sugar is unreliable for either the diagnosis or the accurate monitoring of diabetes and has been largely replaced by blood sugar measurement. Normally, glucose spills over from the blood into the urine once the blood sugar is above 11 mmol/L, but the level can vary from as little as 7 mmol/L to as much as 15 mmol/L. While it may be justified to monitor the occasional patient using urine testing, this would only apply to perhaps the very elderly diabetic who has been admitted to hospital with an unrelated problem and in whom frequent fingerprick testing would be considered unkind and unnecessary. In such a patient it would be reasonable to assume that, if there is little or no glycosuria, then the diabetes is probably under reasonable control. On the Acute Medical Unit the urine test for sugar is most useful as an initial screening test. If heavy glycosuria is found, it is important to look for ketones (see later).

**What about one high blood sugar on admission?** By its nature, the blood sugar in most medical admissions will be a random one rather than fasting. Acute illnesses raise the stress hormones glucagon, adrenaline and cortisone. Their actions counteract those of insulin. This may lead to a temporary diabetic state or may unmask latent diabetes. This effect can be exacerbated by some of the drugs that are used on the Acute Medical Unit:

- corticosteroids: especially dexamethasone or high-dose methyl prednisolone
- diuretics

The action that is taken depends on the circumstances and in particular on the health of the patient. A fit Type II diabetic can tolerate short-term hyperglycaemia relatively well compared with a patient with an acute illness such as a myocardial infarction. An obese new Type II diabetic who has been slaking his increasing thirst with sugary soft drinks may well present with a sugar of 20 mmol/L or more and yet, in the absence of any other complications, this type of patient can often be controlled with dietary advice alone. In contrast, a non-obese patient with marked osmotic symptoms without a high sugar intake will probably need immediate treatment with oral hypoglycaemics or insulin.

Similar considerations apply to Type I diabetics. In particular, single injections of insulin to 'bring the sugar down' are usually unhelpful, as they obscure the pattern of diabetic control and are no substitute for planned management of the diabetes, taking into account the medical condition and the patient's nutritional needs.

In summary: considerations when planning short-term control include:

- Is there a risk of ketosis?
- Will the blood sugar levels directly influence the medical outcome?
- Are there osmotic symptoms (thirst and polyuria) or dehydration?
- What are the risks and consequences of hypoglycaemia?

**What is the importance of urinary ketones?** There are three types of ketones (also known as ketone bodies):

- aceto-acetic acid
- acetone
- beta-hydroxybutyrate

Ketones are acidic substances that appear in the blood when there is excessive breakdown of the body's fat stores. They are used by muscle as an important source of energy when glucose is not available, either because of fasting or because there is no insulin available to drive glucose into the muscle cells.

In fasting states and in dietary glucose restriction, the ketone production is insufficient to cause an acidosis, and there is only mild or moderate ketonuria. This is in contrast to the situation in severe insulin deficiency, in which there is a large rise in blood ketone levels that can lead to a dangerous acidosis (→ Box 6.4).

---

**Box 6.4 – Causes of ketonuria**

- Starvation (extreme dieting, vomiting)   –   small to moderate amounts
- Strict dieting in obese Type II diabetes   –   small to moderate amounts
- Diabetic ketoacidosis   –   moderate to large amounts

Of the three ketones, acetone is largely excreted in the breath, while aceto-acetic acid and beta-hydroxybutyrate are excreted in the urine. Urinary ketones can be detected with Ketostix, which are specific for aceto-acetic acid.

It is vital for nurses to appreciate the difference between starvation (or vomiting) ketosis and DKA. This is a particular issue in the anorexic or dieting Type II diabetic who shows moderate ketonuria: do you rush in with a DKA regimen, or can you reassure the patient and even congratulate them on sticking so rigidly to their diet? This depends on the clinical picture. In general, ketonuria is much more likely to indicate impending ketoacidosis in the thin Type I diabetic than in the obese patient whose diabetes is controlled with oral hypoglycaemics. Moreover, the patient with ketoacidosis is likely to have warning symptoms: thirst, hyperventilation and nausea. The action the nurse would take is also dependent on whether or not there is an acidosis. A diabetic patient with moderate ketonuria may look 'too well' for DKA; check for acidosis. A simple venous blood sample for plasma $HCO_3$ level will reveal if there is cause for concern: if the bicarbonate level is low (less than 15 mmol/L) there is acidosis, if it is normal, then both nurse and patient can be reassured.

Case Study 6.1 illustrates difficulties with blood sugar control in a Type II diabetic. The main problem was steroid-induced hyperglycaemia without ketosis. Metformin is a commonly prescribed first-line oral hypoglycaemic and tends to be used in obese Type II diabetic patients. It was a reasonable choice in this case, although precautions have to be taken when it is used. The main problems concern the risk of lactic acidosis – a life-threatening metabolic disorder. There are a number of situations in which metformin is contraindicated because of this risk, some of which are relevant to the acute medical unit:

● after a myocardial infarction
● in renal failure
● in severe liver disease

---

**CASE STUDY 6.1**   Diabetes in asthma: steroid-induced diabetes and hypertension?

A 42-year-old overweight woman was admitted with a 3-week history of severe thirst and polyuria. Her blood sugar was 34 mmol/L and there were no ketones in her urine. Her blood pressure was 160/115 mmHg.

She had chronic asthma controlled on inhaled corticosteroids. For 8 weeks she had needed high doses of oral steroids 20–30 mg daily to control her worsening symptoms.

Treatment with metformin did not drop her sugars sufficiently nor did it clear her osmotic symptoms. She was therefore treated with short-term insulin while her asthma was controlled and her oral steroids were withdrawn. She was referred to the respiratory unit for review of her asthma and control of her blood pressure.

- in patients who are shocked or critically ill
- in patients more than 80 years old
- in patients who are having i.v. contrast studies

A blood pressure of 160/115 mmHg is unacceptable in a diabetic patient since *any* level of hypertension in a diabetic is associated with accelerated vascular and renal disease. Aggressive blood pressure control reduces the risks considerably and in this patient a target level of 140/80 mmHg would be entirely reasonable. It is likely that, once oral steroids were withdrawn from this patient, both her hyperglycaemia and her hypertension will settle. Short-term insulin was indicated mainly because of the marked osmotic symptoms.

Case Study 6.2 brings out more difficulties associated with the use of metformin in the elderly diabetic. The main problem here relates to the interaction of an acute medical illness and the patient's oral hypoglycaemic drugs, rather than hyperglycaemia itself. This patient presented a complex problem of acidosis but not ketosis and renal failure (high urea and creatinine). The blood sugar was normal. Metformin has caused a lactic acidosis and the two diuretics have combined to produce profound abnormalities in the sodium and potassium levels. Drug side-effects are common in elderly patients, and particular care has to be taken in the case of elderly diabetics, who are prone to complicated acute medical problems.

---

**CASE STUDY 6.2** Complication with metformin in the elderly: lactic acidosis

An 80-year-old man with Type II diabetes presented with a 3-week history of vomiting, breathlessness and diminishing mobility. On admission he was breathless and shivering. His mental test score was 4/10 and his temperature 37.4°C.

Treatment had been metformin 500 mg tds, spironolactone 100 mg bd, frusemide 80 mg od and gliclazide 160 mg bd.

On admission test results were:
BP 150/62 mmHg
WCC 21.8 × 10⁹/L
potassium 8.6 mmol/L, sodium 120 mmol/L, urea 38.2 mmol/L, creatinine 251 μmol/L, sugar 6.4 mmol/L, bicarbonate 5 mmol/L, urine: no glucose and no ketones

---

# PRACTICAL MANAGEMENT OF DIABETES IN ADVERSE CIRCUMSTANCES

Several situations are encountered on the Acute Medical Unit in which it would not be appropriate simply to continue with the patient's usual diabetic regimen and in which the management of the diabetes becomes an important practical problem:

- acute medical conditions that destabilise the diabetes
- acute medical conditions in which hyperglycaemia should be avoided
- diabetic patients who are unable to eat and drink normally

Type I diabetics need insulin at all times, whether they are eating or not; the acutely ill medical patient who is also diabetic is at risk from rapidly changing sugar levels and the development of ketoacidosis. In these patients it is important to ensure tight control with as simple a regimen as possible. Whether Type II diabetics require the same intensive approach depends on the severity of the medical condition, but in many acute situations due priority has to be given to the diabetic control, in addition to treating the immediate medical problem.

## GKI OR GLUCOSE AND A SLIDING SCALE?

There are two techniques that are used to control diabetes in the sick and unstable patient: the careful use of i.v. insulin and glucose, either as a single infusion (bag) containing glucose, potassium and insulin (*GKI*), or as separate infusions of dextrose and a *sliding scale* of i.v. insulin (→ Box 6.5).

In some hospitals, the sliding scale technique is thought to have several disadvantages compared with the simpler GKI 'single bag' infusion:

- the infusions are complicated to administer
- the dependence on separate infusions of insulin and glucose increases the risk of inadvertent swings in the blood sugar

The opposing view is that the advent of sophisticated infusion and syringe pumps has simplified their administration and minimised the risk of error. There are also advantages in having the flexibility of two adjustable infusions, particularly in critical situations in which there is a need for complex fluid regimens.

The safest approach is to use the regimen that is most familiar to the unit and which has been shown to be trouble-free during its use. Whichever regimen is favoured, the key is the attention to detail in setting up and running the regimen, combined with an appropriate level of monitoring.

| Box 6.5 – Pros and cons of GKI and sliding-scale infusions | |
|---|---|
| **GKI** | **Sliding scale** |
| • Simple to use | • Requires volumetric pump and syringe driver |
| • Risk of water overload | • Risk of hypoglycaemia |
| • Insulin + glucose together | • Suitable for complex fluid regimens |

Nurses must appreciate that, whatever their relative advantages and disadvantages, these two techniques do *not* apply to the immediate management of a patient with DKA – in other words, those patients showing the following:

- urinary ketones present in moderate to large amounts
  *and*
- patient is acidotic (low plasma bicarbonate (< 15 mmol/L)/pH < 7.3)
  *and*
- sugars greater than 17 mmol/L

In these patients, the DKA regimen (see later) should be followed, only changing to a GKI infusion (or dextrose and a sliding scale of insulin) once the sugar value is less than 13 mmol/L.

### Glucose–potassium and insulin

**How to manage diabetes with a GKI infusion.** The GKI infusion is the preferred way to control the blood sugars in a number of situations:

- the recovery period in DKA (i.e. once blood sugars fall below 13 mmol/L)
- acute, severe illness in a non-ketotic diabetic patient (e.g. sepsis, stroke)
- post-myocardial infarction hyperglycaemia (once sugars fall below 13 mmol/L)
- Type I diabetics who are nil-by-mouth (e.g. upper gastrointestinal bleeding awaiting endoscopy)

### The intravenous infusion

- 500 ml of 10% dextrose and 10 mmol of KCl (omit the KCl if the serum potassium is more than 5 mmol/L)
- add neutral insulin solution (Actrapid) to the bag according to the blood sugar:

| blood sugar | 2.0–7.0 mmol/L | add 8 units (1 U/h) |
| blood sugar | 7.1–11.0 mmol/L | add 16 units (2 U/h) |
| blood sugar | 11.1–17.0 mmol/L | add 32 units (4 U/h) |

The doses of insulin may need to be reduced for each range of blood sugars if the patient is sensitive to insulin. Substitute doses of insulin for each range would be 4, 12 and 24 units.

Some types of patients need more insulin than usual:

- the extremely obese
- patients on steroid therapy (prednisolone, dexamethasone)
- cirrhosis
- previous high insulin doses, e.g. > 70 units per day

Some patients may need to have the scale 'individualised'. In these situations, it may be necessary to consult with the diabetes team.

*Infusion rate.* 500 ml every 8 h (approx. 60 ml/h) using an alarmed infusion pump.

*Target blood sugar.* Aim for blood sugars in the range 7–11 mmol/L.

*Adjustments.* Check and record the blood sugar with BM stix every hour. If it is necessary to change the insulin dose, make up and start a new bag, but do *not* change the infusion rate, which stays constant at 60 ml/h.

*Blood sugar more than 17 mmol/L?* Stop the dextrose infusion and start isotonic saline at 80 ml/h. Check for urinary ketones and measure the venous bicarbonate. If this is not ketoacidosis, start a low-dose i.v. infusion of neutral insulin (Actrapid) (see below) at 4 units per hour until the sugar falls to less than 17 mmol/L for two consecutive hours. Then restart GKI.

*Blood sugar less than 2 mmol/L?* Stop the GKI and give 10% dextrose 500 ml at 60 ml/h. Check the BM stix every half hour and restart GKI when the blood sugar increases to 4 mmol/L. If the patient becomes clinically hypoglycaemic, seek urgent medical help and prepare to increase the strength of the dextrose infusion.

**Hints on converting from i.v. infusions to subcutaneous insulin**

- Once the patient is stable and able to eat and drink, change to subcutaneous insulin
- Change over in the morning, not at the end of the day
- Plan to give the first subcutaneous injection before breakfast
- If the patient is already on insulin, add 10% to their usual dose for the first few days
- If not previously on insulin, start on 30–40 units of neutral insulin solution (Actrapid) divided into four doses
- Stop the insulin infusion 60 min after the first dose of subcutaneous insulin (i.v. insulin disappears from the circulation in 5 min)

**How good is your subcutaneous insulin injection technique?** Insulin should be injected using an 8-mm needle by pinching up the skin and subcutaneous tissue (*not* the muscle) with thumb and index finger. The injection is given at right-angles (perpendicular) to the skin: '*make a tent and put the insulin in through the front door*'. The fold should be maintained throughout the injection and for 5–10 s afterwards before the needle is removed. During the early hospital stay, the abdomen should be used (for the fastest rate of absorption and onset of action).

    *Note*: The pinching technique does not apply to the new insulin pens, in which the preferred technique is a vertical injection into the skin.

### Glucose infusion and a sliding scale of insulin
**How to manage a diabetic with separate i.v. glucose and insulin infusions.** Sliding scales are used in unstable patients to match the blood sugar with an appropriate dose of insulin. The insulin must always be administered with a

source of glucose, usually 5% dextrose. The aim of a sliding scale is to keep the blood sugar under fairly tight control, while avoiding the risk of hypoglycaemia. The current practice is to use the scale with an adjustable i.v. infusion of insulin rather than with subcutaneous injections, as this gives smoother control. The technique would typically be used in unstable situations such as the critically ill diabetic patient and during recovery from DKA.

When using a sliding scale:

- there should be a dependable and constant supply of carbohydrate as i.v. glucose
- the insulin infusion rate should never be zero
- alter the whole sliding scale if the initial doses do not produce rapid control
- always overlap the infusion with the first dose of subcutaneous insulin by an hour

*The glucose infusion.* Give 5% dextrose 1 L every 8 h. If there is a history of cardiac disease, the volume of fluid should be reduced by using 10% dextrose 1 L over 16 h. Add potassium chloride to give 2 mmol/h, provided that the serum potassium level is less than 5 mmol/L. The potassium should be checked at least 6-hourly.

*The insulin infusion.* Make up an infusion of neutral insulin solution (Actrapid) 50 units in 50 ml of isotonic saline in a 50-ml syringe and driver. The initial hourly rate of insulin should approximate the patient's usual insulin requirement. This can be estimated by dividing the total daily amount of insulin that the patient takes by 24. If this is not known or the patient has not previously been on insulin, estimate the required rate to be 3 units of insulin per hour.

*Target blood sugar.* The aim is to achieve sugar levels in the range 7–11 mmol/L. Allowance may have to be made for any depot insulin already 'on board', onset of action of which may coincide with that of the sliding scale. Check

**Table 6.2  Typical sliding scales: with and without sepsis**

| Blood sugar (mmol/L) | Without sepsis (hourly insulin) | With sepsis (hourly insulin) |
| --- | --- | --- |
| <4 | 1 U | 2 U |
| 4–6.9 | 2 U | 3 U |
| 7–9.9 | 3 U | 4 U |
| 10–13.9 | 4 U | 5 U |
| 14–17.9 | 5 U | 6 U |
| >17 | 6 U and check for ketones | 8 U and check for ketones |

the BM stix hourly while the patient is ill, then reduce to 2–4-hourly once the glucose is stable.

*Adjusting the rate of insulin (the sliding scale).* Adjust the rate of the insulin infusion (1 unit of insulin per hour is 1 ml/h). The example given in Table 6.2 is for a patient who usually takes a total of 72 units of insulin per day (this is equivalent to an i.v. infusion requirement of 3 units per hour). Two sliding scales are illustrated, one with and one without sepsis, to emphasise the need to consider the influence of the underlying illness on the patient's insulin requirements.

Remember to alarm both the insulin *and* the dextrose infusions. If the sugars are 14 mmol/L or less and the dextrose stops running but the insulin continues, there is a risk of hypoglycaemia.

Increase the insulin doses if there is likely to be insulin resistance. Keep the scale under review and if, 3–4 h after starting insulin, the blood sugars remain out of control, the whole scale will need to be reviewed.

*The DIGAMI regimen: an example of controlling the blood sugar in acute illness*
*(→ Fig. 6.1).*
The DIGAMI study itself showed an important survival advantage in keeping sugars within the normal range in patients with acute coronary syndromes who are either known to have diabetes or whose blood sugar at the time of admission is more than 11 mmol/L – findings that may be applicable to other groups such as those with acute stroke. The DIGAMI regimen is an excellent template for the practical approach to the close control of blood sugars in acute severe illness. In contrast to a sliding scale, the DIGAMI regimen uses the *trend* in capillary blood sugar to titrate the rate of administration of insulin, and may give smoother control.

**Managing a case of severe medical problems and hyperglycaemia**
**(→ Case Study 6.3).**
This is the story of acute severe pulmonary oedema with a preceding history of probable recent onset angina. Ischaemic heart disease complicated by a possible myocardial infarction is the most likely primary diagnosis. There is

---

**CASE STUDY 6.3**   Severe breathlessness in a man with Type II diabetes

A 55-year-old man was admitted at 04.00 with a 4-h history of increasing breathlessness associated with chest tightness and copious frothy sputum. He had been a diabetic for 5 years and took a combination of glibenclamide 15 mg once daily and metformin 850 mg twice daily. He was on no other medication. His family gave the additional history that for a month he had complained of chest discomfort on walking from his car to the office. He had also been concerned about his diabetes, his weight was increasing and his GP had not been happy with the results of his recent blood tests.

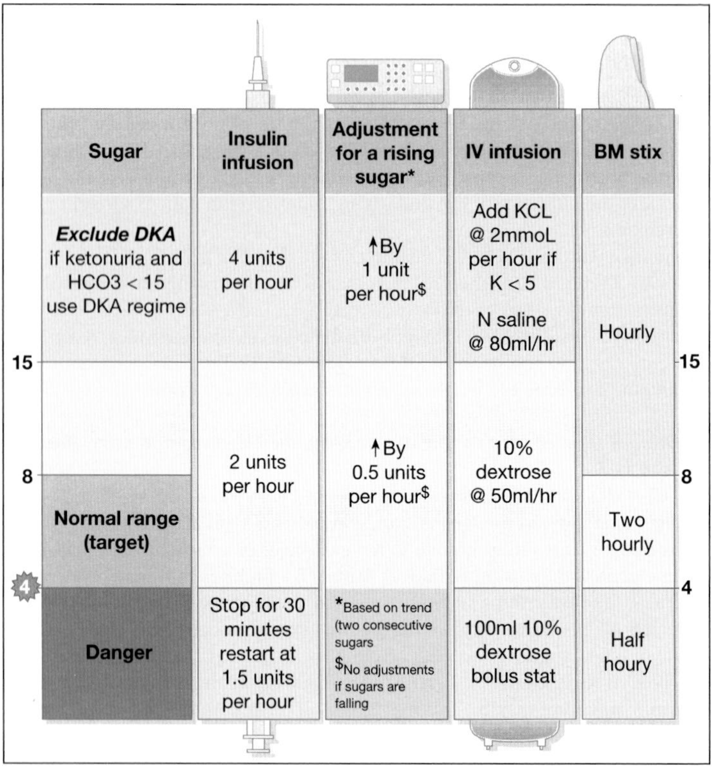

| | Sugar | Insulin infusion | Adjustment for a rising sugar* | IV infusion | BM stix |
|---|---|---|---|---|---|
| | **Exclude DKA** if ketonuria and HCO3 < 15 use DKA regime | 4 units per hour | ↑By 1 unit per hour$ | Add KCL @ 2mmoL per hour if K < 5  N saline @ 80ml/hr | Hourly |
| 15 | | | | | 15 |
| 8 | **Normal range (target)** | 2 units per hour | ↑By 0.5 units per hour$ | 10% dextrose @ 50ml/hr | 8  Two hourly |
| 4 | **Danger** | Stop for 30 minutes restart at 1.5 units per hour | *Based on trend (two consecutive sugars $No adjustments if sugars are falling | 100ml 10% dextrose bolus stat | 4  Half hourly |

**Fig. 6.1**  DIGAMI regimen: an example of blood sugar control in acute medical illness

also a problem with the diabetes: the patient is on maximum oral hypoglycaemic therapy with two drugs, yet his doctor is still worried by recent blood results.

The patient's vital signs of hypotension, tachycardia and breathlessness are all in keeping with acute pulmonary oedema. However, DKA also can present like this. Although the blood sugar indicates that the patient's diabetes is out of control, the absence of ketones in the urine is reassuring at this stage. It will be important to ensure further urine testing remains negative for ketones. The emergency laboratory blood results will also clarify the situation. The finding of heavy proteinuria without signs or symptoms of infection raises the possibility of diabetic kidney damage, which is characteristically associated with both generalised vascular disease and hypertension.

**CASE STUDY 6.3** (continued)

On admission to the Acute Medical Unit, the patient appeared as a distressed, overweight man, sitting forward on the trolley and fighting for breath. He was clammy, with cold extremities.

His skin, feet and pressure areas were all in good condition; there were no signs of infection.

Initial observations were as follows:

- pulse 150 beats/min and irregular
- blood pressure 80/50 mmHg but difficult to hear
- temperature 37°C
- respiratory rate 30 breaths/min
- oxygen saturation on 35% oxygen: **88%**

The patient was conscious and orientated, but was too breathless to speak. The fingerprick blood sugar was 28 mmol/L. A small quantity of urine was obtained; this showed large amounts of sugar and protein, but no ketones.

The investigations confirmed hyperglycaemia without diabetic ketoacidosis. There is mild renal failure. The GP results are helpful: the renal failure has not developed acutely and the patient's diabetes has not been under good control. The $HbA_{1c}$ measures the amount of haemoglobin that has been linked to glucose in the blood; it has become an important indicator of diabetic control because it reflects the levels of blood sugars that have been occurring over the past 2 or 3 months. The higher the $HbA_{1c}$, the higher the recent blood sugars. A 'normal' level of 7.5% or less in the absence of repeated hypoglycaemic episodes is an indication of good control. In this patient, the level of 11% confirms the suspicion of poor control. Reducing the level from 11% will have a progressive effect on reducing the risk of diabetic complications, particularly neuropathy, retinopathy and nephropathy. The immediate priorities are:

- to clear the pulmonary oedema   (symptoms, saturations and respiratory rate)
- to slow the atrial fibrillation   (rate from cardiac monitor)
- to control the blood sugar   (hourly BM stix)

Fluid balance will be critical:

- the patient's heart may not cope with large volumes of fluid
- there is uncertainty about his renal function
- he may need multiple infusions (e.g. inotropic support or nitrates)

The interventions described in the case study resulted in some improvement in the patient's pulmonary oedema and atrial fibrillation. The main problems were persistent hypotension, with a low urine output and continuing hyperglycaemia (but no ketosis). There was uncertainty as to whether or not

**CASE STUDY 6.3** (continued)

Arterial and venous blood samples were taken. The patient's ECG showed atrial fibrillation at 160 beats/min, with acute ischaemic changes, left ventricular enlargement, but no signs of an actual infarct. A portable chest X-ray confirmed pulmonary oedema. The oxygen was increased to 60%. He was given 80 mg of i.v. frusemide and a small dose of i.v. diamorphine. He was started on subcutaneous low-molecular weight heparin.
By this time his blood tests were back:

- Blood gases
  — pH             7.35          not acidotic
  — $pO_2$          8.0 kPa       should correct with increased oxygen
  — $pCO_2$         4.0 kPa       normal (usually low in DKA due to
                                  hyperventilation)
- Bicarbonate      19 mmol/L     not acidotic

- Biochemistry
  — sugar          32 mmol/L     high
  — sodium         144 mmol/L    normal
  — potassium      5.1 mmol/L    normal
  — urea           28 mmol/L     high
  — creatinine     300 μmol/L    high

- The laboratory computer had some GP results from 6 weeks previously:
  — sugar          19 mmol/L     high
  — urea           24 mmol/L     high
  — creatinine     280 μmol/L    high
  — $HbA_{1c}$       11%           high

the patient could be hypovolaemic. High blood sugars like these, particularly if they had been associated with an osmotic diuresis before admission, could have resulted in dehydration.

**CASE STUDY 6.3** (continued)

To bring the patient's atrial fibrillation under rapid control, i.v. digoxin 0.75 mg was given in 50 ml of isotonic saline over 2 h. To control the blood sugar, a low-dose insulin infusion of 50 units of neutral insulin solution (Actrapid®) in 50 ml of saline was started at 3 units (3 ml) per hour. After careful consideration, a urethral catheter was passed to measure the hourly urine output.
Two hours later, the patient was less breathless and felt more comfortable. His observations were as follows:

- pulse                110 beats/min
- blood pressure        85/50 mmHg
- respiratory rate      25 breaths/min
- oxygen saturation     95%
- blood sugar           25 mmol/L
- urine output          20 ml (negative for ketones)

**CASE STUDY 6.3** (continued)

A central line was passed, which showed normal to high CVP readings of between 15 and 20 cmH$_2$O, making it unlikely that the patient was hypovolaemic. He was started on a dobutamine infusion, to improve cardiac function and to increase his blood pressure. His insulin infusion rate was doubled to 6 units/h. He was given a further 40 mg dose of i.v. frusemide.

On this regimen, the blood pressure increased to 110/70 mmHg and his urine output improved to 70 ml/h. Once the blood sugars had decreased to 11 mmol/L, the infusion was converted to a GKI. The patient continued to improve over the following 24 h.

He was transferred to the care of the diabetic team to look at his cardiac status in more detail and to re-assess his long-term diabetic control. Subsequent enquiries confirmed that there had been concerns over previously elevated blood pressures of around 160/110 mmHg, and that he had been considered for antihypertensive treatment 'if the levels did not settle'.

In summary, the patient in Case Study 6.3 presented with pulmonary oedema and atrial fibrillation due to ischaemic heart disease. These were complications of poorly controlled diabetes, diabetic renal disease and inadequately treated hypertension. His management illustrates how care must be coordinated and prioritised to address both the primary medical problems and the diabetes.

### COULD WE (OR SHOULD WE) ASSESS OBESITY ON THE ACUTE MEDICAL UNIT?

At least 75% of all newly diagnosed NIDDM patients are obese, but this is difficult to quantify in the acutely sick patient. Nonetheless, weight loss of 10 kg in this group will halve their fasting blood sugar, reduce diabetes-related death rates by a third, drop their diastolic blood pressure by 20 mmHg, and cut their cholesterol by 10%.

Patients with a BMI (weight/height$^2$) of more than 30 kg/m$^2$ have significantly increased health risks. Similar considerations apply to waist circumference, which is a lot easier to measure in the acute situation: high risk is associated with waist circumferences greater than 102 cm in men and 88 cm in women.

## MANAGEMENT OF ACUTE DIABETIC EMERGENCIES

### DKA

A reasonably sized district general hospital can expect to admit around two cases of DKA per month. Most will be of moderate severity, but a few will be

| Box 6.6 – Causes of DKA | |
| --- | --- |
| Infection | 40% |
| Disruption of insulin treatment | 25% |
| New-onset | 15% |
| Other causes (e.g. infarct, pregnancy) | 20% |

severely ill. Among this population will be the brittle diabetics with recurrent ketoacidosis and often with a history of poor compliance.

### Causes of DKA (→ Box 6.6)

Most cases of DKA are precipitated by infection or some form of disruption to the insulin treatment. This is often due to inappropriate action taken by the patient at the time of an acute illness: usually stopping or reducing insulin because of problems with maintaining oral intake. An important minority of cases of DKA are the first manifestation of new-onset diabetes. There will also be a number of brittle diabetics with recurrent ketoacidosis – predominantly female, socially disadvantaged and poorly compliant, this group often have associated eating disorders. Recently, an increasing problem of ketoacidosis in Type II diabetes is being recognised, particularly in patients of Afro-Caribbean origin. Interestingly, once the episode is over, these patients can return to oral hypoglycaemics or even to dietary treatment alone.

### Underlying mechanism

In DKA there is an acute shortage of insulin. As a result, the liver produces and releases excessive amounts of glucose that appear in the blood (*hyperglycaemia*) and which spill over into the urine (*glycosuria*). The heavy glucose load in the urine pulls in water and electrolytes by osmosis, leading to losses of fluid (*dehydration*), loss of potassium (*hypokalaemia*), and losses of sodium (*hyponatraemia*), phosphate and magnesium. Because there is a shortage of insulin, sugar cannot enter the cells and so the body starts to burn adipose tissue (fat stores) as an alternative energy source. The adipose tissue breaks down to free fatty acids, which are in turn converted into ketones by the liver. Some of the ketones are used by muscles for energy and some are excreted in the urine (*urine positive for ketones*). Ketones are acidic substances, so when excess ketones appear in the blood they produce an *acidosis*. The ketones can be smelt on the breath and measured in the blood and the urine using Ketostix on serum (a simple clotted blood sample) and on fresh urine. The consequences of DKA are illustrated in Fig. 6.2.

### Management

The key to treatment of DKA should be clear from the above discussion:

- adequate insulin replacement
- correction of fluid and electrolyte loss

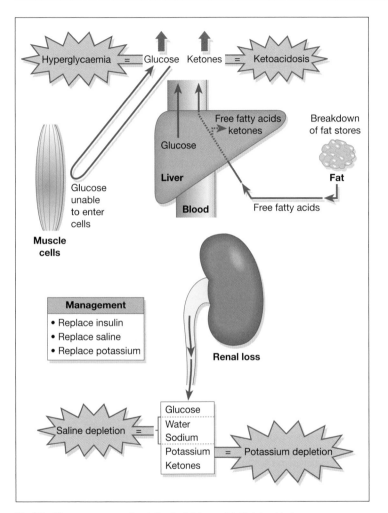

**Fig. 6.2**  The consequences of acute insulin deficiency: diabetic ketoacidosis

Acidosis does not usually need correcting, as it responds to the reversal of the ketosis by insulin, fluid and electrolyte therapy. Case Study 6.4 describes a case of acute severe DKA.

Hyperventilation is a sign of acidotic breathing (the body is trying to correct the acidosis by blowing off carbon dioxide). The patient in Case Study 6.4 had

---

**CASE STUDY 6.4** Acute severe DKA

A woman who had been a diabetic for 30 years, now aged 50, was admitted with a 48-h history of anorexia, headache and breathlessness. Her blood sugar the day before admission was 17 mmol/L. Her husband usually administered her insulin and she had good control, with blood sugars in the range 3–5 mmol/L on twice daily isophane 9 and 7 units and morning soluble 5 units. After a domestic upset, there was some doubt about whether she had received her insulin on the day of admission to hospital. Her husband came home from work to find her nearly unconscious and hyperventilating. There had been one previous admission with DKA 5 years before.

---

not been eating for 2 days and was therefore at risk from ketosis. Missing a single dose of insulin would have been enough to accelerate the onset of ketosis.

The patient had signs of DKA with hypovolaemia (low blood pressure). There were no features of infection. In particular, the chest was clear, there was no skin sepsis and there was no renal angle tenderness. There was no sign of meningeal irritation. Abdominal pain and tenderness are common features in DKA and can be due to acute fatty liver infiltration or pancreatitis. The patient was able to protect her airway (GCS above 8).

Hyperkalaemia is common in DKA, but there is usually a rapid fall as soon as fluids and insulin are given and the potassium enters the cells. Normally, we would administer potassium with the second litre of fluid. In this case, however, there were changes on the ECG showing that the high potassium was putting the heart rhythm at risk. Urgent action was needed to bring the level down. The patient was going to need careful fluid balance – hence the central line and catheter. The nasogastric tube was to prevent aspiration of stomach contents in the event of acute gastric paralysis with distension, a common problem in severe DKA.

**The importance of fluid balance in nursing the diabetic patient.** Nurses must be exceptionally careful monitoring the input and output in acutely ill diabetic patients. In DKA and non-ketotic hyperglycaemia, high volumes of fluid are being given to patients who are in a critical state because of fluid depletion amounting to between 4 and 6 L. However, these patients may well

---

**CASE STUDY 6.4** (continued)

On examination the patient was apyrexial, respiration rate 40/min, pulse 110 beats/min and blood pressure 90/60 mmHg. Oxygen saturations were 99% on air. She was restless and aggressive. Her GCS was 9/15. Examination was otherwise negative, apart from generalised abdominal tenderness. Her breath smelt of ketones.

**CASE STUDY 6.4** (continued)

The ECG showed signs of an acutely raised potassium. The urine showed large amounts of ketones, protein and sugar. BM stix was 55 mmol/L.

Blood samples, including blood cultures, were sent for analysis, and an immediate injection of calcium gluconate was given intravenously. A central line, nasogastric tube and urethral catheter were passed. A portable chest radiograph was performed.

have both cardiac and renal problems due to their diabetes and are at risk from fluid overload. This is critical in the first few hours of admission: typically, a patient with severe DKA may not pass urine for the first hour or two of rehydration, but if this persists they may need catheterisation and even a central venous line to ensure that the fluid input is not overly aggressive. Some DKA protocols recommend 2 L of fluid in the first hour, but this would be too fast for the frail, elderly and those with heart disease. Moreover, over-enthusiastic fluid replacement will wash out ketones and lower the blood sugar, but paradoxically lead to a worsening of the acidosis. An example of judicious fluid replacement of, say, a 7-L deficit (severe dehydration) in a frail patient would be:

2 L isotonic saline over 4 h
1 L isotonic saline over 4 h
0.5 L isotonic saline over 8 h
the remaining 3.5 L over the next 24 h

**CASE STUDY 6.4** (continued)

The following test results came back:

| | | |
|---|---|---|
| ● Hb | 12.9 g/dl | normal |
| ● WCC | 29.7 × 10⁹/L | very high as is common in DKA, even if infection is not present |
| ● Glucose | 58.7 mmol/L | very high (DKA *can* occur at sugars as low as 12 mmol/L, but most are >25 mmol/L) |
| ● Sodium | 127 mmol/L | low due to sodium lost in the osmotic diuresis |
| ● Potassium | 8.6 mmol/L | *very* high; the total body potassium is low, however, and the level will fall rapidly with treatment (known as 'hidden' potassium loss) |
| ● Urea | 14.2 mmol/L | high due to dehydration |
| ● Creatinine | 226 µmol/L | high due to dehydration (normal when tested 3 months prior to admission: always check previous notes for pre-existing kidney function) |

(continued overleaf)

**CASE STUDY 6.4** (continued)

- pH          6.93          severe acidosis (most patients with DKA will
                            have a pH of 7.0–7.2)
- $pO_2$        21.6 kPa      good oxygen levels (on oxygen therapy)
- $pCO_2$       1.6 kPa       low (blown off by hyperventilation)
- Bicarbonate 2.0 mmol/L    low (this increases as the acidosis improves
                            with treatment)

### INSULIN THERAPY

Twenty units of neutral insulin solution (Actrapid®) was given intramuscularly immediately, while an infusion was being prepared and the syringe pump set up. The infusion consisted of 50 ml of 0.9% (normal) saline with 50 units of neutral insulin solution (Actrapid®). This was i.v. at a rate of 6 units (6 ml) per hour. After 6 h, the sugar had fallen to 13 mmol/L; the insulin infusion was stopped and replaced by a GKI infusion.

### INTRAVENOUS FLUID REPLACEMENT

- 2 L of isotonic saline were given in the first hour (via an infusion pump)
- 1 L of isotonic saline was given in the second hour
- 500 ml/h of isotonic saline was then given for 4 h
- The GKI infusion was started at 6 h and the saline discontinued

By 24 h, the patient was feeling well, her urine was showing moderate amounts of ketones only, and she was starting to eat normally. Subcutaneous insulin was re-started at that stage, ensuring a 1-h overlap with the GKI infusion.

Careful fluid management is the key to good treatment. The measure of a well-managed acute DKA is of an accurate fluid balance chart showing hourly input and output, and a flow chart of the blood sugars, potassium, sodium and bicarbonate.

#### What to avoid while treatment is working

*Hypokalaemia.* Patients with DKA may start with a high potassium, but the level drops rapidly once the potassium moves back into the cells when insulin is given. Potassium supplements are usually added to the second litre of saline and continued at 20 mmol/h. Adjustments to the rate of potassium replacement can be made according to the 2-hourly potassium results. An

**CASE STUDY 6.4** (continued)

### POTASSIUM REPLACEMENT

- Potassium was added to the infusion at 20 mmol/h once the serum potassium had fallen to less than 5.0 mmol/L

**CASE STUDY 6.4** (continued)

## BICARBONATE

- 100 mmol of sodium bicarbonate (600 ml of 1.4% sodium bicarbonate) was given through the central line over 30 min

## MONITORING

- Hourly BM stix were continued until the patient could eat and drink normally
- Hourly pulse, BP, temperature, respiratory rate, GCS and urine output until the patient was stable (at least 6 h)
- Hourly oxygen saturations and supplementary oxygen to keep the saturations above 92%
- 2-hourly potassium, sugar, sodium, urea and bicarbonate until the sugar had fallen to 13 mmol/L
- A flow diagram was used to show the progress of the blood tests
- Urinary ketones were checked every 2 h (note that the ketonuria frequently increases initially and may take at least 24 h to clear from the urine)
- Continuous ECG monitor for 24 h (the risk of hyperkalaemia and arrhythmias)

example of the way to adjust the potassium supplements is shown in Table 6.3.

*Hypoglycaemia.* Start GKI as the sugar falls to 13 mmol/L.

*Fluid overload.* The overall fluid deficit will be between 4 and 6 L. In a sick diabetic patient it is wise to use a central line and monitor the CVP. Any infusion should be controlled with a volumetric pump.

*Aspiration.* Care of the patient with altered consciousness. Empty the stomach contents with a nasogastric tube if necessary.

*Intracerebral oedema.* This grave complication is unusual and tends to occur in those patients less than 20 years old. It usually occurs during the first 24 h after initial apparent metabolic and clinical improvement. There is a sudden deterioration in the conscious level (fall in the GCS) with neurological signs

**Table 6.3    Adjustment of potassium level with supplements**

| Potassium level in the blood (mmol/L) | Potassium added to each litre of saline (mmol) |
| --- | --- |
| <3.0 | 40 |
| 3.0–4.0 | 30 |
| 4.0–5.5 | 20 |
| >5.5 | Nil |

such as severe headache, neck stiffness, fitting and bilateral up-going plantars. It may be seen with over-enthusiastic fluid replacement (in these cases the blood appears diluted and the sodium level falls below normal, e.g. to 120 mmol/L) or it can simply occur for no obvious reason in a severe DKA. Diagnosis is by CT scan (and excluding meningitis or stroke) and treatment aims to reduce the raised intracranial pressure with mannitol and dexamethasone.

**A management protocol for DKA**
*Fluid replacement*

1. 2 L of isotonic (0.9%) saline in 4 h
2. 2 L of isotonic (0.9%) saline in 8 h
3. 2 L of isotonic (0.9%) saline in 16 h

Increase the rate if:

- there is persistent hypotension (systolic blood pressure < 90 mmHg)
- the urine output is very high

Reduce the rate if:

- the patient is elderly and frail
- there is a risk of heart failure (e.g. previous left ventricular failure, ankle oedema)

Consider hypotonic (0.45%) saline if:

- the sodium level climbs above 155 mmol/L

*Potassium*

- Give 20 mmol of KCl per hour *once the potassium level is known* (the KCl will therefore usually start with the second litre)
- Do not give KCl while the potassium level is more than 5.5 mmol/L
- Check the potassium level in the blood every 2 h

*Insulin*

- Give 20 units of neutral insulin solution (Actrapid) intramuscularly as soon as DKA has been recognised
- Follow with an insulin infusion at 6 units/h (50 units in 50 ml at 6 ml/h)
- Follow the response with hourly BM stix and 2-hourly laboratory sugar

If there is no fall in the sugar at 2 h:

- *check the i.v. lines and the pumps* (the most common cause for a 'failure' of i.v. insulin therapy)
- double the insulin infusion rate
- double again if no further fall at 4 h

The blood sugar should fall at around 5 mmol/h. If the fall is too rapid,

- reduce the insulin infusion rate

*When the sugar falls to 13 mmol/L*

- Start a GKI infusion aiming for sugars in the range 7–11 mmol/L
- Continue hourly BM stix and 4-hourly urinary Ketostix, but reduce the laboratory measurements

*When the patient can eat his first meal*

- Change to subcutaneous insulin
- Ensure a 1-h overlap between the GKI infusion and the first injection

*When to use sodium bicarbonate*

- Only when there is severe acidosis and hypotension: *pH < 6.9*
- Give 600 ml of 1.4% sodium bicarbonate with 20 mmol KCl over 30 min
- Check gases after 30 min and repeat the dose if pH is < 6.9 and hypotensive
- Avoid extravasation with sodium bicarbonate; use a central line if possible

*General care*

- Catheterise if no urine has been passed within 3 h or if there is hypotension
- Insert nasogastric tube if the conscious level is disturbed (GCS less than 8)
- Administer broad-spectrum antibiotics if sepsis is suspected (e.g. co-amoxiclav and cephalexin)
- Administer low-molecular weight heparin if there are risk factors for venous thromboembolic disease (→ Box 6.7)

## Nursing the patient with DKA

The first 4–5 h are critical in the care of the patient with ketoacidosis. The nurse will be caring for a very sick, distressed and possibly confused patient going through a period of intense clinical activity. The nurse will be combining the technical expertise necessary to administer a complex treatment regimen and the skills needed to meet the personal needs of a patient who is vulnerable, who feels dreadful and who is probably terrified for his life.

### Critical nursing tasks in DKA

**Ensure that the initial infusions are correctly prescribed and administered.** It is critical that there is absolutely no delay in initiating the saline and

---

**Box 6.7 – Indications for anticoagulation in DKA**

- No contraindication
- Severe DKA
- Previous thromboembolism
- Hyperosmolar
- 'Phlebitic' legs

**CRITICAL NURSING OBSERVATIONS IN DKA**

- Is the airway safe?
- Oxygen saturation
- Blood sugar
- Blood pressure
- Pulse (ECG)

**IMPORTANT NURSING OBSERVATIONS IN DKA**

- Glasgow Coma Score
- Temperature
- Test for urinary ketones
- Respiratory rate
- Examine for signs of infection

insulin infusions. The protocol must be followed and the correct amounts of fluid given during the first critical few hours. Particular attention must be paid to the potassium supplements and the subsequent blood levels.

**Monitor the patient's progress.** The hourly observations should chart: a falling pulse, rising blood pressure and increasing urine output as dehydration is corrected. If there is confusion or impairment of the conscious level, the GCS will improve. As acidosis resolves, the respiratory rate will fall and symptoms will improve. The sugar should fall at around 5–10 mmol/L per hour. The potassium should settle between 3.5 and 5.5 mmol/L. Urinary ketones will slowly disappear over 18–24 h and the appetite will return.

 **CRITICAL NURSING TASKS IN DKA**

- Ensure that the initial infusions are correctly prescribed and administered
- Monitor the patient's progress
- Address the patient's physical needs
- Provide reassurance and support
- Initiate plans to prevent this from happening to the patient again

**Address the patient's physical needs.** If the patient is unconscious, the priority is the nursing care of coma. The patient may be in discomfort and possibly in pain. If this is severe, a judgement will be made about the need for effective analgesics. The patient should adopt a comfortable position in bed and due attention should be paid to the pressure sites, *in particular to the heels*. Mouth care will be important because hyperventilation and dehydration will dry out the oral mucosa. There will be nausea, so sucking ice may be preferable to oral fluids. During the first few hours of admission there will be numerous medical and nursing interventions performed, so the patient's physical comfort will need to be continually reassessed.

**Provide reassurance and support.** Initially the patient may feel frightened and powerless. Patients with long-standing diabetes may be worried about relinquishing control to nurses and medical staff who are not part of the usual diabetic team. These fears will need to be addressed and the patient reassured about the temporary need for intensive insulin and fluid therapy. If there is disorientation or confusion, the patient will need support and explanation as the situation improves.

**Initiate plans to prevent this from happening to the patient again.** If your communication and assessment have been effective, it should be clear why this has happened. Involve the diabetic specialist nurse at an early stage and make sure that when the patient is transferred from the acute medical unit it is to the care of a diabetes team.

*Reassurance for patients with DKA*

- Your nausea and vomiting will stop as the drips start to work
- You are breathing quickly to blow off the toxic ketones
- Your breathlessness will improve as your diabetes is brought under control
- The nasal tube is to stop your stomach overfilling with air
- You are getting all the insulin and nutrition that you need in the drips
- Try not to panic on the oxygen mask – you need it to boost your oxygen levels
- Your appetite will return as soon as the diabetes comes under control again
- All the blood tests and close monitoring are needed for the first few hours only
- You can take over blood testing and insulin treatment once you feel well enough
- We are giving you powerful antibiotics to cover any possible infections
- Your heart is fine; the monitor is simply telling us its rate and rhythm
- The blood tests from your wrist are the best way to assess your overall progress

### Answering relatives' questions in DKA

The patient's relatives will be extremely concerned and frightened by the way in which the diabetes appears to have suddenly become a threat to the patient's life. They will need to be reassured.

*Should we have acted sooner?* Examine the relatives' understanding of diabetes. To what extent are they involved in the patient's diabetic care? If the DKA has been precipitated by an intercurrent infection, are they aware of the problems of acute illness in the diabetic? What warning signs did they act on to seek help, and were these appropriate?

*What else could we have done?* Are there areas where they would like more information? The relatives may be frightened by the idea of diabetes, injections, adjusting insulin and so forth. In these circumstances, the diabetic specialist nurse will have an important educational and supportive role, and will need to be involved.

*What will happen next?* You can reassure the relatives that the vast majority of patients with DKA make a complete recovery. There are, however, complications that can occur and the management will have to be particularly intensive for the first 6 h or so. There will be a lot of clinical activity during this time and it is usually helpful to put some constraints on the number of visitors during this period.

**Clinical details from the relatives.** The relatives may also be an important source of urgent clinical information, particularly if the patient is too unwell or confused to give a full history. The relatives can provide important clinical details of the illness and the usual level of diabetic control. The description of the symptoms and how they progressed will help determine the nature of any precipitating infection. Was there headache and fever to suggest meningitis, dysuria and renal tract pain to suggest urinary sepsis, or diarrhoea and vomiting to suggest gastroenteritis? What evidence do the relatives have concerning the usual level of diabetic control and the degree of cooperation and compliance with treatment? Is there a blood-sugar diary card to look at? What is the usual insulin regimen? When was it last administered and when did the patient last eat or drink? On a general note: is there a history of heavy alcohol intake (which can have an impact on diabetic control) and are there any allergies, particularly to antibiotics?

### The importance of patients' and relatives' education in diabetes

The patient in Case Study 6.5 is typical of the diabetic patient who is uncertain what to do when he becomes acutely unwell. There were clear warning signs from his osmotic symptoms that his diabetic control was deteriorating. His acute abdominal symptoms were either gastroenteritis or the first indications of DKA. He should have sought urgent help when he first found urinary ketones, or preferably when he had the combination of

**CASE STUDY 6.5**   DKA – no advice on what to do on sick days

A 17-year-old boy with a year's history of Type I diabetes gave a 2-week history of tiredness, polyuria and high BM stix. He did not seek help or adjust his insulin. Two days before admission to hospital, he developed diarrhoea and continued to vomit all day. He continued his insulin, but was unable to take any fluids. By the evening his urine showed ketones, but he waited a further 12 h before asking for help. On admission he was dry and hypotensive. There were large amounts of ketones in his urine. Test results were: blood sugar 28.5 mmol/L, creatinine 112 μmol/L and urea 8.5 mmol/L. pH was 7.29, bicarbonate was low at 12 mmol/L. He improved rapidly with i.v. fluids and insulin.

vomiting and an inability to keep up with his fluids. Before he was discharged from the Acute Medical Unit, the patient and his mother were given a clear explanation of what had happened and what action they could take in future.

# INFORMATION FOR DIABETICS: WHAT TO DO ON DAYS WHEN YOU ARE SICK

- The main problems occur with gastroenteritis and infections
- When you are ill you may need *more* short-acting insulin than normal
- Your blood sugar can rise even if you cannot eat your normal diet
- While you are ill, check your blood sugar between 2- and 4-hourly and your urine for ketones twice a day
- Adjust your insulin only if you are confident in doing so. (An example of self-adjustment would be a diabetic who is on a bolus regimen totalling, say, 36 units per day who could increase each bolus by 4 units if the sugar values were between 13 and 22 mmol/L)
- If your blood sugar is less than 13 mmol/L, continue with your usual insulin doses
- *Never stop your insulin*
- Keep your carbohydrate intake up with milk and sugar, snacks, ice cream and coke
- Also try to drink 4–6 pints (3.6–5.4 litres) of sugar-free liquid per day
- Seek help if you are ill, *especially if you are vomiting* or if your sugar is continuously > 22 mmol/L or if your urine is positive for ketones
- If the breathing becomes rapid, the vomiting persists and there is drowsiness you, the patient, or your relatives, *must* seek urgent medical attention

## HYPEROSMOLAR NON-KETOTIC DIABETIC COMA

This relatively rare complication is seen in elderly Type II diabetic patients and has a 50% mortality. The patients present extremely unwell, with very high sugars and impaired consciousness levels, but without ketoacidosis. They are usually profoundly dehydrated due to osmotic fluid loss. The history usually involves a precipitating illness – an infection in 80% of cases – with vomiting and thirst that has often been relieved by high volumes of very sugary drinks. The diagnosis is made from the clinical setting and the finding of a high blood osmolality (over-concentrated blood). The osmolality can be calculated by a simple formula using standard blood results:

$$\text{Osmolality} = 2 \times (\text{plasma sodium} + \text{potassium}) + \text{urea} + \text{glucose}$$

The normal osmolality is 275–295 mosmol/kg; in HONK, the level is greater than 350 mosmol/kg.

Management includes CVP monitoring, nasogastric intubation to prevent aspiration and judicious fluid therapy to replace half of a typical 7-litre deficit in the first 12 h, and the remainder over the next 24 h ($\rightarrow$ p. 00; the importance of fluid balance in nursing the diabetic patient).

As the sodium levels are usually very high in HONK, hypotonic (0.45%) saline can be used in place of the initial isotonic saline. Otherwise the treatment is very similar to that for DKA. Because the blood is so concentrated, the patients are at great risk from thrombosis and should be anticoagulated.

## HYPOGLYCAEMIA

The possibility of hypoglycaemia must always be the first consideration when faced with an acute neurological or behavioural disturbance, whether the patient is diabetic or not. It is a major danger for patients who are on insulin.

*Symptoms*
The symptoms of hypoglycaemia present acutely and progress rapidly as the blood sugar drops. Mild symptoms with headache, slight mood changes, excessive sweating of the face and hands or subtle changes in behaviour occur as sugars fall to 3 mmol/L. As the sugar decreases, adrenaline is released, which produces the classical warning signs: sweating, irritability, tremor, palpitations and intense hunger. There may be double vision, aggression and poor cooperation. With severe hypoglycaemia, at sugar levels of 1–2 mmol/L, there may be epileptic fits, confusion, stroke-like symptoms and coma. Untreated, severe hypoglycaemia can result in irreversible damage. In prolonged hypoglycaemia death may occur, but this is a rare occurrence and tends to be associated with deliberate overdosing of either insulin or oral hypoglycaemics.

## Causes

Hypoglycaemia is most common in Type I diabetes as a result of mismatches of insulin, carbohydrate intake and carbohydrate utilisation. Many Type I diabetics now tend to aim for low/normal blood sugars using three- or four-times-daily short-acting insulin. Although these intensive regimens reduce the incidence of long-term complications, they can put the patients at an increased risk from hypoglycaemia. Missed meals, excessive unplanned exercise and (particularly the morning after) an alcoholic binge can all lead to acute hypoglycaemia. Interestingly, islet cell function partially recovers when new diabetics are first started on insulin. This is a temporary effect that lasts only a few months, but the extra natural insulin puts new diabetics at risk from hypoglycaemia during this 'honeymoon period'.

Prolonged hypoglycaemia can occur in Type II patients if they are taking oral hypoglycaemics. It is a particular problem in the elderly if they are inappropriately given long-acting hypoglycaemics such as glibenclamide or chlorpropamide, if they eat poorly and, particularly, if they abuse alcohol.

### Hypoglycaemic unawareness

In some diabetics there are no warning signs of hypoglycaemia on which they can take action – a condition termed hypoglycaemic unawareness. These patients can pass rapidly through a stage of confusion to hypoglycaemic coma. Hypoglycaemic unawareness is seen mainly in diabetics who have frequent hypoglycaemic attacks. These appear to blunt the usual symptoms of impending hypoglycaemia. Even one hypoglycaemic episode will blunt the awareness of a second episode for 24 h or more, so these patients are in a vicious circle. Diabetic autonomic neuropathy will also reduce the body's normal warning response to hypoglycaemia. Therefore, if there is a history of recurrent and potentially dangerous hypoglycaemia, the patient needs urgent referral for detailed assessment of their diabetes, in particular to exclude hypoglycaemic unawareness. Fortunately, awareness can be restored if further hypoglycaemic episodes are avoided.

### Management

Hypoglycaemia is the ultimate medical emergency: the presentation is dramatic, the benefits of treatment are immediate and, most importantly, to miss or to delay treatment is a disaster. Permanent neurological damage from hypoglycaemia, although rare, can be devastating. If you suspect hypoglycaemia, check the BM stix and, if possible, send a laboratory glucose for later confirmation. If the patient is in coma, your priority is to ensure the safety of the patient with regard to his airway, breathing and circulation. If the patient is conscious and cooperative and you diagnose hypoglycaemia, you should give 20 g of quick-acting carbohydrate as:

- 100 ml Lucozade

*or*

- six glucose tablets

*or*

- four teaspoonfuls of sugar

**Intravenous glucose.** A large-bore Venflon will be needed if there is an impaired conscious level, as i.v. glucose will be needed (→ Table 6.4). Give 25 g of glucose as 10, 20 or 50% glucose, but remember: the stronger the glucose the more irritant the solution to the veins. Check the BM stix at 5 and 30 min after treatment has been given. Hypoglycaemia due to oral hypoglycaemics can be prolonged, as some of the drugs have a long course of action. These patients will need careful monitoring for recurrence and may need a 10% infusion of glucose continued for a number of hours.

**Intramuscular glucagon.** If you cannot get venous access, then glucagon can be used. Glucagon is a naturally occurring hormone that has the exact opposite effect to insulin. Give 1 mg of glucagon intramuscularly. It acts more slowly than glucose (in coma consciousness returns in 10–15 min). Glucagon also causes nausea and vomiting and is not very effective in patients who are starved or who have consumed excessive alcohol.

*Always seek the cause for hypoglycaemia*
Case Study 6.6 illustrates why it is important to find out the cause of the hypoglycaemia. Cortisone, like adrenaline and glucagon, is a stress hormone

| Table 6.4 Constitution of glucose solutions | |
| --- | --- |
| *Glucose solution* | *25 g glucose in:* |
| 50% | 50 ml |
| 20% | 125 ml |
| 10% | 250 ml |

---

**CASE STUDY 6.6** Failure to recover from hypoglycaemia

A 35-year-old diabetic was admitted with severe hypoglycaemia. He had been seen by his parents the evening before and had then been found in a confused and barely rousable state in the morning. He had been a diabetic for a year and was quite depressed about its implications for the future. He remained confused and hypoglycaemic for several days, in spite of high-dose i.v. glucose. Initial suspicions that he had taken an insulin overdose could not be substantiated. He was discharged home after eventual recovery, but was admitted a day later with further hypoglycaemia.

Further investigations revealed that he had also developed Addison's disease. He responded well to cortisone therapy and his hypoglycaemia resolved.

**Table 6.5    A guide to infusions and additives in diabetes**

| Infusion / additive | Route | Indications / uses | Risks |
|---|---|---|---|
| Isotonic saline[a] | Peripheral line | Dehydration DKA | LVF (fluid overload) |
| Hypotonic saline | Peripheral line | Hyperosmolar (high sodium) | Overdilution (watch sodium) |
| 5% glucose[b] | Peripheral line | GKI | Overdilution if given >24 h |
| 10% glucose | Large bore | GKI/hypoglycaemia | |
| 20% glucose | Central/large bore | Hypoglycaemia | Hyperglycaemia |
| 50% glucose | Central/large bore | Hypoglycaemia | |
| KCl solution (2 mmol/ml) | Mix *thoroughly* in saline or glucose | Potassium depletion | Potassium overload |
| Sodium bicarbonate 1.26% (600 ml gives 100 mmol of bicarbonate) | Central line | Severe acidosis (pH <6.9) Severe hyperkalaemia (protective action) | Extravasation Sodium overload (LVF) |

[a] Also known as normal saline, 0.9% sodium chloride and physiological saline.
[b] Sometimes also known as dextrose.

that is released in response to hypoglycaemia to try and correct the body's blood sugar. Addison's disease, like diabetes, is another autoimmune disease in which the body produces antibodies against the adrenal gland, the source of cortisone. This patient's natural ability to correct hypoglycaemia was impaired due to his lack of cortisone. Addison's disease and diabetes share a similar mechanism and are known to occur together, like this, in the same patient. This case illustrates the need to follow up any case of hypoglycaemia to establish the exact reason for its occurrence.

In managing all these diabetic emergencies, it is important to be familiar with the various i.v. infusions (→ Table 6.5).

# INFECTIVE COMPLICATIONS IN DIABETES: THE ACUTE DIABETIC FOOT

Acute infection involving the lower limbs and feet are a common cause for emergency admission in the diabetic patient. The feet are extremely vulnerable in diabetes due to the combination of vascular damage, peripheral nerve damage and the diabetic's inherent susceptibility to infection. Half of those with Type II diabetes who are older than 60 years have established peripheral nerve damage. This leads to two major problems in the feet:

- loss of sensation
- muscle imbalance, with resulting foot deformity

If the feet are numb, minor trauma goes unheeded, so that simple abrasions progress to ulceration and infection. Deformity of the feet, and in particular clawing of the toes, puts areas over the soles of the feet at risk from the effects of abnormal pressure loading. Calluses form over the metatarsal heads, which are the main pressure points; these break down and become ulcerated.

As a result of diabetic vascular disease the blood supply to the tissues is poor: they heal badly and may ulcerate, particularly around the ankles. Infections do not clear, and may progress proximally from localised involvement of the feet to the rest of the leg. Ultimately, the tissues may die, with the development of wet or dry gangrene.

*Assessment of the diabetic foot*
The severely infected foot that brings the diabetic patient in as an emergency will characteristically have cellulitis spreading from an area of ulceration. The likely sequence is that a trivial abrasion starts silently and progresses to ulceration. By the time the patient needs admission, the ulcer will have become infected and the whole foot may be at risk. The diabetes may be out of control and if the patient is septic (i.e. infection has spread into the bloodstream), they may also be ketoacidotic.

It is important to recognise that in some patients, particularly the elderly and socially disadvantaged, the acutely infected foot is only part of a picture of generalised self-neglect (→ Box 6.8 and Fig. 6.3).

A reasonable idea of the degree of vascular and nerve damage can be obtained from the patient's history (Box 6.9). Diabetic vascular disease is indicated by a history of exertional calf pain progressing to severe rest pain in the legs and feet, a history of previous bypass procedures, and/or amputation of some of the toes. Diabetic nerve damage is suggested by a history of unpleasant burning, pins and needles or diffuse pain in the feet, all

---

**Box 6.8 – Self-neglect in the elderly diabetic patient**

- Poor vision
- Poor mobility
- Poor motivation
- Multiple medical problems
- Poor skin: sores, excoriation and abrasions
- Hypertension and hyperglycaemia
- Advanced diabetic feet, calluses and foot ulcers
- Obesity
- Superficial candida infection in skin creases, between the toes and in the groins
- Uncut nails with infected nail beds
- Neglected dentition
- Old and dirty dressings/bandages
- Heavy nicotine staining

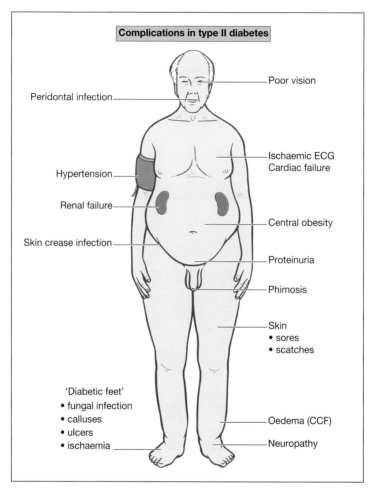

**Fig. 6.3**  Complications of Type II diabetes

of which are worse at night. The feet feel numb, and there may be a previous history of painless damage from ill-fitting shoes or minor trauma.

*How to look at the feet*

1. Remove all old dressings on the lower limbs.
2. Ask the patient if his feet are numb – can he feel you touching his feet?

---

**Box 6.9 – Indications of ischaemic and neuropathic feet in diabetes**

## Ischaemic feet
- History of exertional calf pain and resting foot pain
- Previous lower limb bypass procedures
- Cold, poorly nourished feet, with shiny red skin
- Areas of gangrene/necrosis

## Neuropathic feet
- Burning and tingling feet, particularly at night
- Numb to the touch
- Warm feet
- Callus over pressure points
- Ulcers over pressure points
- Foot deformity (clawed toes)

---

3. What colour is the skin?
   — Red, shiny and hairless skin indicates poor nutrition (ischaemia)
   — Are there any black areas?
   — Are the feet blue and cold, suggesting arterial insufficiency?
   — Are they warm and wet (oedema)? This can indicate nerve damage.
4. Have any foot or leg pulses been found?
   — There may be elements of both arterial and nerve damage.
5. Look at the nails and between the toes (maceration and fungal infection).
6. Are the feet a normal shape?
   — Clawed toes indicate small-muscle damage and make the feet vulnerable to pressure damage, with callus formation over weight-bearing areas.
7. Are there any breaks in the skin or ulcer formation? If there are ulcers:
   — how deep are they? (superficial or penetrating)
   — how big are they? (foot ulcers with an area more than 2 cm² often involve the bone)
   — do they look infected (red, exuding pus and smelling), or are they simply chronic pressure ulcers?

---

**Box 6.10 – Distinction between wet and dry gangrene**

| **Wet gangrene** | **Dry gangrene** |
|---|---|
| • Swollen | • Hard |
| • Moist | • Dry |
| • Blistering | • Demarcation of blackened tissue |
| • Large portion of the foot | • Toes and toe ends |
| • Early debridement/amputation | • Early angiograms/revascularisation? |

8. Is there any cellulitis: tender, red, raised areas around breaks in the skin?
   — The foot may be hot and there may be an obvious collection of pus beneath the skin. There may be a strong odour, suggesting Gram-negative infection. Sometimes gas can be felt as bubbling (crepitus) within the tissues.
9. There may be areas of wet or dry gangrene. The distinction is important (→ Box 6.10).

### Signs of worsening and spreading infection

- The foot becomes increasingly painful and tender
- The patient looks ill
- The skin goes purple and red or black blisters appear
- There is an increase in:
  — pulse
  — temperature
  — blood sugars
  — white cell count
  — respiration rate (acidotic breathing)
- The infection spreads into the leg

Box 6.11 summarises the important points to check for in the acute diabetic foot.

### Management
In the first 24–48 h, the priorities in managing the acute diabetic foot are to:

- control the diabetes
- treat infection
- provide adequate pain relief
- salvage the limb if there is critical ischaemia
- prevent the worsening of any pressure damage

---

**Box 6.11 – Checklist for the acute diabetic foot**

- Is the foot chronically damaged or is there an acute problem?
- Are any skin breaks superficial or penetrating and deep?
- Is there any cellulitis?
- Are the ulcers clean and punched out, or secondarily infected?
- What is the dominant problem: nerve damage, arterial disease, or both?
- Is the patient becoming ketoacidotic?

The infection is identified by taking deep swabs from any ulcers and sets of blood cultures. If there is severe local or spreading infection, broad-spectrum antibiotics are used, e.g. i.v. cefuroxime and flucloxacillin with metronidazole. If MRSA is suspected, i.v. vancomycin and teicoplanin are also used. These will be modified once the results of cultures are known. If the ulcers are deep, the feet are X-rayed to identify any spread of the infection to underlying bone.

If the foot deteriorates or there is wet gangrene, there must be an immediate surgical opinion regarding the need for debridement. Critical (limb-threatening) ischaemia should be suspected if there is a history of severe rest pain, signs of ischaemic ulceration and areas of gangrene. The surgeons must see these patients urgently with a view to immediate angiography and a limb-salvaging procedure (e.g. bypass or angioplasty).

Pressure damage to the heels is a major hazard in these patients, and appropriate protective action is necessary. The position in which the patient is nursed is important, because if the feet are dependent they will become oedematous, and if they are elevated a poor blood supply will become even worse. The patient must be kept on bedrest.

Decisions on longer-term and preventative action and the choice of appropriate dressings and less urgent wound management can be left, to be made later by the diabetic team.

The key points in emergency treatment and management of the acute diabetic foot are presented in Box 6.12.

---

**Box 6.12 – Emergency treatment and management of the diabetic foot**

### EMERGENCY TREATMENT
- Control the diabetes
- Treat sepsis
- Exclude limb-threatening ischaemia

### MANAGING THE INFECTED FOOT
- Control diabetes
- Neuropathic/vascular or both?
- Look at the pressure points
- Avoid pressure damage to heels
- Assess extent and depth of any ulceration
- Deep swabs and blood cultures
- Intravenous antibiotics for cellulitis
- Urgent vascular surgical opinion?
- Improve any local oedema (avoid elevation in ischaemia)

**EXCELLENT DIABETIC CARE**

- Ward protocols for the emergency management of DKA and hypoglycaemia
- Protocol for the use of GKI infusions, with adjustments depending on blood results
- Protocol for the use of separate glucose and insulin infusions, with adjustments
- Management protocol for the acute diabetic foot and acute limb ischaemia
- Planned protocol reviews and updates
- Review of the significance of finding glycosuria, proteinuria and ketonuria
- Appropriate and timely access to the diabetic specialist nurse/medical team
- A system to review techniques for measuring blood sugars and injecting insulin
- A system to calibrate and maintain the blood glucose meters
- An audit of the management of diabetic patients on the Acute Medical Unit
- Educational resources for staff, patients and relatives

## FURTHER READING

DIGAMI (Diabetes Mellitus, Insulin Glucose Infusion in Acute Myocardial Infarction) Study Group 1997 Prospective randomised study of intensive insulin treatment on long term survival after acute myocardial infarction in patients with diabetes mellitus. British Medical Journal 314: 1512–1515

Lebovitz HE 1995 Diabetic ketoacidosis. Lancet 345: 767–772

Mandrup-Poulsen T 1998 Diabetes: recent advances. British Medical Journal 316: 1221–1225

Watkins P 2002 ABC of diabetes, 5th edn. BMJ Publishing Group, London

Watkins P 2003 The diabetic foot. British Medical Journal 326: 977–979

### WEBSITES

A desk-top guide to Type I diabetes mellitus:
http://www.staff.ncl.ac.uk/philip.home/t1dg1998.htm

A desk-top guide to Type II diabetes:
http://www.staff.ncl.ac.uk/philip.home/t2dg1999.htm

# THROMBOEMBOLIC DISEASE

## INTRODUCTION

Almost a tenth of medical emergencies are admitted because of a painful calf with a provisional diagnosis of a DVT or a possible pulmonary embolus. Due to the unreliability of the clinical signs and the anxiety of missing a dangerous clot, these patients have usually been admitted and treated with i.v. heparin infusions until confirmatory tests confirm or refute the diagnosis.

The situation has changed, for two reasons:

- rapid and reliable screening tests are now available for venous thromboembolism
- simplified anticoagulation with once-daily subcutaneous low-molecular-weight heparin is replacing the heparin infusion

There are two important clinical issues:

- differentiating between the various causes of a red, swollen and painful leg: venous thrombosis, cellulitis, varicose eczema and arterial insufficiency
- remembering to consider the possibility of pulmonary emboli in any ill and breathless patient

The overriding consideration in these situations is that a missed diagnosis of venous thromboembolic disease carries with it the potential of a preventable death from a massive pulmonary embolus. It should be remembered that post-mortem studies have shown that 10% of hospital deaths are due to pulmonary emboli; most of them were unrecognised.

# THE NATURE OF THE DISEASE

## THROMBOSIS AND THROMBOEMBOLISATION

*Mechanisms*

Thrombosis refers to the process in which a mass of clot forms inside an artery or a vein. It consists of a dense network of fibrin in which are trapped variable proportions of red cells and platelets. Thrombosis blocks the vessel and impairs blood flow. Arterial thrombosis leads to ischaemic tissue damage (myocardial infarction, stroke and peripheral vascular disease), whereas in venous thrombosis the consequences are due to back pressure and local swelling (oedema). If the clot disintegrates, parts of it can break off, producing emboli that travel onwards – in venous thrombosis through the veins to the lungs (pulmonary embolus), and in arterial thrombosis through the arteries to major organs such as the brain (cerebral embolus), limbs (peripheral embolus), kidneys (renal infarction) and intestine (acute bowel ischaemia).

The trigger for thrombosis depends on whether it occurs in an artery or a vein.

- In the arteries, local damage to the vessel wall, usually in the form of a ruptured atheromatous plaque, initiates thrombosis by the release and activation of clotting factors and the adhesion of platelet clumps to the damaged surface
- In the veins there are three factors that contribute to abnormal clotting and increase the risk of venous thromboembolic disease (DVT and pulmonary embolism):
  — stagnation of the blood flow
  — damage to the vein wall
  — abnormalities of the clotting mechanism

**Stagnation of the blood flow.** Stagnation within the veins is the most important factor in initiating venous thrombosis. Calf muscles act as a venous pump returning blood to the heart. Failure of the calf pump due to enforced immobility (e.g. postoperative bed rest, plaster cast, paralysed limb) leads to venous stasis. This is a particular problem in the elderly, the obese and those with varicose veins: in these patients even 3 or 4 days of immobility can be critical.

*Damage to the vein wall.* Thrombosis is triggered by the activation of clotting mechanisms that occurs when there is damage to the vein wall – indeed, this is the normal mechanism for preventing bleeding at the sites of trauma. Typical situations that lead to vein damage are pressure injuries to the calf from the theatre operating table and the deterioration that occurs in the veins as a result of recurrent venous thrombosis.

**Abnormalities of the clotting mechanism.** There are several inherited and acquired abnormalities of the clotting mechanisms that increase the risk of venous thromboembolic disease (→ Box 7.1). The most common acquired abnormalities are those associated with the oral contraceptive pill, hormone replacement therapy, pregnancy and the presence of malignant disease.

Inherited clotting abnormalities ('thrombophilias') are increasingly recognised as underlying the cause of recurrent DVTs, particularly in younger patients and in those with a positive family history. The most important of several inherited coagulation abnormalities, known as Factor V Leiden, is present in 5% of the population and increases the risk of thrombosis by ten times the normal rate. One in five patients with their first DVT are Leiden Factor V positive. Recent estimates suggest up to half of all patients who present with a venous thromboembolic episode, either DVT or pulmonary embolus, may have a single or multiple inherited abnormalities of their clotting. In these individuals, each episode can be triggered by trivial external events such as minor surgery or immobility. In the future, increasing attention will be paid to identifying these inherited risk factors.

---

**Box 7.1 – Examples of inherited thrombophilia**

- Antithrombin deficiency
- Protein C deficiency
- Antiphospholipid syndrome
- Protein S deficiency
- Factor V Leiden

---

**Multiple risk factors.** In most situations in which the chances of a venous thrombosis are high there are multiple risk factors. Thus in major orthopaedic procedures to the leg there is vein damage and immobility; in pregnancy there is abnormal clotting and stagnation of blood due to intra-abdominal mechanical effects; and in prolonged air travel there is immobility, often associated with a degree of dehydration. The combination of the oral contraceptive pill and the presence of Factor V Leiden increases the risk of a DVT 30-fold.

### Superficial thrombophlebitis

Thrombophlebitis is a painful inflammation of the superficial veins. Classically it is seen with infected venous cannulae, but it also commonly occurs in patients with varicose veins. The clinical picture is of palpable and very tender cords of thrombosed and inflamed veins, with the overlying skin appearing reddened or bruised. Thrombophlebitis is not in itself dangerous; it does not progress to, but may accompany, deep vein thrombosis. Management is based on removing any cause (e.g. an i.v. cannula) and treating the symptoms. Importantly, recurrent unexplained phlebitis is found in patients with unrecognised malignant disease, particularly adenocarcinomas of the gastrointestinal tract and lung.

### Deep vein thrombosis

Deep vein thrombosis is a more serious problem, because of the risk of fatal pulmonary embolus. Most DVTs start in the deep veins of the calf, termed the distal veins, where they cause local pain and swelling.

Although calf vein thromboses do not themselves give rise to emboli, one in five subsequently extend up the leg to involve the proximal veins in the thigh and pelvis – *popliteal and iliofemoral thrombosis*. The risk of a pulmonary embolus from a proximal vein thrombosis is very high, around 50%, and some will be fatal. A significant proportion of the survivors, perhaps one in five, will develop a postphlebitic syndrome in the affected leg, with chronic swelling, varicose veins, skin pigmentation, recurrent thrombosis and venous ulceration.

The management is based on preventing progression of the thrombotic process by using heparin for an immediate effect, followed by warfarin in the medium to long term to lower the risk of recurrence. The aim of treatment is to stabilise the situation. Warfarin and heparin do not dissolve established clot; they are given to:

- prevent extension
- reduce the chances of embolisation
- lower the risk of recurrence

*Pulmonary thromboembolism*

Most pulmonary emboli (90%) arise from the proximal veins in the thigh and pelvis. Depending on their size, emboli that travel to the lung either become wedged in the main pulmonary arteries, where they block the outflow of blood from the right side of the heart, or pass onwards to become trapped in the lung peripheries. The former, termed massive pulmonary emboli, produce a disastrous decrease in cardiac output, leading to sudden death or acute hypotensive collapse. The smaller emboli in the periphery of the lungs produce wedge-shaped areas of lung damage (producing breathlessness and haemoptysis) and give rise to overlying pleurisy (acute chest pain and a fever; → Fig. 7.1).

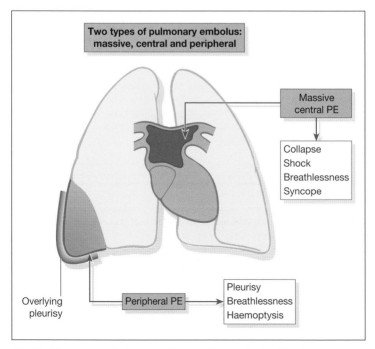

**Fig. 7.1** The two types of pulmonary embolus: massive central and peripheral

Massive pulmonary emboli can move or start to break up either naturally or during the course of cardiopulmonary resuscitation. Thrombolytic drugs such as streptokinase and rt-PA can help to dissolve the embolus and are used in the unstable hypotensive patient. Heparin will prevent further emboli, and as most patients who die survive the first embolus but die from a recurrence within the first few hours, it is important to start treatment urgently. Warfarin is added for longer-term prevention.

The management of smaller peripheral emboli is based on preventing further and possibly bigger emboli by giving heparin and, subsequently, warfarin.

## TESTS TO IDENTIFY VENOUS THROMBOEMBOLIC DISEASE

A number of tests are available to identify venous thromboembolic disease (→ Table 7.1). They are described in more detail below.

**Contrast venogram and pulmonary angiogram.** The venogram examines the veins of the legs and pelvis and the inferior vena cava and is considered to be the 'gold standard' for the identification of venous thrombosis. An invasive test and unpleasant for the patient, its use is confined to difficult cases, particularly those in which active intervention with a vena cava filter is under consideration. The pulmonary angiogram was the 'gold standard' investigation for diagnosing pulmonary emboli, but it has been replaced by the CT pulmonary angiogram.

**Isotope lung scan.** Lung scans are easy to perform and, when used in conjunction with the clinical details, are useful in the diagnosis of pulmonary emboli. Although positive scans are also seen in other conditions and have to be interpreted with care, a normal scan result is very helpful, as it rules out the possibility of a pulmonary embolus.

| Table 7.1 | The value of various tests in the diagnosis of thromboembolic disease | |
|---|---|---|
| *Test* | *Good at:* | *Poor at:* |
| V/Q lung scan | Diagnosing a PE if the chest film is normal | Diagnosing a PE if there is pre-existing lung disease |
| Contrast venogram | The 'gold standard' test | Too invasive for a screening test |
| Impedence plethysmography | Diagnosing a proximal (above knee) DVT | Diagnosing a distal (calf vein) DVT |
| D-dimers | Excluding a DVT if the test is normal. Also positive in PE | False positive result in other conditions, e.g. infection and myocardial infarct |
| Compression ultrasound | Probably the best screening test | Diagnosing a distal (calf vein) thrombosis |

**CT pulmonary angiogram.** The investigation of possible pulmonary emboli has been revolutionised by the introduction of the CTPA. It is superior to both the isotope lung scan and the conventional angiogram. A negative CTPA rules out a significant pulmonary embolus and often gives additional information on alternative causes of the patients symptoms.

**Compression ultrasound.** This looks at compressibility of the vein with an ultrasound probe and also examines venous blood flow using colour Doppler. Compression ultrasound is accurate for thigh vein thrombosis, but not for thrombosis in the pelvis or calf. It is also unreliable at picking up recurrent thrombotic episodes. In spite of these drawbacks, ultrasound is a simple, rapid and very effective diagnostic tool, particularly when combined with clinical assessment and initial screening by the measurement of D-dimers.

**Impedance plethysmography.** In this test, the flow of blood out of the calf is impeded by inflating a thigh cuff. The cuff is then suddenly let down and the flow of blood out of the calf is measured to assess the degree of venous obstruction. The term 'impedance' refers to the technique of deriving a measure of blood flow from sensors placed over the calf.

Ultrasound and plethysmography are reliable for proximal deep vein thrombosis, but are poor at identifying calf vein thrombosis. However, in practical terms (i.e. the risk of pulmonary embolus) thrombosis in the calf only becomes important if it spreads to the thigh – so if the initial clinical suspicion is high it is prudent to repeat either test after a few days, in case a missed calf vein thrombosis has extended proximally to the thigh.

**D-dimer measurements.** D-dimers are fragments of dissolving blood clots that can be identified from a blood sample whenever a thromboembolic process is under way. A positive test is also seen after surgery, in infections, after myocardial infarction and in malignant disease; a positive D-dimer test is not therefore in itself diagnostic. D-dimer tests are most useful for ruling out thromboembolism when the initial clinical assessment suggests a low or intermediate suspicion of the diagnosis. For example a patient who is breathless may have a major risk factor such as recent hip surgery, but has other possible causes of breathlessness such as COPD; in this situation, a negative D-dimer means there is another cause for the breathlessness. When the clinical suspicion is high, D-dimers are not helpful, because a negative result under these circumstances is not reliable enough to rule out the diagnosis (an example would be a patient who is breathless, with no alternative explanation, plus a major risk factor for pulmonary embolus).

# MANAGEMENT OF PULMONARY THROMBOEMBOLISM

The following case studies are used to illustrate management of pulmonary thromboembolism (→ Case studies 7.1–7.4). The classical features of a pulmonary embolus are listed in Box 7.2.

**CASE STUDY 7.1** Acute massive pulmonary emboli

A 35-year-old woman was admitted to hospital having collapsed at home. She had arisen to go to the toilet and collapsed with loss of consciousness for a few seconds. She recovered, but remained clammy with a thready pulse and felt very breathless. The day before, she had complained of a slight pain in the left calf. She was taking a third-generation combined oral contraceptive pill, she was obese and was a smoker. She also had chronic bilateral varicose veins. Three months earlier, she had been admitted with swelling and tenderness of the left calf coming on after exercise, but after equivocal tests had been discharged without anticoagulation.

On examination her pulse was 110 beats/min, blood pressure 104/78 mmHg, oxygen saturations 100% on 6 L/min oxygen. Respiratory rate was 20 breaths/min. The right calf measured 42 cm and the left 46 cm (similar readings to the previous admission). An urgent lung scan showed multiple pulmonary emboli. Seven hours after admission, she collapsed again while walking to the toilet, but on this occasion there was a cardiorespiratory arrest. In spite of prolonged resuscitation and the use of streptokinase, she remained in electromechanical dissociation (EMD) and did not survive.

**CASE STUDIES 7.2** Emboli treated with streptokinase

**CASE 1**

A 54-year-old woman was admitted with a 1-week history of right upper abdominal pain radiating to her back and right shoulder and worse on lying or on deep inspiration. She had become breathless over 2 days.

On admission the patient had a respiratory rate of 16 breaths/min, pulse 80 beats/min and normal blood pressure. The arterial oxygen level was reduced to 88% on air and the chest film showed changes at both lung bases. A provisional diagnosis of diaphragmatic pleurisy due to pulmonary emboli was made and heparin was started.

On the second day the oxygen saturations fell to 76% on air and the pulse had increased to 110 beats/min. Examination and ECG showed increasing strain on the right side of the heart. On the third day there was a sudden attack of near syncope and breathlessness on standing associated with further drops in the oxygen saturation and a blood pressure of 90/60 mmHg. The oxygen saturation remained low at 85% in spite of high-flow oxygen.

The lung scan showed multiple pulmonary emboli. Thrombolysis with i.v. streptokinase was started: 250 000 units over 30 min then 100 000 units hourly for 72 h. Her condition improved, with a fall in the pulse rate and an increase in the oxygen saturations.

A subsequent compression ultrasound showed an extensive right-sided proximal DVT.

**CASE STUDIES 7.2** (continued)

## CASE 2

A 64-year-old woman was admitted with a 5-day history of severe progressive breathlessness and exertional faintness. Two years earlier, extensive investigations for unexplained breathlessness concluded that the diagnosis was hyperventilation.

In her past history there had been extensive plastic surgery to the left calf. On admission she was obese, with bilateral ankle oedema. She was having episodic attacks of breathlessness and pain. Oxygen saturations were dropping to 70% on air. An urgent lung scan showed multiple pulmonary emboli. She was treated with i.v. heparin and then streptokinase, but remained very ill. Combined pulmonary angiogram and venogram showed multiple emboli originating from a left iliac vein thrombosis. A permanent inferior vena caval filter was inserted by the radiologist, to lie in the vena cava just below the renal veins. This prevented further emboli and she slowly recovered.

At review a year later, she remained well, with much improved exercise tolerance and significant weight loss. She was on life-long warfarin.

**CASE STUDY 7.3** Moderate pulmonary emboli

A 67-year-old woman was admitted to hospital with a 1-week history of breathlessness on minimal exertion and 2 days of left-sided pleurisy. She had been immobile for a month with back pain and for 2 days the left leg had been swollen. She had been on tamoxifen for 4 years after a mastectomy for breast cancer, and was an insulin-dependent diabetic.

The lung scan showed multiple emboli; she was given tinzaparin, but because of increasing breathlessness she was also given rt-PA.

**Box 7.2 – Classical features of a pulmonary embolus**

- Pleuritic chest pain
- Breathlessness
- Respiratory rate > 20 breaths/min

There are two problems with the patient in Case Study 7.3 – the management of recalcitrant pulmonary emboli, but also the problem of assessing her swollen leg. The assessment of a painful calf in a patient with diabetes needs care, because the diagnostic possibilities include:

- cellulitis
- critical limb ischaemia
- DVT

**CASE STUDIES 7.4**   Two cases of acute pleurisy – embolus or infection?

## CASE 1

A 50-year-old man was admitted with a 48-h history of very severe right-sided pleurisy, breathlessness and haemoptysis. There was no history of calf pain and no other risk factors. He was sweaty but apyrexial, pulse 110 beats/min, respiratory rate 20 breaths/min, with shallow painful breathing. Oxygen saturation was 90% on air. He was in extreme pain and very anxious. His legs were normal and he was of a slim build. There was fresh haemoptysis. Chest film showed shadowing at the bases of both lungs. His white cell count was normal. He was given i.v. opiate analgesia, immediate oxygen and subcutaneous tinzaparin 12 000 units subcutaneously (175 units/kg). Urgent lung scans were arranged and were of high probability for pulmonary emboli.

## CASE 2

A 45-year-old overweight man was admitted with haemoptysis and severe right-sided pleurisy. He had a week's history of flu-like symptoms culminating in a wheezy sounding productive cough. For 48 h his sputum had been green but then became blood-stained and then brown. His legs had been normal and there were no risk factors apart from obesity. His pulse was 100 beats/min, temperature 38.5°C, saturations 97% on air. There was a brassy sounding painful cough and brown mucopurulent sputum. His calves were normal. Chest film was normal and the white cell count was elevated at 15 000 × 10⁹/L. He was started on antibiotics and analgesiscs (NSAIDs). A lung scan was requested as a precaution and was reported to be normal.

In cellulitis, there is a clear upper limit of demarcation to a swollen red limb. In critical ischaemia due to arterial ischaemia, the leg can be red and swollen, particularly if the patient has been sitting with the leg in a dependent position. Importantly, the limb will be cool, probably pulseless, and will lose its colour when it is elevated.

- Differentiating an acute chest infection with pleurisy from a pulmonary embolism can be difficult. Key symptoms are chest pain, breathlessness and syncope
- Pulmonary emboli can arise from silent DVT
- Oxygen saturations (on air) are commonly below 92% (but can be normal)
- For all pulmonary emboli, the 3-month mortality is 15%, but patients who do particularly badly are:
  — the elderly
  — those with COPD
  — those with congestive cardiac failure
  — those who have underlying malignancy

*Critical nursing tasks in acute pulmonary embolus*
**ABCDE: Immediate resuscitation.** If the patient has collapsed with a cardiac arrest, cardiopulmonary resuscitation is started without delay. A massive embolus can present with a cardiac arrest, typically in the form of electromechanical dissociation (an ECG rhythm trace, but no palpable pulse or blood pressure).

**Ensure adequate oxygenation.** A major embolus cuts off the circulation to the lung, so the patient becomes acutely cyanosed. Immediate high-flow oxygen with a tight-fitting mask and rebreathing bag is indicated to correct this. Intubation and ventilation may be needed in extreme cases.

**CRITICAL NURSING TASKS IN ACUTE PULMONARY EMBOLUS**

- **ABCDE: immediate resuscitation**
- **Ensure adequate oxygenation**
- **Provide an adequate circulation**

**Provide an adequate circulation.** There is an immediate decrease in cardiac output, due to interruption of the circulation by the clot. The blood pressure falls dramatically even though the heart may continue to beat strongly. To help the heart by maximising venous return, the patient must be kept flat with the legs raised. A persistently low blood pressure is an indication for i.v. fluids. *However*, it is unwise to give, say, more than 500 ml of isotonic saline, as the right side of the heart is already under strain and may not cope with a large volume load.

If these measures do not restore the blood pressure, then inotropic support is needed: the options are noradrenaline, dopamine, dobutamine and adrenaline. Drugs such as GTN or frusemide are contraindicated, as they will reduce an already dangerously low blood pressure.

*Important nursing tasks in acute pulmonary embolus*
**Relieve the patient's symptoms.** Chest pain, breathlessness and severe anxiety, the dominant symptoms in a major pulmonary embolus, respond to i.v. opiates: morphine or diamorphine. These patients are often terrified by the sudden onset and will need constant reassurance. Unlike acute left ventricular failure (which in other respects gives a very similar picture to a major pulmonary embolus), the patient's breathlessness is not relieved by sitting up – these patients are most comfortable lying flat.

**Assess the response to treatment.** While resuscitation continues, the pulse, blood pressure and oxygen saturation need to be measured every few

> ### IMPORTANT NURSING TASKS IN ACUTE PULMONARY EMBOLUS
>
> ■ Relieve the patient's symptoms
> ■ Assess the response to treatment
> ■ Anticipate the need for urgent heparin therapy or thrombolysis
> ■ Prepare the patient for further procedures

minutes. Persistent hypotension and tachycardia, in spite of efforts to restore the circulation, suggest that the clot has not shifted and that it continues to obstruct the circulation to the lung. Repeated urgent blood gas measurements will be needed during the initial phase.

**Anticipate the need for urgent heparin therapy or thrombolysis.** If the initial management is successful and the patient's condition stabilises, heparin is used to prevent further, and possibly fatal, emboli. The choice lies between i.v. heparin as an initial bolus, then infusion – and subcutaneous low-molecular-weight heparin. Heparin prevents further clotting and allows the body's natural enzymes to disperse existing clot. In the patient who remains hypotensive and ill, the thrombolytic, rt-PA, can be used to help break up the emboli more rapidly. The recommended treatment is a 50-mg bolus of i.v. alteplase.

**Prepare the patient for further procedures.** Further tests may be needed to confirm the diagnosis, usually a CTPA or an isotope lung scan in medical physics or, less commonly, a pulmonary angiogram. A pulmonary angiogram is primarily diagnostic, but it can help the patient directly if the catheter is used to dislodge the clot or to put thrombolytic drugs such as rt-PA into the pulmonary vessels where the embolus is lodged.

If, in spite of adequate anticoagulation, there are recurrent emboli arising from residual clot in the deep veins, filter devices can be placed in the inferior vena cava. These are effective in preventing further emboli and are usually well tolerated.

*NB*: Prompt heparinisation and subsequent warfarin therapy for 3–6 months reduce the risk of recurrent thromboembolic events and fatal pulmonary emboli by 90%.

### ANSWERING RELATIVES' QUESTIONS IN PULMONARY EMBOLI

*Why did the patient collapse?* A blood clot became dislodged from a thrombosis in the leg and travelled to the lungs, where it became trapped, preventing blood from leaving the heart and reaching the lungs. In effect, circulation of the blood stopped at that point.

*What are the risks from a pulmonary embolus?* The risks of death in a pulmonary embolus are about 5% (reduced from 30% by treatment).

*Is it the clot that is being coughed up?* No. The blood-stained sputum is from lung tissue that has been starved of oxygen because the clot has cut off its blood supply.

*What happens to the clot?* It will break up and dissolve through the body's natural anticoagulants, helped by the treatment he is receiving from us. Warfarin and heparin prevent the clot spreading, whereas streptokinase or rt-PA actually melt any clot away.

*What are the risks of further emboli now that the patient is on heparin?* They are very low indeed (although not reduced to zero). The heparin will be followed by a variable time on warfarin tablets to reduce the risk even further.

# NURSING THE PATIENT WITH A SUSPECTED DVT

The history and examination are unreliable in the diagnosis of venous thrombosis. Seventy percent of the patients who are initially thought to have a DVT will prove to have an alternative diagnosis. Conversely, patients can present with a major pulmonary embolus that has arisen from a completely silent DVT.

There is a high cost for missing a proximal DVT: a 50% chance of a further episode and a 10% chance of a fatal PE within 3 months. The emphasis is therefore on using the combination of key clinical features and further investigations to ensure that the number missed is kept to a minimum.

### Nursing assessment of a possible DVT
**Risk factors from the patient's history.** The major risk factors are:

- lower limb immobility
- major surgery within 4 weeks
- more than two first-degree relatives with a history of DVTs
- active cancer within the previous 6 months
- recently bedridden for more than 3 days

*Lower limb immobility.* After a stroke, a paralysed lower limb often develops chronic ankle oedema, so the diagnosis of a DVT can be difficult, particularly if there is a problem with communication. The risks are similar if a limb is immobilised in a plaster cast.

*Surgery within 4 weeks.* Venous thrombosis is especially common after hip and knee replacements and can occur 4–6 weeks after surgery. Diagnosis can be difficult because of swelling and discomfort due to the surgery itself, but investigations need to be pursued, because 20% of patients undergoing a major lower limb joint replacement will develop a DVT despite prophylactic subcutaneous heparin in the immediate postoperative period.

*Cancer.* Active malignant disease within the previous 6 months increases the risk of DVT. Malignancy, particularly in the lung, prostate and pancreas, can also present as unexplained, often recurrent, venous thrombosis.

*Positive family history.* There is increasing recognition of the importance of a positive history of venous thromboembolic disease in first-degree relatives. The inherited thrombophilias are passed on to half of the offspring, as they are all inherited as autosomal dominant characteristics.

**Other important features in the history**
*Previous DVT/PE.* A previous thromboembolic episode is a major risk factor. The recurrence rate at 5 years is 25%; it is particularly high if there are residual associated risk factors such as malignant disease or immobility.

*Obesity.* Obesity is an important risk factor for both DVT and cellulitis. Commonly, obese middle-aged and elderly medical patients have chronically swollen and oedematous ankles, with areas of pigmentation, old healed varicose ulceration and discrete cellulitic looking areas. These legs can be difficult to assess, in particular to differentiate between acute and long-standing changes.

*Smoking and hypertension.* Heavy smoking and hypertension both increase the risk of thromboembolic disease, particularly in middle-aged overweight females.

**Examination of the legs.** There are three important signs of venous thrombosis in the legs (→ Fig. 7.2):

- local tenderness of the calf or thigh
- swelling of the calf and thigh
- unilateral calf swelling (> 3 cm at 10 cm below the tibial tuberosity)

Three additional signs may be present:

- ankle oedema
- unilateral dilated veins
- calf redness

There is increasing interest in using procedures that combine the results of clinical assessment in the form of a scoring system with the result of a screening test procedure such as the D-dimer tests to determine the next step: immediate discharge, immediate anticoagulation, or further investigation with lung scan, venogram or ultrasound (→ Box 7.3, Fig. 7.3).

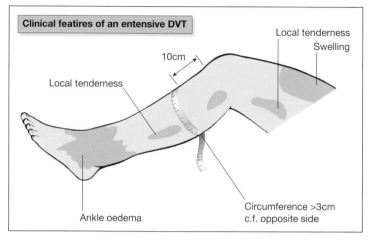

**Fig. 7.2** Clinical features of an extensive DVT

| Box 7.3 – Scoring of the probability of a DVT from clinical features* | |
|---|---|
| **Clinical feature** | **Score** |
| Active cancer (within the previous 6 months) | 1 |
| Paralysis or plaster cast | 1 |
| Bedrest for more than 3 days or major surgery within 1 month | 1 |
| Localised tenderness along the deep veins | 1 |
| Whole leg swollen | 1 |
| Unilateral calf swelling of more than 3 cm | 1 |
| Unilateral pitting oedema | 1 |
| Distended superficial veins | 1 |
| More likely alternative diagnosis | −2 |

| High probability | = 3 or more |
|---|---|
| Moderate probability | = 1 or 2 |
| Low probability | = −2 |

* with permission from Wells et al. Lancet 1997; 350: 1795–1798.

*Other causes of acute calf pain (→ Fig. 7.4)*
**Pain arising from the knee joint.** Mechanical pain from the knee is
suggested by a sudden onset during twisting, turning or crouching. The joint
may be swollen, stiff and tender. The history is particularly important in
rupture of a Baker's cyst, as the signs in the leg can be identical to those
found in a DVT.

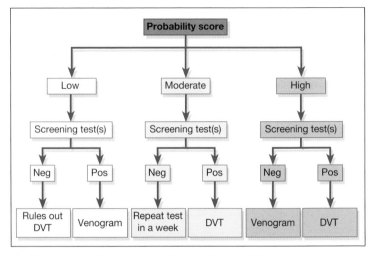

**Fig. 7.3** How probability scores can be utilised to diagnose a DVT

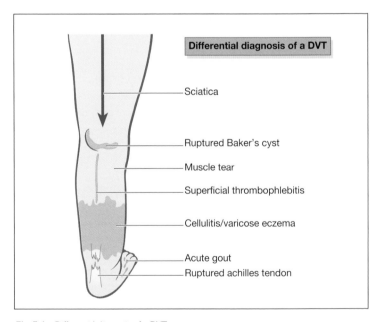

**Fig. 7.4** Differential diagnosis of a DVT

**Muscle tears, ruptured Achilles' tendon.** The history is all important. Torn muscle fibres usually occur during exertion and may be associated with local bruising around the heel and side of the feet. Patients on long-term oral steroids are prone to rupture of the Achilles' tendon, which may occur with surprisingly little effort – even using the stairs.

**Sciatica.** There is a clear relationship in the history to lifting or sudden straining, with the pain commonly radiating from the spine down the back of the leg. With the patient lying on his back, the pain can be triggered by lifting the affected leg straight up in the air.

*Other causes of a swollen painful leg*
**Acutely swollen red legs: illustrative cases** The following case studies illustrate possible diagnoses for acutely swollen red legs (→ Case Studies 7.5–7.7).

**DVT**

| CASE STUDY 7.5 DVT |
| --- |
| Three weeks after a routine right hip replacement, a 55-year-old woman was admitted with an increasingly swollen and painful right leg. There had been mild postoperative swelling, but this had spread from the calf to the thigh. On examination the leg was swollen, oedematous, shiny and warm to the touch, both above and below the knee. The surgical wound was clean and well healed.<br><br>    A diagnosis of iliofemoral thrombosis was made and the patient was started on tinzaparin 175 units/kg subcutaneously once daily. |

- The risk of a post-arthroplasty DVT persists for up to 6 weeks
- Half of the patients will have had a silent pulmonary embolus by the time the DVT presents

| CASE STUDY 7.6 Cellulitis |
| --- |
| An obese 75-year-old man gave a 10-day history of an increasingly painful and swollen right leg. Initially the foot was red and extremely tender, but 3 days before admission the redness spread to involve the whole of the lower leg. He felt ill and shivery.<br><br>    On examination, the pulse was 110 beats/min and temperature 38°C. The right calf and foot were hot, shiny, swollen and very tender. There was a deep purple/red discolouration of the lower leg, with a sudden line of demarcation 3 in (7.5 cm) below the knee. There were some tender red streaks at the back of the calf, spreading upwards towards the buttocks. There was no obvious skin wound, but the spaces between the toes were soggy and inflamed. A diagnosis of acute cellulitis was made, with a site of entry presumed to be the infected web spaces. Intravenous benzyl penicillin 1.2 g i.v. qds and flucloxacillin 1 g i.v. qds were started and the leg was elevated and rested. The web spaces were treated with antifungal agents. Prophylactic tinzaparin 3500 units daily was given in view of the risks of a subsequent DVT. |

**Cellulitis**

Major risk factors for cellulitis are:

- chronic lymphoedema of the leg (chronic brawny non-pitting oedema)
- an obvious portal of entry such as a skin wound
- obesity
- previous leg ulcer

**Necrotising fasciitis.**

*NB*: If the pain from a 'cellulitic' leg is extreme, worsening and seemingly out of proportion to the changes in the leg, it is important to consider the possibility of necrotising fasciitis, a deep, rapidly spreading soft tissue infection.

The main features of necrotising fasciitis are:

- extreme pain and localised numbness
- skin blisters and bullae
- necrotic skin
- hypotension
- WCC $> 15.4 \times 10^9$/L and sodium $< 135$ mmol/L
- history of i.v. drug abuse

Necrotising fasciitis requires urgent surgical assessment with a view to extensive debridement, if the patient is to survive.

---

**CASE STUDY 7.7**   Varicose (gravitational) eczema

An 80-year-old man was admitted with bilateral, red, swollen legs and immobility. His legs had been troubling him for years: he had chronic varicose veins, a previous leg ulcer that had eventually healed, and intermittent ankle swelling. His main complaint was of skin irritation and itch from the legs. He also noticed that both legs would 'break out' and discharge fluid.

On examination, he looked well and was apyrexial. The lower legs were very discoloured by brown pigmentation surrounded by red and inflamed areas. The skin was crusty and flaking and covered in scratch marks up to the knees. There were also multiple small raised blisters, some of which were discharging fluid. The white cell count and blood cultures were negative.

A diagnosis of acute varicose eczema rather than cellulitis was made and after dermatological advice, the legs were cleaned with twice daily 1:10 000 potassium permanganate astringent solution and started on high-potency local steroid cream to the skin.

---

**Varicose eczema.** Cellulitis can be confused with varicose eczema:

- in both conditions the legs are red and inflamed
- crusting and scaling are seen only in varicose eczema
- the skin is shiny and smooth in cellulitis
- if there is doubt, start i.v. antibiotics and seek dermatological help

## MANAGEMENT OF A DVT

*AIM: To prevent extension of the thrombosis and prevent embolisation*

- Identify risk factors before starting therapy
- Baseline FBC, prothrombin time, biochemistry, liver function tests, *consider thrombophilia screen*
- Obtain an accurate weight to determine the dose of low-molecular-weight heparin
- Identify any possible contraindications to anticoagulation therapy
- If thromboembolism is suspected and there is no contraindication:
  — give immediate subcutaneous low-molecular-weight heparin 150–200 units/kg, depending on the heparin preparation
- Confirm the diagnosis (lung scan, compression ultrasound, D-dimers, etc.)
- Give 10 mg oral warfarin loading dose on the same day that the heparin is started
- Subsequent warfarin doses can be predicted using the standard flexible induction dose regimen, which should be available on the ward
- Raise the leg and, in extensive thrombosis, apply class II elastic stockings
- If there is extensive swelling: immobilise for 48 h to allow swelling to reduce, then mobilise in stockings
- Watch for ischaemia
  — loss of sensation
  — pain
  — seek urgent medical assessment if ischaemia is suspected in a swollen leg
- When resting: in bed with leg elevated, *not* down
- Discharge with class II thigh-length hosiery and sleep with foot of bed raised
- Daily walks
- Encourage weight loss
- There is a 6% risk of venous ulceration and chronic disability

Box 7.4 summarises the key points in mobilisation of a DVT in the first 24 h.

---

**Box 7.4 – Bedrest or mobilisation in the first 24 h?**

- Elevate and rest a tense swollen leg due to iliofemoral thrombosis
- Do not elevate a leg that may be ischaemic (be wary in the diabetic patient)
- Rest a leg affected by acute cellulitis
- Mobilise an uncomplicated DVT within the limits of patient comfort
- Do not allow any patient with a swollen leg to sit with the legs dependent. If the leg is elevated or subjected to pressure dressings, watch for ischaemia
  — increasing pain
  — increasing discolouration or pallor of the feet
  — numbness, loss of sensation
  — loss or absence of the pulses

### Anticoagulation therapy

**Intravenous heparin.** Heparin increases the effect of the naturally occurring anticoagulant called antithrombin. There is a wide variation in the response to i.v. heparin, so that the treatment needs careful monitoring, using the APPT in order to individualise the dose. Inadequate initial therapy is associated with a much worse outcome. The aim is to anticoagulate to 1.5–2.5 times the control APPT. Intravenous heparin is continued for at least 4 days and should overlap with warfarin treatment until the INR is in the therapeutic range of 2.0–3.0 for at least 2 days.

Many audits have shown a tendency to undertreat patients with heparin, particularly in the first critical 24 h; this problem can be minimised by the use of a heparin protocol.

**Subcutaneous low-molecular-weight heparin.** Low-molecular-weight heparin has replaced the heparin infusion on most medical units, because it is as effective in treating both DVT and pulmonary embolus. Its simplicity raises the prospect of outpatient treatment.

In contrast to conventional heparin, low-molecular-weight heparin:

- can be given once daily
- has a consistent action in every patient that is determined solely by the patient's weight
- can be given as a fixed-dose subcutaneous injection
- does not require laboratory monitoring

Low-molecular-weight heparin is given for at least 5 days while warfarin is introduced, until the INR is within the therapeutic range (2.5–3.0) for 2 consecutive days.

**Doses (using tinzaparin as an example)**

*Prophylaxis*
**Low-risk surgery.** 3500 units of tinzaparin 2 h pre-op and once daily for 7 days post-op.

**High-risk surgery/high-risk medical condition, e.g. severe DKA.** 50 units/kg 12 h pre-op and once daily for 7 days

*Treatment of thromboembolic event.* 175 units/kg of tinzaparin once daily.

- Weigh the patient
  — 100 kg = 18 000 units per day
  — 80 kg = 14 000 units per day
  — 55 kg = 10 000 units per day

The doses of subcutaneous low-molecular-weight heparins are presented in Table 7.2.

**Warfarin therapy.** Warfarin interferes with vitamin K metabolism and ensures that the naturally occurring clotting factors are manufactured by the

| Table 7.2 Doses of subcutaneous low-molecular weight heparins | | | |
|---|---|---|---|
| *Heparin* | *DVT therapy* | *PE* | *Unstable angina* |
| Enoxaparin | 150 U/kg daily | Unlicensed | 100 U/kg bd |
| Tinzaparin | 175 U/kg daily | 175 U/kg daily | Unlicensed |
| Dalteparin | 200 U/kg daily | Unlicensed | 120 U/kg bd |

liver in an inactive form. Warfarin prolongs the prothrombin time and is monitored by using the INR, a standardised form of the prothrombin time that should be kept in the range of 2.0–3.0, with a target of 2.5 unless there are exceptional circumstances such as recurrent thromboembolic events despite warfarin treatment. Daily INR measurements are necessary in the initial stages of anticoagulation, and the adjusted warfarin dose must be given at the same time each day.

**Over-anticoagulation.** The most common causes for over-anticoagulation are:

- drug interactions
- errors with warfarin therapy
- the development of cardiac failure
- deterioration in liver function

Many drugs increase the effect of warfarin; those most commonly implicated are broad-spectrum antibiotics. Progressive cardiac failure, particularly in the elderly, is often associated with a sudden deterioration in anticoagulant control – INR values of 10 or more are not uncommon. Liver disease itself prolongs the prothrombin time, so clearly its development would have a major effect on the patient who is also taking warfarin.

Once the INR increases above 5.0 there is a risk of bleeding. However, provided that there is no major blood loss, INR values in the range 4–8 can be managed by discontinuing warfarin treatment until the INR falls. If the INR is greater than 8, warfarin should be stopped and if there are additional risks for bleeding (e.g. over 70 years old, previous bleeding, nose bleeds) a small dose (0.5–2.5 mg *orally* of the i.v. preparation) of vitamin K should be given. This will partially reverse the effects of the warfarin.

In the presence of major bleeding, the warfarin is stopped and its effect completely reversed with vitamin K 5 mg by slow i.v. injection. In addition, either FFP 15 ml/kg or, if it is available, prothrombin complex concentrate 50 units/kg, is administered to restore the clotting factors. *FFP is the main source of serious transfusion reactions and should only be considered when there is active and serious bleeding.*

Excessive bleeding on heparin usually responds to stopping the heparin and, if necessary, transfusion. Intravenous protamine sulphate will neutralise heparin at a dose of 1 mg per 100 units given slowly over 10 min, but it only partially reverses low-molecular-weight heparin and no more than 40 mg should be given at any one injection. Treatment can be repeated hourly. FFP is not indicated for heparin overdosage.

*Critical nursing tasks in a suspected DVT*
**In a suspected thromboembolic event, give the first dose of heparin immediately.** Once investigations are under way, the patient may be off the ward for some time during the critical first few hours. The safest course of action is, in the absence of an obvious contraindication, to give the first dose of subcutaneous heparin as soon as the initial assessment is completed.

**CRITICAL NURSING TASKS IN SUSPECTED DVT**

- **Give the first dose of heparin immediately**
- **Ensure there is adequate pain relief**
- **Be vigilant for acute ischaemia**

**Ensure there is adequate pain relief.** A severely swollen leg will cause intense pain. Non-steroidal anti-inflammatory drugs and aspirin are unsafe once warfarin has been started, and paracetamol may not be adequate. Oral dihydrocodeine or tramadol may be sufficient, but in extreme pain subcutaneous morphine 10 mg 2–4-hourly may be needed.

**Be vigilant for acute ischaemia.** Any acutely oedematous leg is at risk from ischaemia as a result of increased soft tissue pressure compromising the circulation to the legs. *Persistent or increasing pain* is the main warning feature, but there may simply be colour change or a loss of feeling in the leg.

*Important nursing tasks in a suspected DVT*
**Care of pressure areas.** The heels and sides of the feet are particularly vulnerable in cases of acutely swollen legs. Inspect these areas regularly, use pressure-relieving strategies, and encourage early mobilisation. Oedematous legs are prone to superficial skin infections, particularly if pre-existing foot hygiene is poor.

**Reassure the patient.** The prospect of a clot breaking off and travelling to the lungs terrifies most patients. They will want to know about mobilisation (to be encouraged once any severe swelling has resolved), about what exactly happens to the clot in the leg and when the swelling will disappear.

**Document all current regular and intermittent medication.** Potential drug interactions will become important once anticoagulation is established.

## IMPORTANT NURSING TASKS IN A SUSPECTED DVT

- **Care of the pressure areas**
- **Reassure the patient**
- **Document all current regular and intermittent medication**
- **Document the target INR (usually 2.5)**
- **Ensure a warfarin loading schedule is followed by the prescribing doctors**

**Document the target INR (usually 2.5).** It is important to oversee the anticoagulant therapy, particularly as the patient may be on and off the ward in the first 24 h having tests, and there may be a delay, with associated uncertainty, before all the tests come back to the ward. This can lead to a delay in anticoagulation or failures in communication among the staff.

**Ensure a warfarin loading schedule is followed by the prescribing doctors.** Table 7.3 details the warfarin loading schedule, depending on INR.

| Table 7.3 Warfarin loading | | |
|---|---|---|
| Day | INR | Warfarin |
| 1 | <1.4 | 10 mg |
| 2 | <1.8 | 10 mg |
| | 1.8 | 1.0 mg |
| | >1.8 | 0.5 mg |

## ANSWERING RELATIVES' QUESTIONS IN DVT

*Why did the thrombosis occur?* There are three reasons that may be important: stagnation of the blood in the leg veins, damage to the walls of the veins that may have triggered it off, and an abnormality in the blood itself that can make it more liable to clot.

*Is it because of the family history?* It is increasingly recognised that, in many patients (especially those with recurrent episodes or unexplained DVT in young people), there is an inherited tendency that could also be present in close family members. Sometimes it becomes necessary to screen family members, because some of these abnormalities can be passed on.

*Was it the result of bad postoperative nursing?* Even with preventative measures (low-molecular-weight heparin, etc.), there remains a significant risk after any surgery, particularly complex surgery and major joint replacements.

*Does the warfarin continue for life?* It depends on the circumstances; for example, if a second DVT is treated with warfarin for 6 months the recurrence rate is 20%, compared with 2% if the warfarin is continued for life.

| Table 7.4 Risk of a thromboembolic event among pill-users | |
| --- | --- |
| | *Rate per 100 000 women per year* |
| Normal non-pregnant | 5 |
| 2nd generation combined pill | 15 |
| 3rd generation combined pill | 25 |
| Pregnant | 60 |

### EXCELLENT CARE FOR THROMBOEMBOLIC DISEASE

- Staff awareness of the critical issues in thromboembolic disease
  - difficulties in diagnosis
  - the importance of immediate treatment
  - preventable mortality and morbidity
  - immediate access to investigation results (e.g. lung scan)
- Staff training in cardiopulmonary resuscitation
- Guidelines for suspected DVT
  - documentation of risk factors
  - use of a clinical scoring system
  - immediate treatment in suspected DVT
- Access to screening tests: simpliRED/ultrasound/lung scanning
- Anticoagulation guidelines
  - the use of low-molecular-weight heparin
  - warfarin guidelines
  - a system for writing up anticoagulation prescriptions
  - managing over-anticoagulation
- Patient information
  - anticoagulation handbook
  - information leaflets
- Clinical audit
  - initial documentation
  - delay to first dose of heparin
  - event monitoring (e.g. sudden collapse from unrecognised PE)

*What about the pill, pregnancy and HRT?*  The risk is increased in all three situations, but particularly in pregnancy. Even so, the overall figures are still low in absolute terms: of 100 000 women on a third-generation pill for a year, only 25 will suffer a thromboembolic event (→ Table 7.4).

The risk of thromboembolism with HRT is lower than that with second-generation oral contraceptives.

*Will it happen again?*  Even with warfarin therapy, there is a risk of recurrence after it is stopped. The rate is around 20% over the following 5 years, but will be less if there was an obvious trigger such as a hip replacement.

*What are the risks of warfarin?*  Standard treatment with warfarin carries an annual risk of haemorrhage of 7% and of death of 0.2%.

*Why is the leg still so swollen – will it ever go down completely?*  Thrombosis damages the valves in the veins that are necessary for the efficient return of blood from the legs to the heart. The leg may remain swollen for some time, and sometimes it may never return to normal. The situation can be helped by regular exercise, the use of support stockings and avoiding sitting with dependent legs.

### FURTHER READING

Donnelly R, Hinwood D, London NJM 2000 ABC of arterial and venous disease: non-invasive methods of arterial and venous assessment. British Medical Journal 320: 698–701
Pout G, Wimperis J, Dilks G 1999 Nurse-led outpatient treatment of deep vein thrombosis. Nursing Standard 13 (19): 39–41

### WEBSITES

BTS Guidelines for the management of Pulmonary Embolus:
    http://www.brit-thoracic.org.uk/docs/PulmonaryEmbolismJUN03.pdf
The diagnosis, investigation, and management of deep vein thrombosis:
http://bmj.bmjjournals.com/cgi/content/full/326/7400/1180

# CHAPTER 8

# DELIBERATE
# SELF-HARM,
# ALCOHOL AND
# SUBSTANCE ABUSE

# DELIBERATE SELF-HARM

## GENERAL PRINCIPLES

Each day an acute admitting ward in an average-sized district general hospital will take in two to three patients with deliberate self-harm. The pressures on medical and nursing time, combined with the problems of finding sufficient beds, often mean that this group of patients is granted a low priority. Although mortality rates are very low, most patients will be discharged without an adequate psychosocial assessment and without any follow-up. This is not acceptable:

- This is a vulnerable population
- Self-harm is invariably associated with considerable emotional distress
- With correct management, the long- and short-term outcomes can be improved
- The contribution of personal culpability for an illness does not influence the management in other areas of health – alcoholic liver disease, lung cancer, chronic obstructive pulmonary disease, HIV – and should not in deliberate self-harm
- The problem is getting larger: the numbers admitted with deliberate self-harm have increased 50% in 10 years

### Principles of treatment
- Appropriate emergency management to ensure the safety of the patient
- Granting the same care, respect and privacy as any other patient
- Proper psychosocial assessment
- Identification of patients at risk from further self-harm
- Where possible, the patient should be given the choice of a male or female member of staff to assess them and provide the care

## WHO COMMITS SUICIDE?

There are 5000 suicides per year in England and Wales: 45% by violent methods, mainly jumping from heights, strangulation and drowning; and 35% by drug overdose, predominantly antidepressants and paracetamol. Interestingly, the rates in both sexes are falling throughout the age range. Numerous factors are said to contribute to this: higher employment rates, recent initiatives to counteract self-harm, and reduction in carbon monoxide levels in exhausts. There is still concern, however, over rates in young males, which, compared with two decades ago, are particularly high.

### Who is at a particularly high risk of suicide?
It is important to be aware of the vulnerable groups, because they will be encountered on the acute medical wards as a result of self-harm or because of their high rates of poor overall physical health.

- Recent acute psychiatric illness, particularly during the first week after discharge
- Schizophrenia, especially in patients who are poorly compliant or lost to follow-up
- History of drug and alcohol abuse
- Any patient who says that they are feeling suicidal, especially if accompanied by feelings of hopelessness
- Patients living in social isolation with no family support
- Several previous episodes of deliberate self-harm (25% of successful suicides have tried before within the past year)
- A single episode of deliberate self-harm carries 1 in 20 rate of suicide within 10 years

## WHICH TYPE OF PATIENTS ARE ADMITTED WITH DELIBERATE SELF-HARM?

The admission rate for deliberate self-harm is 300 per 100 000 of the population per year and is increasing, particularly among males aged 15–24 years.

- The average age is 30 years
- 40% will have taken a previous overdose
- 20% will take a further overdose within a year, particularly those
  — who have a history of alcohol and substance abuse
  — who discharge themselves before the initial assessment has been completed
  — who have had several previous episodes
- Social deprivation and social isolation are common
- Up to 10% will have a serious psychiatric disorder, commonly depression
- There is a strong link with a history of epilepsy, particularly in males
- There is often a history of early parental death or separation
- A quarter will have been in contact with the psychiatric services
- Common triggers are major domestic arguments or a recent separation

*The embarrassed and impulsive*

- The spur of the moment
- Often triggered by a row and alcohol
- Not necessarily a trivial amount, often paracetamol
- Low risk of recurrence or future suicide

*The serious attempt*

- A planned event
- Carried out alone and in secret
- No attempt to get help
- Suicide note
- Admits to the intended outcome
- Even 'trivial' overdoses may represent a determined attempt at suicide

*The recurrent attender*

- Severe personality disorder
- History of drug and alcohol abuse
- History of violence and criminal convictions
- High risk of eventual success

*The high-risk self-harm*

- Older
- Male
- Isolated
- Unemployed/retired
- Alcohol dependence
- Poor general health
- Violent method used
- Repeated attempts
- Suicide note

## WHY DO PATIENTS DELIBERATELY HARM THEMSELVES?

- **To gain temporary respite** – 'I just wanted to get some sleep/escape/to get away for a while'
- **As a cry for help** – 'I didn't know what to do next/where to go/who to turn to'
- **As a signal of distress** – 'Nobody listened/I just couldn't explain what was happening to me'
- **Communicating anger/eliciting guilt/influencing others**
  — 'I did it on the spur of the moment in front of them all'
  — 'This will show her/him what it's been like for me'
- **To end their lives** – 'There's no point in any of it any more'

**Two high-risk patients**
Case Studies 8.1 and 8.2 illustrate different types of self-harm cases.

---

**CASE STUDY 8.1** Overdose

A 40-year-old man was admitted with an overdose of one of the newer less toxic antidepressants.

He complained of feeling generally upset and lonely, but denied significant past illnesses. He was single and lived alone, visiting his father at weekends. He presented as an outwardly cheerful, middle-class articulate man who could not really account for the overdose. Nothing else was noted in the medical or nursing notes.

On subsequent very close questioning, he admitted to previous problems with depression and recalled having ECT in his 20s after a period when he thought he was going mad. He had been treated with antipsychotics at that time. There was a history of progressive social isolation, with only occasional visits away from his bedsit to visit his father.

> **CASE STUDY 8.2**   Violent self-harm
>
> A 75-year-old man with severe ischaemic heart disease, cardiac failure and persistent hypotension was admitted because of self-harm.
>
> He had become increasingly frustrated and angry with an unexplained pain in his lower abdomen, which had been thoroughly investigated. He was feeling low and had been sleeping badly. He went into the kitchen, took the scissors, and made multiple superficial incisions across his upper abdomen to 'relieve the blood congestion'. On admission, he was tearful and frustrated, but embarrassed to have caused so much trouble.

From Case Study 8.1 it is clear that:

- the history needed unearthing
- this patient had a long unrecognised history involving a major psychosis: probably schizophrenia

The man in Case Study 8.2 is at very high risk:

- elderly male
- violent method of self-harm
- features of depression
- failing physical health

In this age group, deliberate self-harm is commonly triggered by disability, social isolation, chronic pain and untreated depression. It is important to recognise symptoms of depression in the elderly:

- anorexia and weight loss
- constipation
- change in sleep
- pattern of mood swings, especially early morning depression
- physical and mental slowing
- suicidal ideas

Because the highest rates of suicide are seen in elderly men, it is generally routine to refer for psychiatric assessment any patient older than 65 years who is admitted with self-harm. Such an act, in the over-65s, signifies significant suicidal intent.

## NURSING THE PATIENT IN SELF-HARM

Acute Medical Assessment Units should have internet access to TOXBASE the UK data base of the National Poisons Information Service. This provides detailed description of the management of individual clinical problems.

*Critical nursing tasks in deliberate self-harm*
**Care of the unconscious patient: ABCDE**

- Is the airway patent and protected? Remove food and vomit from the mouth
- Place the patient head-down in the recovery position to prevent aspiration
- Assess the patient's breathing: measure the respiratory rate

## CRITICAL NURSING TASKS IN SELF-HARM

- **Institute the care of the unconscious patient: ABCDE**
- **Take appropriate blood tests**
- **Consider gut decontamination**

- Document the pulse and blood pressure
- Measure and correct oxygen saturation
- Is the patient hypothermic? This is common with barbiturates and phenothiazines. Use a space blanket to warm the patient
- Is the patient hypoglycaemic?
- Measure the GCS: if less than 8, the airway is at risk
- Expose the patient:
  — As with any unconscious patient, look assiduously for any evidence to suggest a head injury – bruising or bogginess over the scalp and bleeding from the nose or ears
  — Skin blisters are common after overdoses, especially over the fingers, knees, shoulders and hips. Extensive blistering may occur over areas on which the patient has been lying, e.g. lateral aspect of the feet. Bullae should not be punctured – de-roof them once they have burst, and cover with a non-adherent dressing
  — Look for and document any areas of swelling and bruising, particularly in areas exposed to pressure in unconscious patients: underlying tissue damage may lead to complications, for example muscle breakdown (rhabdomyolysis) leading to kidney failure and acute limb ischaemia. Muscle damage is common in overdoses of ecstasy, theophyllines and opiates. Paralysis of a limb (wrist or foot drop) can also occur and is caused by nerve palsies due to the local effects of pressure
  — Examine for signs of self-injury (wrists) and of substance abuse (needle tracks, abscesses)
- Site an i.v. cannula
- Place on an ECG monitor and arrange for a standard 12-lead ECG
- Monitor the oxygen saturations
- Consider a nasogastric tube if the patient is vomiting and may need activated charcoal

- Correct hypotension by nursing the patient head-down and infusing dextrose or saline
- Take blood for measurement of:
  — glucose
  — alcohol
  — paracetamol
  — aspirin
  — liver function tests
  — clotting profile, particularly INR
  — special levels, e.g. theophylline
- Urine – retain for toxicology screen:
  — opiates
  — cocaine
  — amphetamines
  — ecstasy
  — hallucinogens

Assuming, after the initial assessment, that the patient does not need to be transferred to the HDU, steps should be taken to decontaminate the gut.

**Decontamination of the gut**
*Gastric lavage.* Gastric lavage is no longer indicated as a routine in self-poisoning. Occasionally it is used:

- within the first hour of ingestion (particularly with iron tablets or lithium)
- if the airway is secure
- if a potentially life-threatening overdose has been taken

*Activated charcoal*
**Single dose.** A single oral dose of 50 g activated charcoal enhances the elimination of several drugs and is used when anything more than a trivial amount has been taken (accepting the unreliability of the history in this group of patients). It is most effective when given within an hour of the overdose.

It is most useful in:

1. paracetamol
2. tricyclics
3. aspirin
4. theophylline
5. phenytoin
6. carbamazepine
7. digoxin

It is of no value in poisoning with:

1. iron tablets
2. lithium
3. methanol
4. antifreeze

*Multiple doses.* MDAC: 50 g immediately and 50 g every 4 h are given for life-threatening poisoning with:

1. slow-release theophyllines
2. carbamazepine
3. digoxin
4. phenobarbitone

To avoid the risk of aspiration, the airway must be secure before charcoal is used; it may be necessary to administer MDAC via a nasogastric tube.

Repeated vomiting reduces the effectiveness of charcoal treatment, so antiemetics such as i.v. cyclizine 50 mg 4-hourly or i.v. ondansetron may be indicated.

*Experimental and new treatments.* Recent advances in the treatment of self-poisoning include a new antidote for methanol and antifreeze poisoning: 4-methylpyrazole. Whole-bowel irrigation with polyethylene glycol is used for serious overdoses of enteric-coated drugs, iron-containing compounds or sustained-release preparations.

### Important nursing tasks in deliberate self-harm
**Ensure that all the relevant information is available.** If the patient is unable to give a reliable history but there is a strong suspicion of self-harm:

- What is available to the patient?
  — the patient's usual medication, including insulin
  — other tablets and medications at home
  — illicit and recreational drugs
- Is there evidence of self-poisoning
  — empty bottles, blister packs, foil wrappers
  — has alcohol been involved?
- Is there a suicide note?

*Other information from the patient or relatives.* The key pieces of information needed in the patient's history are listed in Box 8.1.

*Confidentiality.* When dealing with the patient's family, the clinical need to know the nature and timing of the overdose must be balanced against the

---

**Box 8.1 – History**

The history must include:

- Mental state
- Past psychiatric history
- Previous self-harm
- Alcohol use
- An assessment of suicidal intent

> ## IMPORTANT NURSING TASKS IN SELF-HARM
>
> ■ **Ensure that all the relevant information is available**
> ■ **Provide a suitable and safe environment in which to recover consciousness**

patient's right to confidentiality. There may be sensitive matters that the patient would not want to disclose to a third party. Common issues in this area include extramarital relationships, serious difficulties at work, unwanted pregnancy and conflict over child custody.

*Relevant medical history*

- Heart disease (tricyclics trigger arrhythmias)
- Liver disease (increases the risk of liver damage with paracetamol)
- Alcohol abuse (liver damage and a marker for high suicidal intent)
- Chronic disability (increases the likelihood of significant depression)

*Psychosocial history*

- The sequence of events that triggered the overdose
- Psychiatric history, especially of depressive illness, drug abuse
- Domestic situation and family support:
  — marital status
  — who else lives in the home
  — names and ages of children and who is caring for them
  — recent bereavements, anniversaries of deaths
  — has the patient a social worker/community psychiatric nurse?
- Previous self-harm
- Are there any vulnerable children/possible abuse? This requires urgent attention
- Job and financial worries
- Alcohol or drug abuse
- Evidence of domestic violence – it is acceptable to ask directly about possible abuse by a partner
- Recent childbirth
- Is there still suicidal intent?

### Provide a suitable and safe environment in which to recover consciousness

- Physical safety is ensured from the use of the recovery position combined with appropriate monitoring of the consciousness level and the vital signs
- It is important to maintain a calm, competent and non-judgemental approach. You are dealing with a very vulnerable group with low self-esteem, high stress levels, guilt about 'wasting everybody's time' and perhaps just extreme embarrassment

- Respect the patient's privacy. Try to encourage medical staff on the Consultant's round to discuss the patient's personal details somewhere other than the foot of the bed
- Organise appropriate communication with the mental health liaison nurse or social services, who can provide effective help
- Listen to the patient. Try and understand why the patient took the overdose at that particular time and with what intent

Case Study 8.3 illustrates the importance of reacting appropriately to the results of nursing observations:

- the combination of carbamazepine and diazepam produced a prolonged period of sedation
- the patient's initial aggression overshadowed the later fall in the consciousness level
- the nursing observations were not acted on with sufficient urgency
- the falling GCS and the increasing respiratory rate should have alerted the doctors of the impending need for ventilation. These patients are better nursed on the HDU

Case Study 8.4 shows that assessment has to be performed with care, if necessary by conforming to a check-list of high-risk factors. However, a check-list cannot replace sympathetic listening. Furthermore, simply asking if

---

**CASE STUDY 8.3** Deliberate self-harm and progressive deterioration in conscious level

A 20-year-old man with financial problems lost his job and on an impulse, took 30 of his father's carbamazepine tablets (a total of 12 g), without any alcohol.

On arrival in AED at 01.30 h, he was agitated and very aggressive and refused oral charcoal. He was given 15 mg of rectal diazepam and admitted.

At 03.00 h his GCS was noted to be 3/15. He remained on the medical ward.

By 04.30 h he became aggressive again and was given a further dose of 10 mg diazepam.

He had improved by 09.30 h, but deteriorated again by 21.15 h the following evening:

- oxygen saturations 80%
- low $pO_2$ (8.0 kPa)
- pulse 120 beats/min

He was given high-flow oxygen and observed

By 05.00 h, his GCS had fallen to 7/15. Oxygen saturations were 86% on high-flow oxygen. His respiratory rate was 20 breaths/min.

Over the next 3 h, his GCS dropped to 6/15. His respiratory rate increased to 50 breaths/min and his pulse to 120 beats/min. He was deemed unable to protect his airway and transferred to ITU for ventilation. X-ray showed an aspiration pneumonia.

After 4 days on a ventilator he made a full recovery.

> **CASE STUDY 8.4**   A previous concealed episode of deliberate self-harm
>
> A 49-year-old woman was admitted to hospital with a significant overdose of
> amitriptyline. She had left a suicide note to her son and had only been found at
> home by luck. She made a good recovery and did not appear depressed on the
> ward. However, on further questioning she admitted that, 2 weeks before
> admission, she had taken 30 nitrazepam tablets but had not told anyone about
> it and her husband had not been aware of her depression.
>    She was considered at high suicidal risk and admitted as an informal patient
> for further psychiatric assessment.

the patient 'feels suicidal' is often enough to identify risk. When time is at a
premium, there are *two key questions* that are known to be an accurate
prediction of genuine depression:

During the past month, have you often been bothered by:

1. Feeling down/depressed or hopeless?
2. Having little interest or pleasure in doing things?

## THE PATIENT WHO REFUSES TREATMENT

This is one of the most difficult areas of clinical practice, even for the most
experienced medical and nursing staff. There are a number of common
scenarios:

- a patient is admitted from casualty, but refuses to stay on the ward
- a recovering patient refuses to wait to see a psychiatrist
- a patient absconds from the ward
- a patient is intoxicated and abusive and refuses to cooperate
- a patient is cooperative, but will not see a psychiatrist
- a patient refuses specific medical treatment for the overdose
- a patient with acute alcohol withdrawal discharges himself

In all such cases, a balance must be struck between *the duty of care* that we
owe to our patients, and *a respect for their autonomy*, which is based on their
competence *at the time* to make a decision.
   Within the decision-making process, there are two components to this
competency:

- understanding and retaining the details of proposed treatment – its
  benefits, its risks and the consequences of turning it down
- having the ability to weigh up the alternatives in coming to a decision

It is important to understand that it is the *ability of the patient to participate in
the decision-making process*, and *not* the *quality* of the decision, that is
important. A competent patient can refuse treatment even if the decision

seems irrational or abnormal or lacking common sense and perhaps may even result in his death.

An assessment of competency (or '*capacity*', as it is termed legally) will, in difficult cases, require the expertise of senior medical staff, although it is clear that in most acute situations the combination of emotional distress and the effects of drugs or alcohol makes it fairly obvious when a patient is not competent to make such important decisions. The patient's capacity must be carefully documented in the records.

*If* the patient is not competent to make a decision about treatment *and* the treatment would 'save life and limb' (e.g. i.v. *N*-acetylcysteine [Parvolex] in severe paracetamol poisoning), then such measures can be given against the patient's wishes under what is termed, in England and Wales, *Common Law*.

The Mental Health Act can be used on medical wards to detain and, in some situations, treat a patient against his wishes. However, this would only apply in exceptional circumstances: the laws are complex, they rely on careful psychiatric assessment and the laws themselves vary within the UK. In England and Wales, Section 5(2) of the Mental Health Act can be invoked to detain a medical inpatient against their will for an emergency period of 72 h. Certain criteria must be met:

- The capacity to make a decision should be impaired because of a psychiatric disorder
- In the case of an overdose, the law allows life-saving treatment to be administered against the patient's wishes if the act of deliberate self-harm was itself a direct consequence of a psychiatric disorder
- The Mental Health Act can also be used to detain a patient *with a mental disorder* against his will if he is a danger to himself or to others

Using the Mental Health Act is not ideal: it takes time and organisation and, for an emergency Section on the medical ward, the consultant physician has to be there in person. By their nature, these acute problems arise at extremely unsocial hours – usually at 02.00 or 03.00 h.

The skill in dealing with such patients is to try and avoid the situation from arising by:

- avoiding confrontation
- maintaining a supportive and non-judgemental approach
- establishing a good relationship with the patient
- using persuasion and negotiation rather than coercion or bullying
- avoiding predictions of the time when a drip comes down/when a psychiatrist visits/of discharge
- within the confines of patient confidentiality, involving the relatives

In difficult situations, these principles should be followed:

- act reasonably and in the best interest of the patient
- involve senior nursing and medical staff at an early stage
- give the patient options should they change their mind

- document events and outcomes in detail
- use common sense

If a patient absconds or discharges themself, it is important to consider *who* needs to be informed and *when* would be the most appropriate time to do it:

- the next of kin
- the GP
- social services
- community psychiatric services
- the health visitor (if children are involved)
- the police
- the probation officer

Case Studies 8.5 and 8.6 illustrate the kinds of difficulties that may occur in cases of self-harm.

---

**CASE STUDY 8.5**  Substance abuse, deliberate self-harm and absconding

A 25-year-old known heroin user was admitted to hospital with an overdose of diazepam and slashed wrists, soon after leaving prison. He was described by the police as a violent man and had struck his wife because of suspicion that she had been unfaithful. On admission, he was conscious, but had slurred speech and was drowsy.

Soon after admission, in the middle of the night, he walked out of the ward taking his drip and drip stand with him, to stay with his friends near the hospital. The police were informed and persuaded him to return. By 03.00 h he was threatening to walk out again, saying that he was going to kill himself.

**What were the options?**

- **Let him go again**. He exhibited several high-risk features for suicide: substance abuse, male, etc.
- **Detain him under common law**. He is under the influence of the diazepam overdose and is probably not competent to make decisions. He is a danger to himself.
- **Section 5(2) of the Mental Health Act**. There is no mental illness immediately obvious.
- **Persuasion**. After a long talk with a senior doctor, he calmed down. It transpired he was virtually illiterate, was depressed about his hopeless employment prospects, and had been denied access to his children because of his behaviour. His marriage looked unlikely to survive the effect of his prison sentence. He was referred for some form of problem-solving based therapy.
- **Negotiation.** Typically for this type of situation, the problem of smoking on the ward became a major issue. Agreeing to let the patient find an acceptable place to smoke can defuse tension and also form the basis of negotiation to try and encourage the patient to stay on a voluntary basis.

> **CASE STUDY 8.6**   Detention under the Mental Health Act
>
> A 40-year-old man was admitted to hospital having taken a trivial amount of nitrazepam. He had cut his left arm (to 'let out the badness'). He was hearing voices that were telling him to kill himself, and he was demanding to leave hospital. He was pacing the room and wringing his hands in agitation, saying he just wanted to be left in peace to go home and die.
> He had previously had ECT and had been on various psychotropic drugs.
> In the early hours he continued in his efforts to leave the ward, and there were practical problems in obtaining psychiatric help. The security staff were called and the consultant physician came in. After evaluating the situation, the consultant signed Form 12 [Section 5(2)] which, after being received by the manager of the mental health services, detained the patient against his will for 72 h to allow a psychiatric assessment to be made. A mental health nurse was seconded to look after the patient until the morning, when he was transferred to the mental health unit.

## SPECIFIC OVERDOSES

Three type of drugs make up 85% of the overdoses: of these, paracetamol and antidepressants are particularly toxic.

| | |
|---|---|
| Paracetamol | 45% |
| Benzodiazepines | 20% |
| Antidepressants | 20% |

### BENZODIAZEPINES

Benzodiazepines, unless taken as part of a more toxic cocktail, depress the conscious level, but not sufficiently to put respiration at risk unless the patient also aspirates. Management is based on maintaining respiration and keeping a secure airway. The specific antagonist i.v. flumazenil reverses benzodiazepine coma immediately, but the drug has potential problems:

- the effects of a single dose soon wear off
- if tricyclic antidepressants may also have been taken, flumazenil is contraindicated: the surge in excitability associated with sudden benzodiazepine reversal may trigger a life-threatening tricyclic-induced cardiac arrhythmia
- the sudden reversal of benzodiazepine coma may trigger acute agitation – this will need careful management

### PARACETAMOL POISONING

Paracetamol poisoning is common and dangerous. There are 70 000 cases per year in the UK, and of these 200 will die due to liver damage – paracetamol remains the most common cause of acute liver failure.

**How does it cause liver damage?** Paracetamol is handled by the liver through two biochemical pathways. After a normal-sized dose, 90% is converted to harmless by-products, but 10% is converted by the p450 enzyme system to a highly active and toxic compound, NAPQI. NAPQI is deactivated in the body by glutathione.

In overdosage, the first pathway is swamped and large quantities of paracetamol are sent down the p450 route to produce NAPQI. Glutathione stores are eventually exhausted in mopping up excessive NAPQI. Once this happens, NAPQI starts to destroy the liver.

These simple biochemical pathways explain three important facts:

- Chronic alcoholics and malnourished patients have low glutathione levels and are therefore particularly susceptible to paracetamol toxicity
- N-*acetylcysteine (Parvolex)* and *methionine*, which replenish glutathione stores, will act as effective antidotes in paracetamol poisoning
- Drugs that increase p450 levels (anticonvulsant therapy, anti-TB treatment, St John's Wort) send more of the paracetamol down the 'toxic route' and increase the toxicity of paracetamol

**How much is a significant overdose?** For most patients *12 g* of paracetamol (24 tablets) or more than *150 mg per kg* body weight can produce severe liver damage.

- In susceptible patients – the malnourished (especially patients with HIV, cystic fibrosis and eating disorders) or alcoholics – half this amount can be dangerous
- Liver toxicity may occur even if the tablets are ingested over the course of several hours
- You cannot rely on the patient's story for the quantity or the timing of the overdose
- Patients will often have taken combination tablets (e.g. dextropropoxyphene and paracetamol) or a cocktail of drugs and alcohol that may each need treatment in their own right

*Clinical picture of severe paracetamol toxicity*
**0–24 h**

- Minimal immediate symptoms
- Mild nausea and vomiting within a few hours
- Liver function tests normal in the first 12 h, abnormal by 18 h

**24–48 h**

- Right upper abdominal pain with continued vomiting
- Liver tenderness
- Progressively deranged liver function tests (ALT and AST levels > 1000 IU/L indicate severe damage)
- Prolonged prothrombin time
- Loin pain, haematuria, proteinuria and deteriorating kidney function

**Days 3 and 4**

- Maximum liver damage on fourth day
- Jaundice
- Increasing confusion with grade 3/4 hepatic encephalopathy

*Immediate management*

- It is critical to establish the exact timing of the overdose. Focus on the history:
  — time tablets purchased
  — time tablets swallowed
  — time help arrived
  — could the overdose have been staggered over several hours?
- What else was taken? *Co-proxamol* (325 mg paracetamol and dextropropoxyphene) is frequently taken in self-poisoning. Dextropropoxyphene is an opioid and, especially when mixed with alcohol, can cause sudden and severe respiratory depression with coma, pinpoint pupils and cardiovascular collapse. Coma management and reversal of the drug's effect with naloxone is the immediate priority; patients may subsequently develop liver damage from the paracetamol
- Is this a susceptible patient?
  — eating disorder, HIV, cystic fibrosis or malnourished
  — chronic alcoholic
  — epileptic medication/anti-TB drugs
  — underweight (toxic dose [150 mg/kg] in a 50-kg patient is 15 tablets)
- Consider activated charcoal
  — overdose taken within an hour
  — methionine is not going to be used (charcoal inactivates methionine)
- Take blood for measurement of paracetamol levels (if overdose taken within an hour or so of admission, wait 4 h before testing, but if more than 24 tablets taken, still consider immediate antidote). Determine baseline LFTs and clotting, particularly if a substantial overdose or of uncertain timing
- Start *N*-acetylcysteine (Parvolex) treatment if indicated. Repeat LFTs and prothrombin time at the end of the infusion (20 h).

*Late presentation (8–24 h) or staggered ingestion over several hours*
The situation is urgent, because any delay progressively reduces the effectiveness of *N*-acetylcysteine (Parvolex) and patients who present late tend to have more serious overdoses. If more than 150 mg/kg or 12 g have been taken, it is safest to start treatment while awaiting the blood results. The following factors are considered:

1. history (toxic dose of > 150 mg/kg per day)
2. symptoms (abdominal pain and vomiting)
3. blood levels (of little value in staggered overdoses)

4. prothrombin time
5. liver function tests and creatinine
6. blood gases

The place of *N*-acetylcysteine (Parvolex) at times in excess of 24 h is uncertain, but it should be given if the prothrombin time, creatinine or liver enzymes are abnormal or if the blood gases show an acidosis.

**Who gets i.v. N-acetylcysteine (Parvolex) or methionine?** A single paracetamol blood level measured at 4 h or more after the overdose will predict who is at risk from liver damage. Blood levels from earlier than 4 h are of no value in assessing the risk of liver damage. The graph of the blood levels of paracetamol against time since the overdose is used to determine who needs the antidote (→ Fig. 8.1). The timing of the overdose is therefore critical to the management of the patient. Patients with a paracetamol value that falls above the 'normal treatment line' joining 200 mg/L at 4 h to 6.25 mg/L at 24 h have a 60% chance of serious liver damage that *N*-acetylcysteine (Parvolex) or methionine will completely prevent.

The second 'high-risk treatment line' on the graph joining lower levels is used in patients who are particularly susceptible because of malnourishment etc.

● The graphs only apply for tablets taken as a single dose: overdoses stretching over hours or days are difficult to evaluate using blood levels
● When in any doubt – *TREAT AND TREAT WITHOUT DELAY*!

*N*-acetylcysteine (Parvolex) and methionine are most effective if given within 12 h of the overdose, but Parvolex works up to 24 h and possibly longer. It is the treatment of choice on the Acute Medical Unit, but methionine is useful in particular situations:

● the patient refuses a drip
● the patient insists on leaving hospital, but would take methionine with him

*N-acetylcysteine (Parvolex).* The patient *must* be weighed, so that the correct dose can be given:

1. 150 mg/kg in 200 ml of 5% dextrose over 15 min
2. 50 mg/kg in 500 ml of 5% dextrose over 4 h
3. 100 mg/kg in 1000 ml of 5% dextrose over 16 h

*Double-check the correct dose of* N*-acetylcysteine (Parvolex) is drawn up: 1 ml contains 200 mg of Parvolex – 1 ampoule contains 2000 mg*

In cases of severe overdosage the infusion will be used beyond 24 h (at a rate of 150 mg/kg per 24 h) until the prothrombin time decreases to less than 20 s. If there is severe liver damage, the patient must be kept very well hydrated and broad-spectrum antibiotics such as i.v. cefuroxime are used.

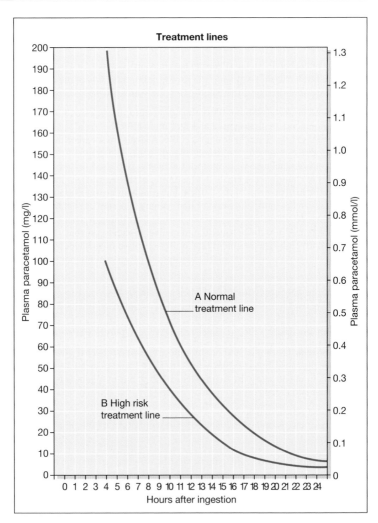

**Fig. 8.1** The use of plasma paracetamol levels in the decision to use N-acetylcysteine (Parvolex)

There is a 1 in 20 risk of a rash/wheeze/itching or some other generalised reaction within an hour of starting *N*-acetylcysteine (Parvolex). The infusion should be stopped for 60 min while the reaction settles before restarting at 50 mg/kg over 4 h. If the reaction is severe, i.v. antihistamines and hydrocortisone should be given.

**Oral methionine.** Methionine is an alternative to *N*-acetylcysteine (Parvolex) and is easier to give – the dose is 2.5 g immediately and 2.5 g every 4 h for three further doses. However:

- patients are frequently vomiting at the time it needs to be given
- it is only helpful within 10–12 h of the overdose
- it is inactivated by oral charcoal

**When to discharge.** Patients should be discharged only:

- after psychosocial assessment
- after completion of *N*-acetylcysteine (Parvolex), provided that the liver enzymes, creatinine and prothrombin time are normal
- *and* if there are no symptoms

There is a poor prognosis 24 h after the overdose if:

- prothrombin time is more than 24 s
- pH < 7.3
- creatinine is > 300 mmol/L

Clear instructions, as outlined in Box 8.2, should be given to the patient who discharges themself.

---

**Box 8.2 – Clear written instructions to patients who go home or self-discharge after paracetamol**

- Return if there is:
  — abdominal pain
  — persistent vomiting
  — confusion
- Consider oral methionine

---

## ANTIDEPRESSANT OVERDOSE

There are two important types of antidepressants used in deliberate self-harm:

- The older tricyclic antidepressants (e.g. dothiepin, amitriptyline, protriptyline)
  — these are dangerous and cause coma, convulsions and cardiac arrhythmias
  — dothiepin is the most dangerous, particularly as it is available in 75-mg tablet strength
- The new generation of antidepressants SSRIs
  — drugs like fluoxitine, while safer than tricyclics, can cause the 'serotonin syndrome' – acute confusion, fever, muscular rigidity and twitching

*Management*
The patients initially show features of atropine-like poisoning, with a dry mouth, blurred vision and dilated pupils. In severe toxicity, e.g. more than

750 mg of a tricyclic drug, the patient becomes increasingly drowsy over a period of 4 h or so. A dose of 2 g or more produces severe toxicity lasting several hours.

The tricyclic overdose provides the classical example of patients who 'were fine' in casualty but can deteriorate at a frightening rate when they reach the ward – often in the critical interval between the initial nursing assessment and the time when they are seen by the junior doctor.

The main dangers are:

- **Respiratory depression**. The GCS, respiratory rate and oxygen saturations should be monitored hourly in these patients, more often if they are showing any signs of toxicity. Blood gases are checked: tricyclic poisoning can cause a dangerous acidosis that needs correction with i.v. bicarbonate.
- **Cardiac arrhythmias**. Patients must be monitored and cared for near the nursing station. The first sign of trouble may be a cardiac arrest in ventricular fibrillation. A standard ECG recording may show warning signs of cardiac toxicity (the QRS complexes are slurred to more than the width of four small squares). Arrhythmias can be abolished with i.v. sodium bicarbonate which can be given prophylactically if there are warning ECG changes – conventional antiarrhythmic drugs can make the situation worse by depressing cardiac function.
- **Convulsions**. These are treated with intravenous diazepam or lorazepam.

Patients remain at risk for at least 12 h after admission and are prone to arrhythmias if they mobilise prematurely. Dothiepin, in particular, has been associated with a significant number of in-hospital deaths.

### Immediate management of tricyclic overdose
**Gastric lavage?** There is little point in lavage unless large amounts of the drug have been taken within the hour. Indeed, by pushing the tablets further down the gut, lavage may increase absorption.

**Single-dose activated charcoal.** A single dose of 50 g of activated charcoal reduces absorption if given within an hour of ingestion. If there are signs of significant drug toxicity, a further dose can be given at 2 h.

## CARBON MONOXIDE POISONING

### Basic mechanisms
Carbon monoxide is odourless, colourless and extremely dangerous. It binds to and poisons circulating haemoglobin, preventing it from taking up, or releasing, oxygen. As a consequence, patients suffer hypoxic damage to their heart and central nervous system.

The gas has two important sources:

- incomplete combustion of carboniferous domestic fuel (gas, coke, coal, wood) associated with faulty installations or accidental fires

- car exhaust fumes (catalytic converters reduce the content of carbon monoxide)

*Clinical picture*

**Acute exposure.** Headache, nausea and dizziness progress to collapse and loss of consciousness. In severe poisoning with coma, there may be skin blistering and pressure-induced muscle damage (rhabdomyolysis). The limbs are spastic and there may be acute heart damage, pulmonary oedema or increased intracranial pressure.

**Subacute exposure.** Slower onset of nausea, vomiting, headaches and drowsiness. The clinical picture can mimic flu or gastroenteritis – a source of confusion. As with gastroenteritis, a whole household can be affected if exposed to the same source.

*Assessment and management*

- ABCDE: care of the patient with an impaired conscious level:
  — airway management
  — assess cardiac function and monitor the heart rhythm
  — monitor oxygen saturations
  — monitor blood gases and venous blood for COHb levels. Severe toxicity is associated with COHb levels greater than 20% (heavy smokers reach levels of 8–10%)
- Give immediate high-concentration oxygen – 100% oxygen is indicated for significant toxicity. This will need a tightly fitting mask with an inflated face-seal (seek anaesthetic advice, as the standard re-breathing masks are inadequate)
- Consider *hyperbaric oxygen* (oxygen given in a specialist unit at 2.4 times normal atmospheric pressure), especially in cases of:
  — pregnancy
  — COHb more than 20%
  — signs of neurological dysfunction
- If this is accidental domestic exposure, the local environmental health department should be involved to assess the safety of the house

# ALCOHOL ABUSE

## PROBLEMS OF ALCOHOL ON THE ACUTE MEDICAL UNIT

Estimates suggest that around 20% of acute medical admissions are directly or indirectly the result of alcohol abuse (→ Fig. 8.2). Acute alcohol intoxication is potentially dangerous in terms of respiratory depression and aspiration, and must be managed carefully. It is equally important to recognise chronic alcohol dependence – those patients who, while they

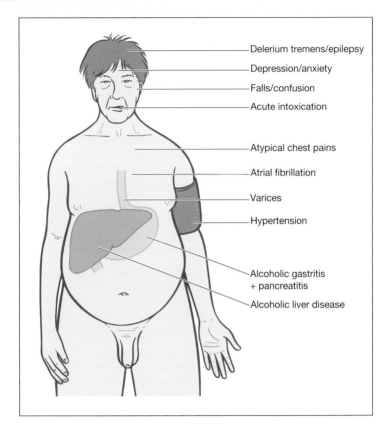

Delerium tremens/epilepsy

Depression/anxiety

Falls/confusion

Acute intoxication

Atypical chest pains

Atrial fibrillation

Varices

Hypertension

Alcoholic gastritis
+ pancreatitis

Alcoholic liver disease

**Fig. 8.2** The medical complications of alcohol abuse

would not necessarily concede to being 'alcoholic', have drinking patterns that cause repeated problems to themselves and others.

- Acute alcohol intoxication – common in young adults
- Alcohol as a component of deliberate self-harm – alcohol and paracetamol or antidepressants/benzodiazepines are commonly taken in combination. The risks are of respiratory depression and aspiration. The associated intoxication makes history-taking difficult and often results in a very uncooperative patient
- Alcohol dependence as a cause of deliberate self-harm – either in the patient or in his close family/partner
- Acute alcohol withdrawal syndromes – delirium tremens, anxiety states, fits, acute thiamine deficiency

- Alcohol-induced disease:
  - alcoholic gastritis
  - acute variceal bleeding
  - alcoholic liver disease
  - pancreatitis
- Other alcohol-associated medical conditions:
  - unexplained vomiting
  - atypical chest pain (often after binges)
  - binge-associated acute atrial fibrillation
  - hypertension
  - unexplained falls and confusion in the elderly
  - depression

### How to take a drinking history

Although patients with alcohol-related problems do not usually welcome detailed enquiries into their drinking habits, an acute drink-related crisis in their health or personal life is often followed by a period of reflection and self-examination. During this time the patient may accept for the first time that alcohol may be the root cause of his problem.

It is surprising how often the bland question *'Do you think you may have been burning the candle at both ends?'* leads to important disclosures and an initial acknowledgement of the critical issue.

It is important to establish the levels of consumption and of dependence.

**The amount and pattern of drinking**

1. How *often* do you drink (include 'stiffeners' added, particularly by the elderly, to tea and coffee)?
2. How *much* do you drink on a usual day (a unit is half a pint, a glass of wine or a single of spirits)? A regular consumption of more than 4 units a day puts the patient 'at risk'.
3. Have you had more than 5 units any day in the past month?
4. Have you had home, health or work problems in the last year due to drink?
5. Has anyone (including yourself) been harmed by your drinking?
6. Do you use alcohol to help solve your problems?
7. Has anyone suggested that you cut down?

**The level of dependence**

1. Do you have difficulty in controlling the amount that you drink once you start?
2. Do you have difficulty cutting down?
3. Do you have withdrawal symptoms (including early awakening and episodic anxiety)?
4. Are you drinking to avoid withdrawal symptoms?

These questions are distilled into a shortened form: the CAGE questionnaire. Two or more positive answers to the four questions suggests alcohol dependence.

- Have you felt you should **C**ut down?
- Have you been **A**nnoyed by criticism of your drinking?
- Have you felt **G**uilty about your drinking?
- Do you ever have an **E**ye-opener in the morning to steady your nerves?

CAGE can be used on the patient to confirm any suspicions of alcohol dependence raised from an initial drinking history. The nature of the questions, however, means that it is not good for identifying problems in young adults or in the elderly.

### Acute alcohol-withdrawal syndrome

Case Studies 8.7 highlight some features of acute alcohol-withdrawal syndrome.

- It is important to recognise the clinical features of alcohol withdrawal in any patient admitted to hospital ($\rightarrow$ Box 8.3). Timely sedation with benzodiazepines will prevent the onset of convulsions or progression to delirium tremens. The most effective regimen is to control the agitation, sweating and tremor with 'symptom-triggered dosing' using oral diazepam 10–20 mg every 2 h up to a maximum of 100 mg in 24 h. Antiemetics may also be required.
- Patients with an alcohol-withdrawal syndrome are often very apprehensive or frightened. They may be acutely disturbed and

---

**CASE STUDIES 8.7**  Acute alcohol-withdrawal syndrome

#### CASE 1

A 35-year-old man was admitted, having had a grand mal fit. He had discharged himself from AED a week before after a similar episode. He had been drinking cider heavily for 15 years, and since losing his father 6 months previously he had been drinking up to two bottles of vodka per day and had started antidepressants. He had recently had a normal endoscopy and colonoscopy for morning vomiting and episodic diarrhoea. On examination, he had severe shaking and sweating and was extremely agitated and anxious.

His liver enzymes were high and his alcohol levels were zero. His MCV was 103 $\mu m^3$. He was started on a regimen of chlordiazepoxide and high-dose parenteral vitamins. Within 36 h he was much improved, but insisted on discharging himself, with a promise that he would stop drinking 'through his own efforts'. He continued on a reducing regimen of chlordiazepoxide.

#### CASE 2

A 40-year-old man was admitted to hospital after a series of grand mal convulsions. He was a club steward on holiday in the area. While working, he would drink 'constantly' throughout the day and evening, but would always stop completely on holiday. He was treated with thiamine and a benzodiazepine withdrawal regimen, and made a full recovery.

---

**Box 8.3 – Symptoms of alcohol withdrawal**

- Tremor
- Sweating
- Apprehension
- Nausea and vomiting
- Weakness and syncope
- Insomnia
- Auditory and visual hallucinations
- Fitting
- Severe confusion

---

hallucinating. It is important to nurse them in a well-lit room and provide a calm, reassuring environment.

- Severe acute alcoholic agitation can be managed with i.v. diazepam 5–10 mg over 2 min. An infusion of chlormethiazole (Heminevrin) is the traditional treatment for acute withdrawal states, but it carries a risk of respiratory depression. When taken long-term, chlormethiazole can itself lead to dependence and has in general been replaced by the benzodiazepines.
- If the patient looks poorly nourished or is confused and unsteady on his feet, an acute Wernicke Korsakoff Syndrome (WKS) may be developing. WKS is a serious acute brain disturbance caused by thiamine deficiency and can be triggered in hospital by a carbohydrate load such as an infusion of dextrose. The clinical picture can be confused with that of acute intoxication, but the damage is permanent unless treated urgently with i.v. thiamine (in the form of high-dose vitamins B and C combination [Pabrinex]: two pairs of ampoules three times a day for 3–5 days, each pair infused in 100 ml of normal saline over 30 min).

*Acute alcohol intoxication*

- There is an increasing problem with young people binge-drinking out of doors, encouraged by the ready availability of 'designer drinks', including types of fortified wines and strong white ciders (→ Case Study 8.8)
- The main problems are hypoglycaemia, respiratory depression, airway protection and, in severe cases, fitting
- The units of measurement are confusing and can lead to misinterpretation:
  — UK driving limit      16 mmol/L (80 mg/100 ml)
  — Severe intoxication    76–98 mmol/L (350–450 mg/100 ml)
  — Potentially fatal      > 98 mmol/L (> 450 mg/100 ml)

The management is that of any metabolic coma, with a number of important exceptions:

- Alcoholics are prone to head injuries while intoxicated:
  — take a history from any witnesses

---

**CASE STUDY 8.8**   Acute alcohol intoxication

A 16-year-old boy was admitted with a GCS of 3 and an unrecordable blood sugar, having been found lying in an outdoor play area. He had been drinking white cider and vodka out of doors with his friends. He recovered uneventfully over a period of 12 h, with attention to his airway and correction of his blood sugar.

---

— observe carefully for signs of trauma (bruising behind the ears, boggy swelling, etc.)
— monitor the GCS – it is not appropriate to assume the patient will simply 'sleep it off'
— failure to recover fully after a head injury may indicate impending WKS
- A cocktail of drugs and alcohol may have been taken – a situation that is particularly dangerous in opiate abusers
- In severe intoxication, start i.v. dextrose 10% 250 ml. If i.v. dextrose is being used in a chronic alcohol abuser, combine it with thiamine to avoid triggering the WKS. The management of severe intoxication in the familiar 'hardened' drinker who is unkempt and malnourished (and often disruptive) should include at least one pair of thiamine and vitamin C (Pabrinex) ampoules daily for the first 3 days.

*Alcohol, dextropropoxyphene and opiates*
The combination of dextropropoxyphene-containing tablets such as co-proxamol with alcohol can, in overdosage, be a particularly potent cause of severe respiratory depression. A similar situation occurs with methadone and alcohol. The interactions are unpredictable and, because all these drugs induce vomiting, these patients are also at particular risk from aspiration. Intravenous naloxone reverses the depressed conscious level, but single doses wear off within a short time, so the conscious level needs to be monitored regularly.

# SUBSTANCE ABUSE

## ECSTASY

Ecstasy, or MDMA, has been a commonly used recreational drug for the past decade, particularly in the clubbing scene. Its amphetamine-like properties provide hyperstimulation, which, combined with the exertion of prolonged dancing, can result in:

- dehydration and electrolyte disturbance
- hyperarousal – agitation, tachycardia, hypertension
- muscle breakdown (rhabdomyolysis) and kidney failure
- hyperthermia up to 40°C
- convulsions
- acute liver failure
- severe acidosis

*Management*
Reassurance and adequate i.v. fluids are the main measures. Hyperthermia is managed by active cooling and with i.v. dantrolene 1 mg/kg repeated as needed, to a maximum of 10 mg/kg. Acute agitation and convulsions respond to benzodiazepines. Acidosis may need correction with sodium bicarbonate.

## LIQUID ECSTASY

Liquid ecstasy is the drug GBH. Case Study 8.9 illustrates abuse of this substance.

---

**CASE STUDY 8.9**   Liquid ecstasy

Two women aged 24 and 21 years who were at a night club each took four bottle-capfuls of a pink aniseed-flavoured liquid that they knew to be GBH. Within a few minutes they developed euphoria that progressed over an hour to drowsiness and coma. They were carried out by bouncers and the paramedics were called.
  On admission:

|  | Case one | Case two |
|---|---|---|
| GCS | EI VI MI | E2 V2 MI |
| Pulse | 30 | 42 |
| Blood pressure | Unrecordable | 70/40 |
| Respiratory rate | 6 | 8 |
| Pupils | Normal and reactive | Pinpoint |
| Treatment | Atropine | Atropine |
|  | Charcoal | Charcoal |

  The anaesthetists were called and oropharyngeal/nasopharyngeal airways were passed. Activated charcoal was administered down a nasogastric tube. Atropine 1 mg increased the pulse and blood pressures and both patients regained consciousness within 3–4 h. According to the women, the desired effect is usually generalised tingling and a floating euphoria. This was the first time they had not spread the doses over 3 or 4 hours.

## DYSTONIC REACTION AND PSYCHOTROPIC DRUGS

Case Study 8.10 describes abuse of psychotropic drugs. The picture is typical of the abnormal posture and muscle spasms that occur in acute dystonic reactions to a variety of psychotropic drugs, including haloperidol, and various antiemetics, including metoclopramide. Problems with substance abuse are widespread in the prison population.

---

**CASE STUDY 8.10** Dystonic reaction

A prisoner with a previous history of psychosis and i.v. amphetamine abuse found a packet of tablets in a copy of a novel in the prison library. He took them for a buzz. A few minutes after taking them, he developed what he thought was a fit, with intense spasm of his jaw and neck and arching of his back.

He was taken to casualty, and after an intramuscular injection of procyclidine 10 mg his symptoms improved rapidly.

---

## HEROIN ABUSE

Heroin abuse is an increasing problem, particularly among the young, and is associated with several major health-related and psychosocial problems (→ Case Study 8.11):

- HIV
- hepatitis C and B
- superficial and deep soft tissue sepsis
- venous thromboembolic disease
- opiate overdose (often combined with temazepam, alcohol and diazepam)
- social isolation
- crime

---

**CASE STUDY 8.11**

A 17-year-old single girl was admitted with acute asthma because her inhalers had run out. She had been smoking heroin for 2 years but in the last month her boyfriend, who was now in prison, had introduced her to intravenous heroin. She was using 1 g a day, which she funded by shoplifting. She had been thrown out by her mother and did not get on with her father. She wanted to sort out her life and her asthma.

---

*Methods of heroin ingestion*
*Chasing the dragon.* An increasingly popular way of taking heroin, 'chasers' are younger, show less dependence and are less involved in the heroin

culture than the more traditional i.v. user. Heroin is heated on tin foil and inhaled. Alternatively, it is smoked as a cigarette – 'tooting'.

*Mainlining.* In contrast to chasers, injectors are older and more likely to be male. They show high dependence and are likely to be using the drug in higher doses and on a daily basis. They are unlikely to have non-users as friends, and are steeped in heroin 'culture'. This group is increasingly turning to methadone treatment programmes.

Many established users will have been injecting opiates for years: the average age at a methadone maintenance clinic will be around 35 years, with most starting to inject opiates at around the age of 20 years. More than 70% of these long-term addicts will test positive for the hepatitis C virus, around 50% will be positive for hepatitis B, and a significant proportion will be HIV positive. At least half will have shared injection apparatus.

### Heroin overdose

Overdose may be due to simple error (especially if alcohol is also involved), to inadvertent ingestion of a particularly pure batch of heroin, to loss of tolerance following abstinence or to a deliberate act of self harm. Patients are usually deeply comatose, with pin-point pupils. Treatment is with i.v. naloxone, the specific antidote, but reversal can be dramatic, leading to acute agitation, aggression and violence.

### Methadone therapy

Addicts who are admitted to medical wards often claim that they are 'registered' and as such they are 'entitled' to methadone or even to diamorphine.

- Only doctors who hold a special Home Office licence may prescribe diamorphine for the treatment of drug addiction.
- Since 1997, addicts are no longer registered with the Home Office (although there are voluntary anonymised regional and national Drug Misuse Databases for patients who first present with drug misuse).
- The addict will demand methadone in hospital because he realises that he is dealing with inexperienced staff who may comply with his wishes.
- Methadone can be abused and has a high value on the black market, particularly in tablet form (which can be crushed and injected) and in ampoules.
- The current recommendations for a methadone treatment programme are:
  — only methadone syrup, not tablets, should be prescribed
  — daily prescriptions should be given
  — the effective maintenance dose should not exceed 50–100 mg of methadone daily

Methadone programmes are carefully supervised and managed with a system of daily supply and directly observed ingestion. Apart from using methadone syrup (not tablets or injectable forms), effective treatment programmes monitor drug ingestion with blood and urine testing (the prevailing ethos for treating drug addiction is one of 'tough love').

Methadone treatment is not universally popular and some institutions, notably the prison service, use dihydrocodeine, in long-acting preparations, to aid withdrawal. Buprenorphine is a useful alternative heroin substitute, particularly as it has a low risk of causing respiratory depression if taken in excess. A typical regimen would be a rapidly tapering course of sublingual buprenorphine, starting at 4–16 mg per day, to be followed up longer term by the opiate blocker, naltrexone.

### Nursing assessment of the addict

- What drugs: how and in what quantity?
- Is the patient known to the Drugs Advisory Service?
- Is there a child at risk or is the patient pregnant?

## SPECIAL RISKS TO MEMBERS OF THE STAFF

The three most common work-related injuries in hospital staff are caused by falls, needle stick injuries and violent incidents.

### NEEDLE STICK INJURIES

Human immunodeficiency virus, HBV and HCV are blood-borne infections that put at risk those nurses who are exposed to the blood of infected patients.

### The nature of the risk

A needle stick injury with HIV-infected blood carries a small but significant risk (1 in 300) of HIV infection in the recipient. Hepatitis is more easily transmitted than HIV: if the blood is from a patient with hepatitis, the risk can be as high as 1 in 10. The risks are lower after exposure of broken skin (e.g. severe eczema on a nurse's hands) or mucous membranes (eyes or mouth) to infected blood or blood-stained body fluids.

*Nurses must be aware of the risks and systems of care should assume that blood-borne infection could be present in any or every patient. There must be a well-publicised local policy from Occupational Health, consistent with the most recent Department of Health Guidelines.*

It is vital that staff know what to do in the event of a needle stick injury:

- Who do you contact during the day?
- Who do you contact at night and at weekends?
- Where are the starter packs for HIV prophylaxis?

- Could the system deliver HIV prophylaxis within 1 h of the incident?
- What blood specimens need to be taken from the patient and the staff member?
- Who can give expert advice?

### Outcome

The outcome of the incident depends on four factors:

- type of exposure
- status of patient (HBV positive/HBC positive/HIV positive)
- immunity of staff member (hepatitis B immunisation)
- effectiveness and timeliness of the emergency measures

### What constitutes significant exposure?

- Needle stick or blood-contaminated sharps
- Bite causing skin puncture
- Mucocutaneous exposure to blood or blood-stained body fluids

### What emergency action should be taken?

1. Irrigate and wash and encourage any skin breaches to bleed
2. Report the incident
3. Attend the relevant department immediately (Occupational Health or the AED)

The important emergency interventions are the immediate (ideally within 1 h) institution of triple-drug antiretroviral therapy in a definite HIV exposure, and instituting accelerated anti-hepatitis B vaccination or a booster dose of vaccine in the case of definite exposure to hepatitis B.

### Risk assessment to identify the patient's infectivity

1. Hepatitis B (positive for hepatitis B surface and E antigens: HBsAg, HBeAg)
2. Hepatitis C
3. HIV positive
4. Known to have HIV risk factors

*Blood testing of patient and storage of blood from staff member.* If there has been significant exposure, the patient should have his HbsAg checked urgently. If there are risk factors for hepatitis C or HIV, consent should also be sought to check these: the possible outcomes are therefore:

1. urgent testing of the patient (10 ml blood for HBsAg, HVC, HIV and storage)
2. storage with delayed testing should it be necessary
3. baseline tests on the nurse and storage for later testing

**Documentation.** Document the incident using an official incident form.

## HOSPITAL-ACQUIRED METHICILLIN-RESISTANT STAPHYLOCOCCUS AUREUS INFECTIONS

Hospital acquired MRSA is an increasing problem leading to unnecessary deaths and disability. Health-care workers infect themselves by handling MRSA-positive patients and from touching adjacent contaminated surfaces. The staff then spread the organism from one patient to another. Spread is prevented by effective isolation, careful room cleaning and the use of universal precautions, of which by far the most important is thorough and frequent hand-washing.

## VIOLENT INCIDENTS

The most common forms of violence on the acute medical wards are those seen in severely agitated patients with confusional states who strike out, grab or scratch the medical or nursing staff, whom they misinterpret as posing a threat. Less common, but more dangerous, is the physical aggression that accompanies severe paranoid states due to an acute physical or psychiatric illness. The combination of drug or alcohol intoxication with a paranoid illness is particularly dangerous.

The principles of management are:

- do not take risks
- any patient showing an obvious paranoid state should be asked if they are carrying any sort of weapon
- ensure your own safety and that of the patient
- seek immediate help from other staff members
- use the absolute minimum of force to control the situation

*Prevention*

- Recognise the causes:
  — acute anxiety and fear
  — alcohol and drug-withdrawal syndromes
  — delirium
  — dementia
  — major psychosis, e.g. paranoid schizophrenia
- Recognise the warning signs:
  — agitation
  — shouting and pacing the room
  — misinterpreting nursing interventions as personal threats
  — threats of violence and previous violent behaviour
  — paranoid ideas, fearing for their life
  — delirium/clouded consciousness

*Management*

The acutely disturbed and potentially violent patient should be cared for only by an appropriate number of trained, experienced and easily identified (uniformed) staff. It is critical that a medical assessment is made at an early stage to detect reversible causes of acute confusion, e.g. hypoxia, infection, drug toxicity. The patient should be nursed in a quiet, well-lit room in which he cannot harm himself. It can be calming to an acutely disturbed patient if you exhibit a relaxed but attentive manner and avoid anything that could be misinterpreted as being confrontational. Listen, explain and reassure. Remember that any physical contact may be misinterpreted as threatening behaviour, so explain very clearly what it is you are planning to do in terms of nursing observations and monitoring. If the situation deteriorates, you must obtain immediate help from the medical and security staff and, if serious violence, say with a weapon, is threatened, the police.

There are situations in which common sense dictates that the patient should be restrained for their own safety: a clear example is someone with a severe toxic confusional state who has become acutely paranoid and is trying to escape through a window. Patients who are mentally disordered and putting themselves *or others* at risk can be treated under Common Law without consent.

To calm an acutely disturbed or aggressive patient intramuscular sedation can be used and repeated when necessary:

| | |
|---|---|
| Midazolam | 7.5–15 mg |
| *or* | |
| Haloperidol | 5–10 mg combined with 50 mg of promethazine |

If sedation is administered, the patient must be monitored carefully to prevent aspiration, respiratory depression and hypotension.

If, as a last resort, temporary restraining force is needed, there must be a sufficient number of experienced staff to apply it to an absolute minimum, ensuring the patient comes to no harm. Under these situations, it is essential to involve senior nursing and medical staff and subsequently to complete detailed nursing documentation.

## FURTHER READING

Hassan TB, MacNamara AF, Davy A et al 1998 Management of deliberate self poisoning in adults in four teaching hospitals: descriptive study. British Medical Journal 316: 831–832

Hassan TB, MacNamara AF, Davy A, Bing A, Bodiwala GG 1999 Managing patients with deliberate self harm who refuse treatment in the accident and emergency department. British Medical Journal 319: 107–109

House A, Owens D, Patchett L 1999 Deliberate self harm. Quality in Health Care 8 (2): 137–143

Roberts D, Mackay G 1999 A nursing model of overdose assessment. Nursing Times 95 (3): 58–60
UK National Poisons Information Service 1995 National guidelines: Management of acute paracetamol poisoning. Paracetamol Information Centre in collaboration with the British Association for Accident and Emergency Medicine, London

**WEB ADDRESS**

Guidelines for acute alcohol withdrawal:
  http://www.rcplondon.ac.uk/pubs/books/ActNHSai/alcoholNHSappx.pdf
NICE Guidelines for Self-Harm 2004:
  http://www.nice.org.uk/page.aspx?o=20034
TOXBASE: The UK on-line poisons information service:
  http://www.spib.axl.co.uk/

# THE 'SOCIAL ADMISSION'

## INTRODUCTION

Many acute medical assessment units have now abandoned the concept of age-related admission policies: on most units, 10–15% of patients will now be aged 80 years and over. This group of patients calls for particular skills in assessment and management, not least in the area of prioritising their care. Characteristically, the medical histories are complex, they involve several systems, and it is often difficult to establish which of their many conditions contribute most to the reason for admission.

The label of 'social admission', while acknowledging the issue of the home circumstances, is a disservice to this group of patients, as it inevitably means that less effort is paid to establishing exact diagnoses. In fact a pure 'social' admission – one in which the patient is medically stable but in which the care input has failed – is a rare event and the term is generally *unhelpful*:

- it suggests a non-urgent or elective admission
- it denies a medical cause for admission
- it discourages a full medical assessment
- it implies a 'social' solution to the problems
- it suggests the patient can soon be shifted to hotel-type care
- the term falls into the same category as the unhelpful 'bed blocker' or even 'off legs and unable to cope', in which the emphasis suggests the unwelcome nature of the admission, rather than the challenge of returning an elderly person to their home with improved health

## COMMON ERRORS AND OMISSIONS IN THE ADMISSION OF ELDERLY PATIENTS

### Failure to obtain an adequate history
- Simple communication failure – patient too ill or too deaf to communicate
- Acute confusion/delirium
- Long-standing confusion
- Inadequate referral details, particularly from the deputising service or from a nursing home

### Failure to establish a correct drug history
It is important to establish:

- what the patient's doctors have prescribed
- what the patient has actually been taking
- when any changes in medication occurred

Common problems with the drug history include:

- new treatments that do not appear on a repeat prescription list
- tablet bottles that contain a mixed assortment of drugs
- medications that the patient does not consider to be a drug

- eye drops and skin treatments
- Etidronic acid (Didronel PMO; 'fizzy drink')
- monthly (e.g. B$_{12}$) or weekly (e.g. methotrexate) treatments
- insulin
- non-compliance with multi-drug regimens (more than three different medications)
- failing to mention p.r.n. drugs, especially analgesics
- confusion concerning the doses of diuretics and the correct use of inhaled medication

*Failure to make an adequate review of the patient's previous hospital records*
Re-admissions in this age group are common. Hospital notes are helpful, but they can be difficult to track down. Some of the patient's problems may have been identified already: examples include septicaemia due to known kidney stones or gallstones, recurrent angina or dizzy episodes due to arrhythmias, and falls due to alcohol abuse.

## Inadequate nursing and medical assessment

- Failure to assess the musculoskeletal system
- Missed crush fracture of the spine
- Missed fracture of the long bones
- Missed joint infection
- Missed shoulder injury following a fall
- Missed broken skin over pressure areas
- Failure to diagnose 'silent' myocardial infarction
- Silent pneumonia
- Silent septicaemia
- Faecal impaction as a cause of worsening confusion in a patient with dementia
- Failure to take an alcohol history (alcohol problems in the elderly present with depression, confusion and falls)

# TAKING THE HISTORY

## TAKING A HISTORY FROM THE PATIENT

Elderly unwell patients often have considerable difficulty in recalling the time course of the symptoms that brought them into hospital. For many, the point at which new symptoms took over from the chronic symptoms of generalised ill health and multiple pathology will be far from clear. For many elderly patients the process of giving a history, often more than once when they are already feeling unwell, can be a considerable ordeal. The tendency is for staff to rush them rather than sit and listen (→ Case Study 9.1).

---

**CASE STUDY 9.1**   Failure to give adequate time to a patient

An 84-year-old man was admitted under the chest physician with immobility due to painful feet. He was frustratingly slow to give a rambling history, but after having successful dermatological treatment to his cracked and fissured soles he slowly mobilised. He was referred for rehabilitation and seen briefly at the end of very rushed ward rounds as '... and just the sore-foot man waiting to go to elderly care'. On a less hectic round he mentioned that he, too, had worked in a hospital and proceeded with a detailed account to a chastened chest consultant about the 20 years he had spent nursing in one of the country's earliest cardiothoracic surgical units, how fierce the matron was and, in his day, how precise the bed alignment had to be prior to consultant ward rounds.

---

- Every patient has his or her own life story and, with patience, you will learn more from them than they will from you
- Piece together the history and try and find something of the person rather than simply the 'admission problem'
- In the elderly, you are more likely to encounter atypical symptoms in commonplace conditions: dizziness as a presentation of myocardial infarction; 'off legs' as a result of a urinary tract infection; acute confusion as a side-effect of a change in drug treatment
- It is important that efforts are not duplicated and that the patients are not subjected to unnecessary repetition
- It is critical to obtain a history from a third party; a close relative, a professional carer or from the patient's GP

*Pain*

It can be difficult to separate symptoms from different systems. The problem of referred pain and the inability of some elderly patients to describe and localise their pain clearly can make it challenging for the listener. Examples include band-like abdominal pain attributable to collapsed thoracic vertebrae, upper abdominal pain due to acute myocardial ischaemia with cardiac failure, and diffuse abdominal pain due to a strangulated femoral hernia. To complicate the issue, many patients have pre-existing chronic pain from joint degeneration, from poorly controlled angina and from chronic arthritis of their spine.

## TAKING A HISTORY FROM A THIRD PARTY

The patient's description of the home circumstances and his level of dependence must be supported by evidence from other sources. Without a detailed background, the assessment is seriously flawed:

- the patients may be unforthcoming because of confusion, anxiety or depression

- the patients may minimise their disability
- carers may have a different perspective on the situation
- late information cannot contribute to the critical initial diagnostic process and will probably delay the eventual discharge

### Where to go for information

1. Relatives
2. The previous hospital medical and nursing notes
3. GP – early liaison with primary care will save a lot of time
4. Community nurse
5. Nursing home staff
6. Health visitors
7. Neighbours
8. Home care services
9. Social services

### Dealing with relatives

- Many relatives fear that an elderly person may be written off at an early stage and may therefore be defensive about their normal level of dependence. Just because someone is 85 years old, it is wrong to assume that either the relatives or the patient will take a philosophical view about having had a 'good innings'. Some of the most serious allegations of substandard care concern this area. Relatives often assume that, in the chaos of an acute unit, the elderly are given lower priority.
- Be sure who you are dealing with and what input they have in the care of the patient. It is not helpful to have an early detailed discussion with a niece who happens to be on the ward, before speaking to the daughter who has been sacrificing her sanity and her marriage to look after her confused elderly father for the past 5 years.
- Be sensitive to family dynamics, particularly in the issues of chronic dependence and dementia. The admission may have been the culmination of months of severe family stress in trying to cope with an increasingly difficult situation. The elderly spouses of patients with dementia often show evidence of significant stress-induced ill health. A straightforward and tactful information-gathering exercise is all that is needed in the early stages.

### Liaising with the medical staff

Communication with the admitting doctors is of paramount importance in the management of the elderly. Apart from minimising the ordeal for the patient of repeating the same information to different staff members, there is critical information that *must* be shared at the outset:

- the patient's baseline level of dependency
- the presence and time course of any confusion

- the list of current medication
- any suspicion of a head injury or a fracture
- the relatives' main immediate concerns
- any particular risk of falling

### EXCELLENCE IN COMMUNICATING WITH THE RELATIVES

1. Establish the depth of personal knowledge. Is the history from a third party due to personal familiarity with the patient, or is it hearsay?
2. When was the patient last well, and from that point how did the symptoms first develop, giving an approximate order?
3. What is the level of dependence and when did this change?
4. Establish the usual mental state and if there is a component of confusion/loss of short-term memory – when did it first develop, and how has it progressed or changed over time?
5. When you are doing your assessment, try to picture the patient in their own environment.

## FALLS

Falls are a common and important cause for acute medical admission. Almost 10% of patients aged 70 years and over will attend the Accident & Emergency Department at least once per year with injuries caused by a fall and a third of these will be admitted to hospital. Apart from a 10% risk of a fracture, falls have long-term consequences, particularly if they are recurrent:

- they lead to loss of confidence
- they are a threat to independence, particularly when they are recurrent
- hospital admission after a fall often triggers a slow general decline

In spite of their importance, patients are often not adequately assessed to establish the causes or the effects of their fall. Many will have attended on several previous occasions: a first-time faller has a greater than 50% chance of falling again within 12 months. In a significant proportion, the cause is reversible or the risk factors can be reduced.

### THE CAUSE OF FALLS

Fig. 9.1 and the following case studies illustrate the many factors that increase the risk of falls.

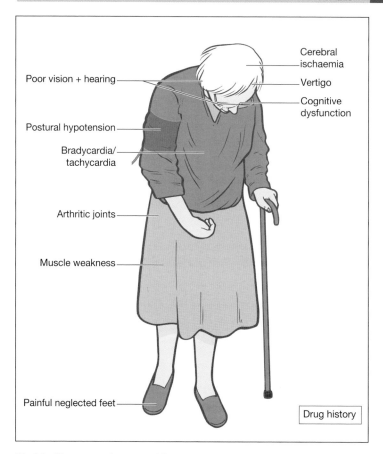

Poor vision + hearing

Postural hypotension

Bradycardia/
tachycardia

Arthritic joints

Muscle weakness

Painful neglected feet

Cerebral
ischaemia

Vertigo

Cognitive
dysfunction

Drug history

**Fig. 9.1** The patient with recurrent falls

Most falls are caused by a combination of *internal* problems with balance, vision and posture, and *external* factors such as loose rugs, poor lighting and cluttered living space. The fall may be triggered by new medication leading to dizziness or confusion, or the effects of an intercurrent acute illness such as anaemia, heart failure or infection. Case Studies 9.2 illustrate such falls.

Patients will be admitted after a fall if:

- they fail to make a full recovery
- they have injured themselves
- they are in need of care that is not available at home
- a serious medical cause for the fall is suspected

**CASE STUDIES 9.2** Causes of falls

## CASE 1

A 90-year-old-woman was started on the antidepressant, dothiepin: one tablet in the morning and two at night. She was also already taking atenolol 100 mgHg a day, beta-blocker eyedrops and bendrofluazide. She had fallen and lain against the radiator, suffering a full-thickness burn to the right shoulder. On admission, her systolic blood pressure fell by 30 mmHg when she stood up from lying, associated with unsteadiness. She was otherwise well.

- Drug treatment is a common and treatable factor in falls
- Half of all elderly fallers cannot get back on their feet unaided

## CASE 2

An 86-year-old woman was visiting her daughter at Christmas. She tripped in her bedroom and was in the line of a fan-heater. She was unable to move and suffered extensive burns to both lower legs.

- Falls are more common in unfamiliar surroundings, particularly those encountered when staying in cluttered or poorly lit spare rooms. People become used to their own frayed carpets and unsafe stairs, but these pose a threat to an elderly guest.

## CASE 3

An 83-year-old man was admitted having been found on the floor with extensive occipital bruising. He had signs of a chest infection, but with treatment made a good recovery. Mobilisation, however, was very slow. He had generalised stiffness, a tremor and was very reluctant to move his feet due to fear of falling. A diagnosis of Parkinson's disease was made and he was started on treatment.

Falls are common in Parkinson's disease:

- patients tend to topple backwards
- they are slow to correct any imbalance
- there is often an associated postural hypotension

## ASSESSMENT AFTER A FALL

*Critical nursing tasks in assessment after a fall*
**Ensure the safety of the patient: ABCDE.** Assess the vital signs and, if the patient is acutely ill, correct oxygen saturation, exclude hypoglycaemia, examine the pulse for bradycardia or tachycardia and measure the core temperature (hypothermia or fever). Always search for postural hypotension: *a fall in the systolic blood pressure of 20 mmHg or more on standing upright* (postural changes can be identified in the immobile from recordings taken when the patient sits up with the feet dependent over the side of the bed).

## CRITICAL NURSING TASKS IN ASSESSMENT AFTER A FALL

- **Ensure the safety of the patient: ABCDE**
- **Look for injury**
- **Has this been a stroke?**
- **Arrange for an urgent ECG and cardiac monitor**

**Look for injury.** Pain is the main clue to injury, although acute confusion can mask pain completely. Note the sites of pain – they will need to be X-rayed if there is tenderness, deformity or swelling. Inspect the scalp for bruising, look behind the ears (Battle's sign; → p. 104). Is there bruising around the hips? Look for pain on moving the wrists, shoulders, hips and elbows. Pleuritic pain may be due to fractured ribs. Deep pain in the lower back or groin is seen after pelvic fractures. If the patient has been lying in one position, there may be soft tissue pressure damage (bruising, discolouration and swelling) or burns.

**Has this been a stroke?** Examine for one-sided weakness, facial droop or an obvious speech disorder. Confusion must not be confused with dysphasia. If a stroke is suspected, check the safety of the airway and of the swallow.

**Arrange for an urgent ECG and cardiac monitor.** This is to exclude a myocardial infarction or arrhythmia as the cause of the fall.

### *Important nursing tasks in assessment after a fall*
**Obtain an adequate history**

- What were the circumstances? A fall, often forwards and causing facial injury, in which there is no warning and no loss of consciousness, suggests a *drop attack*. A 'draining away', particularly on standing with greying vision and fading voices, suggests *syncope*. It should be remembered that the elderly may not realise that they have lost consciousness and can have significant postural hypotension in the absence of symptoms. Dizziness with the room spinning, especially if triggered by sudden turning or neck extension, suggests *vertigo*. If the patient has acute vertigo and cannot stand without support, and particularly if there is also slurring of the speech and focal weakness, a posterior circulation stroke is the likely cause. Head injuries, particularly in males, are frequently associated with excessive alcohol intake.
- What is the drug history? The main culprits are nitrates, diuretics and antihypertensives – all causing postural hypotension – and psychotropics, notably long-acting benzodiazepines (e.g. nitrazepam), anticonvulsants and antidepressants, affecting balance and causing drowsiness.

### Assess mobility

- Establish the patient's existing mobility and cross-check their account with that of a relative; patients often overestimate their usual level of function.

---

**IMPORTANT NURSING TASKS IN ASSESSMENT AFTER A FALL**

- ■ Obtain an adequate history
- ■ Assess mobility
- ■ Assess cognitive function
- ■ Speak to the carers and close family

---

- For a more objective assessment, there are three simple tests that can be tried once the patient has recovered from the immediate effects of the fall.
  1. 'Get up and go' – The patient who can rise from a chair, stand steadily, walk across the ward, then turn and return to the chair without help does not have an immediate problem with mobility or balance.
  2. Can the patient stand on one leg for 10 s? This will give a rapid global assessment of balance, power in the lower limbs and difficulty with weight bearing due to, say, problems with arthritic knees.
  3. Does the patient stop walking when he talks? Patients who are beginning to find mobility an increasing problem, for whatever reason, have to marshal their resources when dealing with the challenge of walking. This is apparent if a conversation is started while the patient is on the move – they will stop walking in order to talk.

**Assess cognitive function** This is an important part of any assessment in the elderly patient, but in the particular case of recurrent or unexplained falls, cognitive impairment will have a profound effect on the plans for discharge.

The AMTS (→ Box 9.1) is simple to administer: a score of less than 7, assuming this is not due to a simple communication problem, suggests

---

**Box 9.1 – The abbreviated mental test score (AMTS)**

1. How old are you now?
2. What time is it now (to the nearest hour)?
3. I will give you an address and ask you to repeat it later on: 42 West Street
4. What year is it now?
5. Can you tell me where you are now?
6. Can you tell me who (two persons) these people are?
7. Can you tell me the date of your birthday (day and month)?
8. What were the dates of the First World War?
9. Who is on the throne at present?
10. Can you count from 20 to 1 backwards?

cognitive impairment. The next step is to establish from the relatives' history whether this is a recent or long-standing problem.

**Speak to the carers and close family**

- Obtain an overall picture of the patient in his home, with an emphasis on mobility, vision and the immediate domestic environment. Confirm the drug (and alcohol) history. Check the input from family and professional carers.
- Has there been evidence of cognitive impairment: memory loss and difficulty with complex tasks?

*Additional assessment on examination*

- Look at the feet and lower limbs. Examine for generalised arthritis, particularly of the knees. Knees that are swollen, arthritic and stiff are often associated with thigh muscles that are weak and wasted through disuse. Is there generalised weakness of the legs? Are the feet well cared for or are they misshapen, with overlapping toes, bunions, painful fissures and huge uncut nails?
- Assess the hearing and vision. Sensory deprivation leads to loss of balance, a loss of the compensatory mechanisms needed to maintain equilibrium, and a reduction in the level of self-confidence. Ensure hearing aids and glasses are brought in soon after admission.
- Evaluate and localise any pain and ensure appropriate analgesics are prescribed and given.

## ANSWERING RELATIVES' QUESTIONS IN PATIENTS WHO FALL

*Will everything be all right?* You should be guarded about the prognosis until more information is available. The outlook after a fall can be poor: for example, a fall followed by a lie on the floor for an hour or more carries a 6-month mortality rate of 50%.

*Why do the falls keep occurring?* The majority of elderly patients who fall will fall again. However, while some risk factors cannot be corrected some, such as drug side-effects and environmental factors, can be addressed.

*What can we do to prevent it?* Our assessment will identify any reversible medical cause for the falls, and part of the rehabilitation will involve an evaluation of the situation at home.

*Shouldn't he now be in a nursing home – we cannot possibly take him into our house?* One of the outcomes of this admission will be an assessment of the domestic situation, to assess the patient's personal needs and to look at what support is available. Any eventual discharge will take all these factors into account as well as your views and those of the patient.

*Does he need all those tablets?* We will take this opportunity to re-evaluate all his medication – what he is prescribed, what he actually takes and what he really needs.

*Why did he fall in the ward?* Patients who are unsteady on their feet are more likely to fall in unfamiliar surroundings, particularly if an acute illness has led to confusion. We will try and prevent further falls by treating the underlying problems and in the meantime it may be helpful to bring in glasses/supportive footwear/usual walking aids.

*Can't you use sedation or cot sides?* Sedation or physical restraint are the absolute last resorts – and only then if the patient is a danger to himself. Their use causes increasing confusion and there is no evidence that they are effective in preventing falls; indeed, they may slow down mobilisation.

*What are the chances of this happening again in hospital?* Recurrent falls are quite common at this age, even if all possible precautions are taken. There is always a balance to be struck between safety and encouraging the patient to maintain his independence. There are effective ways of reducing the chances of falling again: a detailed risk assessment of all the factors which may be contributing to the falls, leading to a management plan to reduce these and special targeted exercise programmes to improve balance, gait, posture and muscle strength.

## EXCELLENT CARE FOR PATIENTS WHO FALL

- Are the staffing levels appropriate for the dependence levels in your patients?
- Are your elderly patients assessed according to a protocol?
- How much unnecessary duplication is there?
- Are the relatives and carers interviewed on admission?
- Do you use an AMTS as routine in assessing the elderly?
- Can you identify the 'high-risk faller'?
- Is there a protocol for the prevention of falls/use of cot sides?
- Have you audited falls on the acute ward?
- How safe is your ward for the elderly unsteady?
  - bed to chair or commode
  - chair to bathroom
  - how cluttered is the space around the beds?
  - how well do their pyjama bottoms fit!
- How soon after admission do you start planning for discharge?

# IMMOBILITY

Increasing immobility can have many important causes, as the following case studies illustrate (→ Case Studies 9.3–9.6).

---

**CASE STUDY 9.3** Advanced malignant disease presenting as increasing immobility

An 86-year-old woman presented with an 8-week history of increasing immobility, anorexia and reduced fluid intake. She had previous admissions to elderly care for respite care. She denied any particular complaints and said she was able to walk with a stick.

On initial assessment, she appeared frail and cachectic. Her MTS was 4/10. She had a productive-sounding cough and evidence of left lower lobe pneumonia.

The initial diagnosis was 'poor mobility and a chest infection'.

Immediate blood tests showed that she was anaemic and also had abnormal liver function tests. An ultrasound showed a large right-sided renal cancer, with secondary spread to the liver.

- When elderly patients become ill, their history cannot be relied on.
- Malignant disease rather than 'frailty of old age' is often the cause of progressive deterioration.
- Early investigations mean that an appropriate management plan can be instituted soon after admission.

---

**CASE STUDY 9.4** Infection as a cause of acute immobility

A 78-year-old widower took to his bed because he was too weak to walk. His only complaint was of burning on passing urine. He was unable to recall any of his medication, but his daughter later provided a list, which included prednisolone, oral nitrates and atenolol.

Coliform bacteria were cultured from his urine and blood. Within 4 days of starting antibiotics, he was feeling well and was fully mobile.

Infection, particularly urinary infection, can lead to generalised ill health. It is important to identify those regular medications that must not be stopped suddenly. These may include:

- steroids (acute steroid insufficiency)
- beta-blockers (rebound angina)
- anticonvulsants (recurrence of fits)
- benzodiazepines (withdrawal syndromes)

---

**CASE STUDIES 9.5** Immobility due to drugs

### CASE 1

An 85-year-old woman with Alzheimer's disease came up to casualty and had her dislocated shoulder reduced under sedation with i.v. diazepam. Two days later, she was admitted with an impaired conscious level, having taken to her bed with an aspiration pneumonia. She had a productive cough and GCS of 5. She responded to physiotherapy and i.v. antibiotics.

- Patients' psychosocial circumstances must be assessed fully before discharge.
- There is a major risk in sending an elderly infirm woman with dementia home from hospital immediately after sedation.

### CASE 2

A 73-year-old diabetic woman with a previous history of strokes was admitted with a gradual deterioration, lethargy and increasing immobility. She was a 'dead weight' and her husband was unable to cope. Nothing specific found. She was transferred to elderly care where she was noted to be on two sedatives, antidepressants and nitrazepam. These were gradually withdrawn. She made a spontaneous recovery and was rapidly (over 3–4 days) able to mobilise with a zimmer frame and support.

- In any immobile patient, the drug history is critical.
- A third of admissions in the elderly are related to drug toxicity.
- Polypharmacy increases the chances of interactions, drug duplications and non-compliance.

---

'*Off legs and unable to cope*' is the commonplace label for immobility, and should be ignored. Immobility is either part of a slow global deterioration in function or, more commonly on the admitting ward, it occurs suddenly over days or weeks and signifies an acute illness of some form.

The common causes of recent onset immobility are:

- stroke
- Parkinson's disease
- heart failure
- acute exacerbation of COPD
- musculoskeletal disease (arthritis and osteoporosis)

These may be accompanied or triggered by:

- depression or grief
- anxiety, especially associated with a fear of falling
- pain
- underlying cognitive impairment

**CASE STUDY 9.6**  Difficulties in predicting the outcome in the elderly immobile

An 80-year-old man with a known history of chronic heart failure and atrial fibrillation was admitted with sudden generalised deterioration and confusion.

On assessment, his MTS was unrecordable, he was unable to stand unsupported and was incontinent of urine. His speech was slurred and he was slumped in bed with a respiratory rate of 30 breaths/min. Blood pressure was 235/122 mmHg and his oxygen saturations were 85%. His initial blood tests showed dehydration. The diagnosis was 'acute confusion'.

Two hours after admission he was found on the floor, having fallen from his bed and bruised his shoulder. The next morning on reassessment he appeared dysphasic rather than confused and was slumped to one side with definite evidence of unilateral weakness. Further blood tests showed high digoxin levels but nothing else of note.

By 24 h, his GCS had fallen from 15 on admission to 6, and his respiration had become laboured and irregular (Cheyne–Stokes respiration). An urgent CT scan showed a large cerebral bleed related to his severe hypertension. A diagnosis of stroke complicated by aspiration pneumonia was made. He was started on i.v. ampicillin and metronidazole. The neurosurgeons advised that there was no indication for surgery.

By the eighth day of admission, he was sitting up cheerfully in bed with mild functional impairment and was starting to mobilise. His blood pressure was controlled with cautious use of antihypertensives.

- Stroke presents as confusion.
- Dysphasia may be mislabelled as confusion.
- Always look for evidence of weakness down one side (the family will often notice this first).
- Outcomes are difficult to predict in the elderly, who can have excellent powers of recovery (patients who reach 80 years old have a proven track record of survival!).

*Critical nursing tasks in assessing immobility*
**Immediate safety of the patient: ABCDE**

- Exclude hypothermia: a core or tympanic membrane temperature < 35°C
    — hypothermia causes confusion and incoordination
    — triggers include alcohol and psychotropic drugs
    — it can result in dehydration and pneumonia
    — active rewarming is indicated

**Assessing the cause: establish the full history**

- From the patient *and* a third party
- Establish the sequence of events: acute/chronic/acute on chronic
- A comprehensive list of medications

**CRITICAL NURSING TASKS IN ASSESSING IMMOBILITY**

■ **Ensure the safety of the patient: ABCDE**
■ **Establish the full history**

- What is the patient's normal level of mobility?
  — how did the immobility develop: progressive/sudden onset/stuttering?
  — is there musculoskeletal disability?
  — how are hearing, sight and balance?
  — are there recurrent falls?
  — have you access to previous nursing or medical notes?

*Important nursing tasks in assessing immobility*
**Assess the overall condition**

- Does the patient look well for their age (grooming/foot care/state and cleanliness of the skin)?
- Is there evidence of neglect (underweight/poor hygiene/chronic changes to the skin and feet)?

**Is the patient in pain?** Pain, particularly on movement, leads to immobility and commonly arises from the musculoskeletal system – either chronic arthritis or vertebral collapse. Severe osteoporosis is a major cause of increasing immobility, with loss of height, spinal deformity and severe pain from fractures of the thoracic and lumbar vertebrae. When bones are osteoporotic, even minor falls can lead to fractures of the hip, wrist, pelvis and ribs.

**IMPORTANT NURSING TASKS IN ASSESSING IMMOBILITY**

■ **Assess the overall condition**
■ **Is the patient in pain?**
■ **Look at the areas of risk**
■ **Look for evidence of malnutrition and dehydration**
■ **Examine the patient's mobility**
■ **Is there any evidence of urinary incontinence?**
■ **Should the patient be catheterised?**

**Look at the areas at risk**

- Examine skin creases and groins
- Record any changes over the pressure areas
- Remove any dressings and note the findings
- Examine and record any areas of bruising, redness or tenderness

**Look for evidence of malnutrition and dehydration.** The risk factors for malnutrition are:

- poverty
- depression
- social isolation
- dementia
- recent bereavement
- anorexia
- ill-fitting dentures and sore mouth

There may be signs of vitamin and protein deficiency – but the main clue remains the patient's weight: *a BMI (weight in kg/height in metres squared) of less than 19 indicates likely malnutrition* (to estimate height in the bed-bound or those who have lost height, double the distance from finger tip to mid sternum). These patients should be referred immediately for nutritional assessment and dietetic support.

**Examine the patient's mobility**
*Note*: Remember the risk of postural hypotension.

- What do you anticipate from the history you have already?
- Is the patient well enough to try and stand?
- Can the patient sit up unsupported with good balance?
- Is there any obvious one-sided weakness in the face, arms or legs?
- Can the patient lift each foot, in turn, 3 in (8 cm) or more off the bed?
- Can the patient sit on the edge of the bed unsupported?
- Can the patient transfer to a chair?
- Can the patient 'get up and go'?

**If there is evidence of urinary incontinence, what is the time course?**
*Long-standing incontinence.* Chronic incontinence is common in the elderly, particularly those with cognitive impairment: one in five nursing home residents are incontinent during the day. However, even in established incontinence, there may be reversible causative factors such as immobility or overuse of diuretics. The acute admission provides an opportunity to review possible underlying causes.

*Recent onset urinary incontinence.* There are four mechanisms that can interact to result in acute urinary incontinence:

- **Impaired cognition** – this is seen in delirium, stroke and over sedation, all of which are potentially reversible

- **Reduced mobility** – an elderly patient with bladder irritability may have to urinate every hour or so. Any cause of sudden immobility can therefore result in incontinence
- **Excessive fluid challenge** – overuse of diuretics or the excessive osmotic diuresis from uncontrolled diabetes can both overwhelm an ageing bladder and lead to temporary incontinence
- **Bladder instability** – a common problem in the elderly, the additional effect of urinary infection or faecal impaction on the bladder will produce urgency and incontinence

**Should the patient be catheterised?** Catheterisation is associated with short-term complications, impairment of early mobilisation and reduced chances of regaining continence. Situations in which it may be justified include:

- terminal illness when there is distress from bladder distension or incontinence
- to allow healing when incontinence has produced skin excoriation or ulceration
- in critical illness in which measurements of the hourly urine output are required
- patients in coma

## CONFUSION

Cognitive impairment is a common and challenging problem on the Acute Medical Unit, with current estimates that, among those over 65 years admitted as an emergency, it will be a significant issue in 20%. In half of these the picture is of chronic confusion (dementia) and in the remainder there will either be an acute confusional state (delirium) occurring *de novo*, or a combination of long-standing confusion with a sudden worsening, coinciding with the admission to hospital.

*Delirium*
Delirium is an acute confusional state with the following features:

- a fluctuating conscious level – the patient is unable to stay awake or is difficult to arouse
- a reduced level of attention – questions have to be repeated
- disorganised thinking – rambling, incoherent and slurred speech

Delirium occurs in around one in five elderly patients after admission to hospital:

- it carries a significant mortality
- it can mask pain and acute illness
- it delays rehabilitation and discharge
- it can take weeks to resolve

There are six important risk factors:

1. existing cognitive impairment
2. visual and hearing impairment
3. immobility
4. acute physical illness
5. dehydration
6. sleep deprivation

There are five major causes on the Acute Medical Unit:

1. infection
2. hypoxia
3. metabolic upset (particularly dehydration)
4. major organ failure
5. drug therapy

**Principles of management**

- Make an immediate comprehensive assessment (→ Fig. 9.2)
- Establish exact baseline health and functional status
- Treat any acute medical condition
- Prevent deterioration in existing function through enforced immobility, lack of communication, unfamiliar surroundings
- Prevent infliction of harm through unnecessary drug therapy, neglect, falls or premature discharge from hospital

---

**CASE STUDIES 9.7** Confusion

## CASE I

An 83-year-old woman was admitted from a nursing home. The background was of a diagnosis of Alzheimer's disease with 2 years' progressive memory loss. Before her recent deterioration, she was fully mobile and able to dress, but she needed some help with personal needs and was failing to recognise close family members. For 48 h she had taken to her bed with increasing restlessness and confusion.

The patient was admitted to the Acute Medical Unit at midnight. She was not initially assessed, and at 01.00 h she fell from the bed onto the floor, sustaining extensive superficial grazes above her eyes and an abrasion to her face. Subsequent examination revealed a lady with an abbreviated MTS of 3/10 and evidence of recent urinary incontinence. She was restless and unable to give an account of herself, but was apyrexial. By the next day her respiratory rate had increased to 25 breaths/min, she had a wet, productive-sounding cough and remained incontinent of urine. She was sitting anxiously picking at the bed clothes and was clearly distressed but unable to say why.

With physiotherapy she produced green sputum. The head wounds healed uneventfully and she slowly returned over the subsequent few days to her previous state.

The diagnosis was of an initial urinary infection complicated by a fall.

*(continued overleaf)*

**CASE STUDIES 9.7** (continued)

### Should cot sides have been used?

Probably not: there is little evidence that cot sides are helpful in acute confusion, indeed, they increase the potential height of any fall. The main value of cot sides is in combination with pillows to maintain a safe position, in patients with a depressed conscious level.

### History

It is important to obtain a history from a nursing home and relatives, although it is common for elderly women to have no close relatives available at the time of admission.

### Should antibiotics be used blindly?

Antibiotics should not be given blindly in acute confusion and incontinence on the assumption that there may be a urinary tract infection. Treatment should be reserved for proven infection associated with any of the following:

- fever
- dysuria
- lower abdominal pain
- new incontinence
- frequency/urgency

Pneumonia can be difficult to recognise in the elderly, but an increased respiratory rate and a productive cough are sufficient evidence of infection to start antibiotics.

### Alzheimer's disease

Patients with Alzheimer's disease have a low threshold for developing a super-added confusional state in response to even minor acute illnesses. Patients should not be sedated but they must be maintained in a safe environment to reduce the risk of self-injury through falling.

### CASE 2

An 82-year-old woman with dementia was admitted to hospital 'off legs and vomiting'. No history was available from the patient as her MTS was 1/10. She was weak, incoherent and febrile. The day after admission, she became poorly responsive and more febrile. The patient then rallied and became brighter, but her speech was noted to be incomprehensible. She was, however, said to be 'back to her normal self'. The patient was transferred to elderly care for rehabilitation. There she required full nursing care. On medical review, she was found to be dysphasic, with some receptive problems. The new diagnosis of a stroke was discussed with her son, who with great frustration said the family had been saying that all along but no one was listening.

Care must be taken with the label of dementia and particular attention must be paid to the preadmission functional level and to the family's account of their relative's normal state of health and of how the illness developed.

**CASE STUDIES 9.7** (continued)

## CASE 3

A 72-year-old woman was admitted with coffee-ground vomiting and hallucinations. She was also mildly dysphasic. The history was limited, but her hallucinations were addressed at the expense of her vomiting, and a referral was made to the psychogeriatricians, who felt her social circumstances needed sorting out. She was transferred to elderly care, where a subsequent endoscopy showed pyloric stenosis and significant ulceration.

The hallucinations had coincided with initiating opiate analgesia. This was stopped and at a later date fentanyl patches were effectively introduced for what turned out to be severe post-herpetic neuralgia. She mobilised well and after a successful home visit was discharged from hospital.

This patient did not undergo a comprehensive initial assessment. In her case there was a combination of physical conditions and cognitive impairment – these are impossible to sort out without full background information from a third party. In particular, there must always be a full drug history, which should include any sedation, anticonvulsants and analgesics, as these may accumulate, causing toxicity and contributing to confusion.

## CASE 4

A 94-year-old woman who lives alone was found on the floor unable to get up. Apparently she had fallen before. On admission she was confused, with a productive cough, a temperature of 38.5°C and an MTS of 2/10. The oxygen saturations were low, at 88%, and she had signs of a chest infection. She was treated with i.v. fluids and antibiotics, but remained confused.

Six days after admission, her neighbour brought in her hearing aid. Her MTS improved immediately to 8/10 and she complained of persistent severe back pain. The fall had resulted in a crush fracture of a thoracic vertebra. With analgesia, she was able to cooperate with physiotherapy and started to make a good recovery. On further assessment, she had a long-standing tendency to fall backwards, which was probably related to the development of mild Parkinson's disease.

- Always look for hearing problems when assessing confusion
- Have hearing aids brought in urgently
- Recurrent falls usually have a clear cause
- Falls followed by enforced immobility on the floor can lead to serious complications (and carry a significant mortality rate):
  — hypothermia
  — unrecognised fractures
  — pressure damage to soft tissue and muscle
  — pneumonia
  — deep vein thrombosis

Case Studies 9.7 present some of the problems encountered with confused patients.

*Critical nursing tasks in assessing the confused elderly*
The critical nursing tasks in the acutely confused elderly patient are similar to those in a seriously ill younger patient. Although there are differences in the way in which problems present, the essential priorities are the same: addressing basic resuscitation using the system ABCDE and maintaining the immediate safety of the patient.

Fig. 9.2 summarises the assessment of acute confusion.

**What must have immediate attention?**
*Hypoxia*

- The most common cause of hypoxic confusion in the elderly is pneumonia with sputum retention. The chest sounds wet on coughing, but the patient is often too weak to expectorate. Chest pain after a fall may be due to fractured ribs and can severely inhibit deep inspiration and coughing. The pain must be addressed before the patient can have effective chest physiotherapy. It is important to recognise that the pneumonia may be complicating another event: a fall with an unrecognised fracture or a stroke with aspiration. The only signs of pneumonia may be an increased respiratory rate and confusion; the temperature may be normal or only increase after admission.
- The other main cause of hypoxic confusion is acute LVF, which can be very difficult to distinguish from pneumonia or even COPD. Examination can be unhelpful in this age group, and chest films are difficult to interpret. Initial emergency management will often be a compromise by targeting both the heart and the lungs: combining nebulised bronchodilators and antibiotics with diuretics and nitrates.

*Management of hypoxia*

- Sit the patient up
- Encourage the patient to cough. If it sounds productive, arrange urgent physiotherapy. Ensure there is effective analgesia, without the risk of further sedation or confusion

**CRITICAL NURSING TASKS IN ASSESSING THE CONFUSED ELDERLY**

- **Identify and correct hypoxia**
- **Exclude hypoglycaemia**
- **Consider head injury**

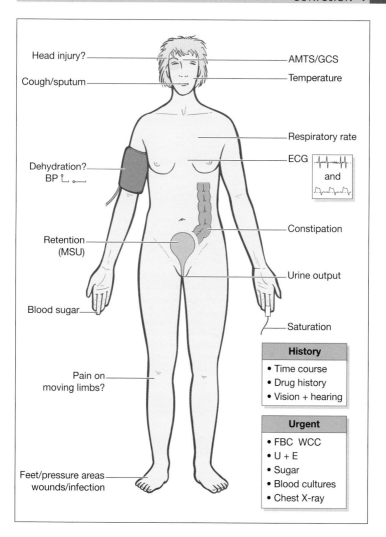

**Fig. 9.2** Assessing the patient with confusion

- Administer oxygen to increase saturations to 90%
- Organise an ECG to exclude an acute myocardial infarction or arrhythmia (acute atrial fibrillation is very common in this age group)
- Patients should be catheterised if intensive diuretic therapy is planned, particularly as the confused patient is likely to be incontinent: it is kinder for the patient and the output can be accurately assessed during the critical first 24–48 h

*Hypoglycaemia.* In this age group, hypoglycaemia is seen only in diabetic patients on insulin or (and) oral hypoglycaemics, and occasionally after a heavy drinking binge. Longer-acting oral hypoglycaemics such as glibenclamide and chlorpropamide are particularly dangerous in the elderly. If drug interaction with the oral hypoglycaemics is suspected (and it should be whenever a patient is taking four or more drugs), contact the ward pharmacist for advice.

*Head injury.* Head injuries are a very important cause of reversible confusion – a trivial injury can result in a subdural haemorrhage and the history will not be forthcoming in a delirious patient. If there is a fluctuating conscious level or a progressive fall in the GCS, it is vital to consider a CT scan before the situation becomes irretrievable. Even the very elderly can benefit from neurosurgical intervention in the appropriate circumstances. Important clues, apart from the all important history, are facial bruising, scalp wounds, bruising behind the ears and 'raccoon eyes'.

*Hyponatraemia.* Hyponatraemia (a low serum sodium) is a less pressing but nonetheless important and common cause of confusion in the elderly. It is often due to excessive urinary salt loss from diuretic therapy, particularly if the patient also loses excessive fluid, say from acute diarrhoea. The signs in these patients are of hypovolaemia (high pulse rate and postural hypotension) and treatment is with saline. This is not the only cause of hyponatraemia: in some patients it can be due to inappropriately high levels of ADH – a hormone that stimulates the kidneys to retain salt-free water and hence dilute the blood. ADH secretion is vital as the normal response to dehydration, but in this group of patients the trigger for ADH secretion is either an adverse drug reaction (especially psychotropics) or, occasionally, cancer of the lung. Treatment of inappropriate ADH secretion is with fluid restriction.

### Important nursing tasks in assessing the confused elderly

**Assess the degree of cognitive impairment.** The AMTS is a tried and tested method to identify cognitive impairment. Provided the patient can hear and is not dysphasic, a score of 7 or less signifies significant impairment. It does *not* distinguish between acute and chronic confusion; for this a full history is also required.

**Exclude infection and dehydration.** The main sources of infection are the chest, the urine and the soft tissues. Generalised infection, and even septicaemia, may have very non-specific findings in the elderly:

---

**IMPORTANT NURSING TASKS IN ASSESSING THE CONFUSED ELDERLY**

- ■ Assess the degree of cognitive impairment
- ■ Exclude infection and dehydration
- ■ Subcutaneous fluids
- ■ Assess constipation
- ■ Make an assessment of the social circumstances and dependence

---

- increased respiratory rate of > 15 breaths/min
- tachycardia
- hypotension
- mild confusion

Patients with infected wounds may be confused because of the development of septicaemia or spreading soft tissue infection. Any wound should be fully exposed in a good light to determine and document its depth and extent, and to look for elements such as critical limb ischaemia or gas gangrene. In difficult cases it is preferable for the wounds to be exposed to a combined team of nursing staff and doctors. A management plan can then be produced on admission, rather than taking dressings down three or four times during the first 24 h for a selection of doctors and nurses of varying expertise and experience.

- If there are skin breaks, wounds or ulcers that concern you, ensure that these are all accessible and highlighted on the consultant's ward round.

Dehydration can be difficult to identify without blood tests showing increases in the urea and creatinine. The most reliable signs are:

- postural hypotension
- tachycardia
- decreased level of consciousness
- urine output of less than 50 ml/h

**Subcutaneous fluids.** It can be difficult to give sufficient fluids to an acutely confused patient. Drinks will be refused and infusions will be pulled out. Subcutaneous fluids are often the key, particularly in the first 48 h until the patient improves. Up to 1.5 L of isotonic saline or 5% dextrose can be given every 24 h. In the very agitated patient, siting the 'butterfly' posteriorly below the shoulder blade can reduce the risk of its being pulled out.

**Assess constipation.** In the elderly, faecal impaction causes acute confusion, worsens existing cognitive dysfunction and is a reversible factor in urinary incontinence. It can be suspected from a full history and stool chart, but can only be diagnosed by a combination of a rectal examination and an abdominal X-ray.

**Make an assessment of the social circumstances and dependence.** Gain information (from both patient *and* carers – do not let the carers leave the ward until they have been seen, or telephone them at the end of the initial clerking for further information).

1. Does the patient live alone?
2. Does the patient care for someone else?
3. What is the degree of family and/or neighbour support?
4. Is the property secure?
5. Are there pets at home?
6. What are the levels of input?
   — district nurse
   — warden
   — social services and meals on wheels
   — home help
   — voluntary help
   — social worker

# DEMENTIA

Dementia commonly complicates acute medical conditions in the elderly: it obscures the immediate diagnosis, impairs recovery and has an obvious impact on planning for the patient's discharge.

Sixteen percent of all women and 6% of all men who reach an average life expectancy will develop dementia – a rate equivalent to around one in five people over the age of 80 years. Of these, 80% will have Alzheimer's disease, in which there is a progressive continuous deterioration; 10% will have multi-infarct dementia, in which the deterioration is stepwise punctuated by a series of mini-strokes; and 5% will have dementia against a background of Parkinson's disease, in which the picture is complicated by immobility and drug-induced side-effects, often with hallucinations.

In some cases there will be another psychiatric disorder present: depression, acute anxiety or an alcohol-related problem. This will need to be recognised and addressed.

## The diagnosis of Alzheimer's disease
As Alzheimer's disease progresses, the history becomes less reliable due to memory loss. It is unusual for patients to complain directly of memory disturbance – the first indications are usually the onset of problems with complex tasks and difficulties with the challenge of new or unexpected events: specific common examples include:

● managing medication
● using the telephone
● using transport
● coping with a household budget

*Complications of dementia that can occur in the Acute Medical Unit*

**Psychoses.** These usually take the form of acute paranoia and can be triggered by any acute medical illness. Classically, they are seen after acute myocardial infarction. Patients become intensely suspicious of the staff and often accuse them of being plotters or poisoners. Mobile patients may actively try to flee from the ward to escape this 'persecution'. Acute paranoid states need urgent psychiatric assessment and the warning signs require urgent action.

**Aggression.** This is also seen in dementia as a complication in acute illness, and may be a result of drug toxicity or dehydration. Treatment with sedation is usually unhelpful in the acute situation. Traditional management with haloperidol 2 mg every 8 h leads to drug accumulation, Parkinsonian side-effects and over-sedation. If there is no alternative for a severely disturbed patient, a short-acting benzodiazepine such as lorazepam is the drug of choice. Any prescription for sedation must be reviewed at least every 12 h to ensure the patient is not oversedated.

*Nursing observations for a patient who has required sedation*

- Hourly conscious level: GCS
- Is the airway safe (use the recovery position)?
- Respiratory rate (< 8 breaths/min: oversedation? > 20 breaths/min: developing pneumonia?)
- Pulse and blood pressure
- Oxygen saturations: maintain at > 90%

Any sudden change in behaviour is likely to have a cause – metabolic disturbance, pain, drug toxicity, or an acute event such as pneumonia or myocardial ischaemia.

## NURSING HOME ADMISSIONS

Dependence levels in patients who are admitted from a nursing home vary tremendously. One patient may have been bed-bound and totally dependent for all their needs for a number of years, whereas another from the same home may be mobile and dependent on nursing care only for specific areas of needs. The majority will be dependent for several basic functions, at least half will have cognitive impairment, and as many will have chronic urinary incontinence. *The exact level of baseline dependence must be established from the home in every case.* Particular care is needed in patients who have come to the nursing home within recent weeks – there may not have been time to identify any reversible causes of confusion or ill health. Their admission to the nursing home may have been triggered by an unrecognised but reversible physical illness.

Common problems in this group of patients are:

- falls
- dehydration during acute illness
- pressure sores and contractures
- delirium
- incontinence
- hearing problems
- visual problems
- depression
- dementia

During influenza outbreaks, many nursing home residents are admitted with cardiac failure, increasing breathlessness, wheeze and toxic confusion caused by pneumonia.

It cannot be assumed that every admission from a nursing home is for terminal care (→ Case Studies 9.8). However, one of the current features of

---

**CASE STUDIES 9.8** Admission from nursing homes

### CASE 1

An 85-year-old woman was admitted from a nursing home. She had been mobile with a walking frame, but had a 3-day history of increasing breathlessness. She remained very distressed and it was impossible to differentiate between bronchopneumonia and LVF. She was treated with oxygen, a combination of antibiotics, frusemide and low-dose opiates, on which she settled. She recovered fully.

### CASE 2

An 81-year-old woman was admitted from a nursing home. She had been to the pain clinic within the previous 3 months because of unremitting backache and been started on fentanyl patches. She had become progressively dependent, and 1 month before admission had been transferred from a rest home into a nursing home, where she had continued to deteriorate and had taken to her bed.

On examination she had a GCS of 15, but was lying rigidly in bed continually moaning, yet denying on direct questioning any discomfort or pain. Assessment was very difficult; there was no evidence of drug side-effects despite the fentanyl, and she appeared to have adequate levels of pain relief. She was screened for sepsis, the nursing home was contacted to make absolutely sure there were no other drugs that may have given a Parkinson's disease-type of side-effect, and her fentanyl was reduced slightly in case this was an opiate-induced state.

None of this made any difference, but a rectal examination 24 h after admission revealed severe faecal impaction. She was treated with Micralax enemas and stool softeners with a good result and appeared less distressed. Nonetheless, she remained very dependent and was eventually transferred back to the nursing home.

nursing home care is that frail patients are seen out of hours by on-call deputising medical services and admitted to hospital. There may be pressure from relatives that 'something must be done', equally there may be dismay that a seemingly natural progression towards death is punctuated by an unnecessary trip to an unfamiliar noisy ward in the middle of the night. It is critical to speak to the relatives immediately the patient is admitted.

- What is the level of dependence?
- What is the time course of the deterioration?
- What are their expectations of the outcome?
- Have they any particular concerns or worries (this often involves uncontrolled pain/seeing their relative suffer)?
- Have they an opinion on what the patient may want?
- Has the patient been discharged from hospital recently?

It is far better to treat a patient aggressively in the early stages, particularly while the normal level of functioning or degree of reversibility is unclear.

# ETHICAL ISSUES AND THE ELDERLY SICK

This is a very difficult area, in which even the most experienced medical and nursing staff can be left feeling very uncertain as to whether the correct decisions have been made. The fundamental issue for the individual patient is how far to pursue medical and supportive treatment or, having started them, whether they can be withdrawn:

- Cardiopulmonary resuscitation?
- Ventilatory or renal support?
- Surgery?
- Antibiotics?
- Artificial nutrition?
- Fluids?

## Who should decide?

- **The patient?** The patient has the basic right to give consent for treatment, but in the very situations in which the decisions are most hard to make – the elderly with delirium, dementia or severe illness – the patient is least able to contribute. Advance directives and living wills are virtually unheard of in the UK, and it is very unusual for a patient to have had prior discussions concerning his resuscitation status even if he has undergone repeated hospital admissions.
- **The doctor?** Although the medical staff have traditionally adopted this role, this may not be ideal. Their paternalistic role has become less acceptable to the public. Studies also show that doctors may systematically underestimate pre-existing quality of life in their patients, as well as being poor at predicting the patient's own wishes concerning treatment.

- **The patient's advocate?** This is an onerous task – weighing up the burdens and benefits of any proposed intervention and trying to predict what the patient would have wanted can prove too much for many close relatives; indeed, it may be unfair to burden some with such a difficult decision. Often, they may simply want reassurance that 'everything possible is being done'.

Most of these very difficult issues can be resolved with effective sharing of information between the health professionals and the family (→ Box 9.2). This can be particularly important within the first 48 h of admission, when the medical condition can change rapidly. It can be very helpful to contact the family, or to have them on the ward, at the times that key assessments are completed:

- soon after admission
- after the registrar's ward round
- after the Consultant's round

---

**Box 9.2 – Providing clear information to the family**

- What is the diagnosis and what is the prognosis?
- What are the goals of management?
    — simple prolongation of life (e.g. nutritional support in irreversible coma)
    — maintaining or improving function (e.g. successful defibrillation)
    — providing comfort (e.g. subcutaneous morphine in advanced cancer pain)
- What are the prospects for reaching these goals with and without treatment?
- What is the burden associated with treatment?
    — discomfort and side-effects (e.g. trauma of intubation and ventilation)
    — survival with severe disability (e.g. post-arrest anoxic brain damage)
    — what are the alternative treatments (e.g. oxygen and physiotherapy but not ventilation)?

---

*Withholding versus withdrawing treatment?*
The decision to withhold treatment may be appropriate if the treatment would do more harm than good – prolong suffering, increase discomfort or shorten life. Withdrawing treatment can be more difficult unless it is clear that the original treatment goals – say to improve ventilation and relieve respiratory distress – cannot be reached. It is therefore important for everyone – carers, family and patient – to be clear what can and cannot be achieved by the intervention in question, before it is started.

Like many difficult issues on the ward, the key is to keep open the best possible lines of communication between the medical and nursing staff, the relatives and, most importantly, the patient.

## FURTHER READING

### FALLS

Downton JH 1993 Falls in the elderly. Edward Arnold, London

Oliver D, Britton M, Steel P et al 1997 Development and evaluation of evidence based risk assessment tool to predict which elderly patients will fall. British Medical Journal 315: 1049–1053

Shaw FE, Kenny RA 1997 The overlap between syncope and falls in the elderly. Postgraduate Medical Journal 73: 635–639

Tinetti ME 2003 Preventing falls in elderly persons. New England Journal of Medicine 348: 42–49.

### CONFUSION

Brown TM, Boyle MF 2002 Delirium: clinical review. British Medical Journal 325: 644–647

Lacko L, Bryan L, Dellasega C, Salerno F 1999 Changing clinical practice through research: the case of delirium. Clinical Nursing Research 8 (3): 235–250

# CHAPTER 10

# MULTISYSTEM FAILURE

# SHOCK: THE BASIC MECHANISMS

Shock is the clinical condition in which a generalised reduction in tissue perfusion reduces the blood supply to vital organs, notably the kidneys and brain. Untreated, shock leads to cell death and multiple organ failure. It is therefore important to recognise the early warning signs and start immediate corrective action. Restoring the blood pressure and improving oxygenation are the priorities in shock; establishing its exact cause may have to wait.

In the *early stages*, the extremities are cool as blood is diverted to more important areas, the pulse increases and the blood pressure starts to fall.

Once *established*, shock causes a cold clammy skin, tachycardia and increased respiratory rate. Oxygen saturations decrease. The urine output is reduced due to impaired blood flow to the kidneys. The release of lactic acid from ischaemic, poorly perfused tissues leads to an acidosis. Acidosis in turn impairs cardiac function and leads to further falls in the blood pressure.

In *severe shock*, reduced perfusion to the brain leads to agitation, restlessness and eventual coma. By this stage, the reduced blood supply to the kidneys means there may be little or no urine output.

The classical features of shock are listed in Box 10.1 and illustrated in Fig. 10.1.

There are three forms of shock: cardiogenic shock, hypovolaemic shock and redistributive (low-resistance) shock.

### Cardiogenic shock

In cardiogenic shock, the heart as a pump fails to propel blood around the circulation. The common causes of cardiogenic shock are:

1. **Heart muscle damage** – a myocardial infarction severe enough to damage a large part of the left ventricle will reduce the cardiac output sufficiently to produce shock.
2. **Severe arrhythmia** – an acute rapid arrhythmia, most commonly atrial fibrillation, can reduce the blood pressure enough to cause shock. This commonly occurs in the setting of a pre-existing acute illness such as DKA or pneumonia.

---

**Box 10.1 – The classical features of shock**

- A systolic blood pressure of less than 90 mmHg
- A tachycardia
- An increased respiratory rate (above 20 breaths/min) and reduced oxygen saturations
- Mottled, cool and clammy skin
- Evidence of hypovolaemia: dry mouth, dry axillary skin, postural hypotension, thirst
- Low urine output (less than 0.5 ml/kg per h)
- Confusion or agitation progressing to coma

---

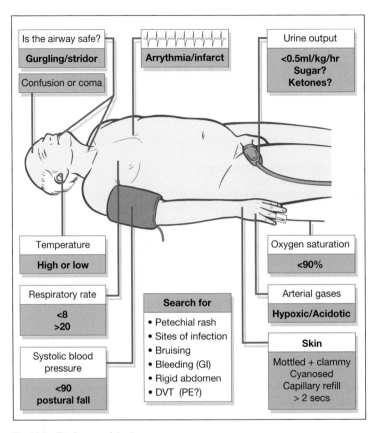

**Fig. 10.1** The features of shock

3. **Valve disease** – acute valve failure is an important reversible cause of cardiogenic shock. Sudden mitral regurgitation can complicate myocardial infarction and acute aortic incompetence can complicate bacterial endocarditis.

4. **Output obstruction** – this is seen in massive pulmonary embolus: the output from the right side of the heart is suddenly cut off by a clot lodging in the main pulmonary arteries, leading to sudden profound shock.

*Hypovolaemic shock*

Hypovolaemic shock is probably the most important type to recognise; it is relatively easy to treat and is rapidly fatal if allowed to progress. In hypovolaemic shock, there is a reduction in the circulating blood volume due to either external fluid loss or 'internal loss' by fluid being sequestrated within the body's internal compartments.

Common medical causes of acute external fluid loss are:

- upper gastrointestinal bleeding
- severe diarrhoea and vomiting
- diabetic ketoacidosis

Internal fluid loss is seen in:

- acute pancreatitis
- severe paralytic ileus

*Redistributive (low-resistance) shock*

Redistributive shock is due to the effect of circulating toxins disturbing the normal distribution of blood flow within the body. Some vessels, notably those in the skin, open up and provide little or no resistance to blood flow. Other vessels shut down in a pattern in which organs such as the kidney are starved of blood. In contrast to the other forms of shock, in redistributive shock the overall resistance to blood flow is reduced: the cardiac output is therefore high, the pulse is bounding and the peripheries are warm. The patient appears flushed and warm rather than grey and clammy. Without treatment, however, the progression is the same as that in other forms of shock – to kidney failure and to increasingly severe acidosis.

The main causes of redistributive shock are:

- sepsis, especially from gut and renal tract infections
- anaphylaxis

# ACUTE SEVERE HYPOTENSIVE COLLAPSE

Clinically, patients with shock present to the Acute Medical Unit as a problem of acute severe hypotensive collapse. Given this clinical situation, there are five groups of conditions to consider:

1. cardiorespiratory collapse (→ Case 1 in Case Studies 10.1)
2. massive pulmonary embolus
3. septicaemia (→ Case 2 in Case Studies 10.1)
4. hypovolaemia (→ Case 3 in Case Studies 10.1)
5. anaphylaxis

## IMPORTANCE OF IMMEDIATE RESUSCITATION

Resuscitation from hypotensive collapse is frequently inadequate on the Acute Medical Unit and instituted too late. Several problems can arise:

## CASE STUDIES 10.1

### CASE 1

A 70-year-old woman is admitted with collapse.

#### Initial observations

She is coughing frothy sputum and cannot lie flat. She has pulse 160 beats/min, blood pressure 90/60 mmHg, saturations 80%, respiratory rate 35 breaths/min, and temperature 37.4°C.

- This is pulmonary oedema due to acute heart failure – cardiorespiratory collapse
- She needs to be sat up and given immediate oxygen
- Her low blood pressure and high pulse are due to the heart problem

### CASE 2

An 80-year-old man with a urinary catheter is admitted with confusion and rigors.

#### Initial observations

He is hot and delirious, with rigors. He has pulse 115 beats/min, blood pressure 70/40 mmHg, saturations 82%, respiratory rate 30 breaths/min, and temperature 38.5°C.

- This is septicaemic shock
- He needs urgent oxygen, i.v. fluids and immediate antibiotics
- Progress can be judged from the blood pressure and urine output

### CASE 3

A 50-year-old man has collapsed after vomiting a large amount of fresh blood.

#### Initial observations

He is cold, clammy and very restless. He has pulse 130 beats/min, blood pressure 100/50 mmHg lying and unrecordable on sitting, saturations 88%, respiratory rate 40 breaths/min, and temperature 36.5°C.

- This is hypovolaemic shock
- He needs urgent oxygen, a large cannula, rapid i.v. fluids then blood
- Progress can be judged from the falling pulse rate and increasing blood pressure

- there are delays before the patients are first seen
- priority may not be given to the sickest patients
- abnormalities in the basic vital signs – *oxygen saturation* and *blood pressure* – are not corrected
- the results of urgent investigations are either not seen or ignored

These deficiencies in the first critical hours of admission have an impact on the patient's chance of recovery, especially, as in Case Study 10.2, where there

---

**CASE STUDY 10.2**

A patient came in at 13.30 h and was clerked in at 16.30 h. Although the nursing notes record a blood pressure of 90/40 mmHg, this is not recorded in the doctor's clerking. Blood gases were taken on admission, but the results were not recorded in the notes. The chest X-ray showed a right upper lobe pneumonia.

At 19.30 h the registrar was asked to see the patient because of persistent hypotension. A blood pressure of 60/40 mmHg was noted, as were the abnormal blood gases and a high creatinine (indicating a renal problem). Intensive i.v. fluids were started.

The patient had a central line put in at 01.30 h, 12 h after admission, and was transferred to the ITU. Noradrenaline was needed to restore the blood pressure. By the second day, the whole of the right upper lobe had consolidated due to the rapid progression of pneumococcal pneumonia. The pneumococcus bacterium was grown in two sets of blood cultures taken on admission.

---

is sepsis. Once the condition deteriorates to septic shock, the mortality rate approaches 50%. In this case, the priority should have been to correct the oxygen saturation and try and restore a blood pressure within the first half hour of admission. The admitting nurse and doctor must share their information from the initial assessments in order to draw up an effective management plan. There are critical time intervals between the admission and the first:

- dose of antibiotics
- treatment with oxygen
- initiation of i.v. fluids
- correction of the blood pressure

*Resuscitation of the patient with hypotensive collapse*

It is important to identify the patient who needs a high priority for resuscitation. This is done by the triage system, ABCDE. In these critically ill patients, resuscitation will commence before the full diagnosis is apparent.

**Rapid assessment in the critically ill: the importance of ABCDE**

*AB: the airway and breathing.* If the patient can respond appropriately to 'Are you okay?', then it can be assumed that the blood is reaching the brain and that the upper airway is clear.

*Look.* A respiratory rate of < 8 breaths/min (depressed respiration) or > 20 breaths/min suggests a serious problem.

- Remember that an increased respiratory rate is seen in any cause of shock, even if the lungs are normal.
- Measure the oxygen saturation: a level below 90% indicates severe hypoxia.

- Does breathing look like hard work or is the patient tired and losing interest?
- Does this look like acute asthma?

In LVF, the patient will be sitting upright and coughing frothy sputum.

***Listen.*** Gurgling indicates aspiration and needs urgent aspiration of the mouth and oropharynx (attempting to aspirate the larynx or trachea may trigger laryngospasm) with a rigid Yankauer suction catheter.

- A crowing sound or a harsh inspiratory stridor suggests acute upper airway obstruction, which is seen in acute epiglottitis or severe tonsillitis
- Snoring suggests an unsafe airway and is seen in coma or stroke
- Wheezing occurs in COPD, asthma, LVF and massive pulmonary embolus

***Feel.*** A finger sweep may be needed to clear an airway or obstruction. Well-fitting dentures can be left, as they will make it easier to apply a mask and maintain an airway.

*C: The circulation.* An impalpable pulse suggests a systolic blood pressure of less than 80 mmHg. Hypotension is the major finding in shock and, if severe, will be associated with an increased respiratory rate, anxiety and confusion due to reduced blood flow to the brain. Other features of a low blood pressure will be cool and clammy skin, reduced capillary refill and a low hourly urine output (< 0.5 ml/kg per hour). Capillary refill time provides an important assessment of the state of the circulation: after digital pressure has been applied to a finger tip for 5 s, the capillaries should refill in less than 2 s – a delay indicates an impaired circulation and is a useful sign, especially in hypovolaemic shock.

   *Important: An increased pulse rate may only appear as a late sign of shock, especially in otherwise fit young patients, and occasionally the response to a major internal bleed may be a slowing of the pulse. An increase in respiratory rate is frequently the first sign in shock.*

*D: Disability.* Check the consciousness level quickly using the AVPU score (*a*lert, responding to *v*oice/*p*ain, *u*nresponsive; → Chapter 4: Acute neurological problems; p. 104). Use the GCS for a later more detailed assessment if the conscious level is impaired.

   Shocked patients are restless and often uncooperative due to impaired circulation to the brain.

*E: Exposure.* Examine for sites of infection, sites of soft tissue damage and for the characteristic rash of meningococcal septicaemia. Shock complicated by extensive bruising suggests DIC, in which clotting becomes deranged. A leg swollen from the ankle to the groin would suggest an extensive iliofemoral DVT and a possible pulmonary embolus. Anaphylaxis is associated with an urticarial rash and swelling of the face, lips and tongue.

## Common examples of the critically ill

*Cardiac arrhythmia.* A man comes in with very rapid atrial fibrillation and hypotension after suffering a painless myocardial infarction at home.

*Massive pulmonary embolus.* An obese woman in her 20s collapses with breathlessness, syncope and hypotension a week after a caesarean section.

*Anaphylaxis.* A young man with nut allergy collapses with wheeze and hypotension after inadvertently consuming peanuts during a Chinese meal.

*Gastrointestinal bleed.* A man in his 40s vomits a pint of fresh blood and passes a large melaena stool. He comes in with hypotensive collapse.

*Acute abdomen.* A woman aged 35 years, known to have gallstones, comes in with a 12-h history of increasing abdominal pain, hypotension and signs of acute pancreatitis.

*Septicaemia.* An elderly lady has a week's history of vomiting and diarrhoea and is admitted to hospital with hypotension and renal failure. Her blood cultures yield *Salmonella*.

*Pneumonia.* A 35-year-old man becomes increasingly breathless and confused during an influenza epidemic. He is hypotensive and hypoxic. The chest film shows pneumonia.

*Soft tissue infection.* A 60-year-old woman with multiple sclerosis is admitted with hypotension and drowsiness. She has necrotic infected sacral pressure sores and positive blood cultures.

**Recognition of a deteriorating patient.** Chapter 1 outlined the basis of using simple nursing observations in scoring systems which can be used to recognise the patient who is deteriorating and is at risk. The scores are used to document clinical progress and to trigger corrective measures, particularly through the involvement of Critical Care Outreach Teams.

The assessment aims to recognise what is initially reversible that, unless corrected, will progress to:

1. persistent hypotension
2. increasing acidosis
3. kidney failure
4. cardiorespiratory failure
5. cardiorespiratory arrest

Box 10.2 summarises the clinical findings that need urgent attention on the Acute Medical Unit.

*Critical nursing tasks in assessing hypotensive collapse*
**Maintain the safety of the patient.** Secure the airway and maintain oxygenation.

---

**Box 10.2 – What needs immediate action in the Acute Medical Unit**

*N.B. Patients who have a cardiac arrest often go through a warning period of unrecognised deterioration in their vital signs.*

**Threats to the airway**
- Impending obstruction: anaphylaxis with swollen tongue, epiglottitis
- Unsafe airway: impaired consciousness level or stroke

**Respiratory failure**
- Respiratory arrest
- Respiratory rate low (< 8 breaths/min) or very high (> 30 breaths/min)
- Poor arterial gases: $pO_2$ less than 8.0 kPa on at least 60% oxygen
  $pCO_2$ more than 6.5 kPa
  pH less than 7.2

**Circulatory failure**
- Pulse less than 40 or greater than 140 beats/min
- Systolic blood pressure less than 90 mmHg
- Urine output (i.e. circulation to the kidneys) of less than 30 ml/h

**Falling level of consciousness**
- GCS of less than 12 or a fall of 2 or more

---

**Measure the respiratory rate and the oxygen saturations.** Choose the most appropriate oxygen delivery system to bring the saturations above 90%. When there is doubt, administer continuous high-flow oxygen at 15 L/min through a tight-fitting mask with a reservoir bag. The doctors will do urgent blood gas measurements to:

- assess the adequacy of the oxygen therapy
- look at the degree of acidosis (low pH and low bicarbonate)
- use the $CO_2$ levels as a measure of adequate ventilation
- measure the blood lactate levels (high) as evidence of poor overall tissue perfusion

*These critical results must be communicated to the medical staff.*

**Measure the radial and apical pulse rates.** If the pulse is weak, use the monitor or an ECG trace. Rapid atrial fibrillation will give a deficit between the apical and radial pulses.

**Measure the lying blood pressure and look for any postural decrease.** Hypotension will, in general, require i.v. fluid replacement or drugs to support the heart. A patient with a systolic blood pressure of less than 90 mmHg will show signs of reduced blood flow to the brain – restlessness, confusion and a reduced conscious level. Reduced blood flow to the kidneys results in reduced hourly urine output.

**Ensure large-bore venous access.** Venous access must be obtained immediately, as the priority in shock is often the need for urgent fluid replacement.

**Obtain an immediate 12-lead ECG.** This will exclude myocardial infarction and acute arrhythmias as the cause of the hypotension.

## CRITICAL NURSING TASKS IN ASSESSING HYPOTENSIVE COLLAPSE

- Maintain the safety of the patient
- Measure the respiratory rate and oxygen saturations
- Measure the radial and apical pulse rates
- Measure the lying blood pressure and look for any postural decrease
- Ensure large-bore venous access
- Obtain an immediate 12-lead ECG
- Keep the relatives on the ward

**Keep the relatives on the ward.** You may require urgent information concerning:

- the recent history (in the elderly, any sudden deterioration can be due to sepsis)
- previous health and levels of dependence, history of substance or alcohol abuse
- details of medications and allergies
- information to inform future discussions regarding resuscitation status

*Important nursing tasks in assessing hypotensive collapse*
**Monitor the heart.** For the best trace, use adhesive electrodes placed over bony prominences. The skin should be shaved and cleaned with alcohol. The red electrode should be placed below the right clavicle, the yellow one in the same position on the left, and the green electrode below the left rib margin.

**Assess the site and severity of any pain.** Examples of pain in sudden hypotensive collapse are:

- severe chest pain: myocardial infarction or pulmonary embolus
- severe abdominal pain: perforation/acute pancreatitis/leaking abdominal aneurysm

**Reassure the patient about the management plan and initiate symptom relief**

- Make sure that you supply adequate analgesia. There is no place for withholding analgesia on the basis that it may mask the development of complications – pain needs pain relief
- Relieve breathlessness: give oxygen and sit the patient up if he wishes (unless hypovolaemic)
- Ensure the mask is comfortable and tight-fitting and that the patient understands that he is to keep it on
- Prepare the patient for possible further procedures:
  — blood gas sampling (wrist arterial puncture)
  — central venous line placement (via internal jugular or subclavian veins)
  — urinary catheterisation
  — further tests (endoscopy, CT, ultrasound). It is critical that resuscitative measures are not compromised while the patient is off the ward

---

### IMPORTANT NURSING TASKS IN ASSESSING HYPOTENSIVE COLLAPSE

- **Monitor the heart**
- **Assess the site and severity of any pain**
- **Reassure the patient about the management plan and initiate symptom relief**
- **Explain**
- **Speak to the relatives**
- **Access further information**

---

**Explain.** Explain what has gone wrong and what will be the signs of improvement, e.g.:

| | |
|---|---|
| Acute LVF: | less dyspnoeic, falling pulse, good diuresis |
| Upper gastrointestinal bleeding: | less thirsty, less light-headed, no further vomiting, clearing of melaena |

**Speak to the relatives**

- Explain what they will see: drips, monitors, urinary catheters, masks
- Explain the management plan
- Explain the signs of improvement or deterioration
- Forewarn the relatives that the patient may need to be transferred to an HDU/ITU

**Access further information.** Obtain the previous hospital records and any previous laboratory results urgently.

An example of the immediate management of hypotensive collapse in a man with abdominal pain is given in Case Study 10.3.

---

**CASE STUDY 10.3** Hypotensive collapse

A 30-year-old man was admitted with a 3-day history of upper abdominal pain. He was reluctant to give many details and denied any significant past history, but he was clearly in considerable discomfort and was very agitated. His wife was with him and added that he had been drinking a litre of strong cider a day for several years and that, 6 months previously, he had been investigated for alcohol-related liver damage and told that he should stop drinking for good.

Initial assessment was of a wasted man lying restlessly in bed with severe upper abdominal pain. His GCS was 15 but he scored only 7/10 on an abbreviated mental test score. His respiratory rate was 30 breaths/min and oxygen saturations 88%. His pulse rate was regular at 120 and his blood pressure was 90/70 mmHg lying and 70/50 mmHg sitting up. On general exposure there was scattered bruising and he appeared moderately jaundiced. His abdomen was distended, tense and silent but only moderately tender. The BM stix was satisfactory at 7.0 mmol/L.

1. He was given high-flow oxygen at 60% with immediate improvements in his saturation to 98%
2. Venous access was obtained with difficulty and blood was taken for:
   — FBC – to look for bleeding (low Hb) and infection (high white cell count)
   — platelets – he is bruised, and alcoholics have low platelet counts
   — biochemistry:
     • to check for dehydration (U&E)
     • to exclude acute pancreatitis
     • to check the liver function tests
   — Clotting – bruising can indicate a serious coagulation disturbance
3. Arterial blood gases were taken to look at the oxygen level and to identify acidosis (a common problem resulting from hypotension in the setting of an acute serious illness)
4. While awaiting initial results a small dose of i.v. opiates was administered to provide immediate pain relief and he was reassured that further analgesia would be available once the test results had been seen.

The investigations showed a very high amylase (1500 IU), abnormal liver function and early kidney failure. Combined with the clinical assessment the overall picture was of acute pancreatitis complicated by *redistributive shock*:

• hypotension
• confusion
• hypoxia
• poor kidney function due to hypotension

**Basic management plan**
• Administer continuous oxygen immediately
• Provide effective analgesia

*(continued)*

**CASE STUDY 10.3** (continued)

- Bring up the blood pressure urgently
  - assess the i.v. fluid requirements with a central venous pressure line
  - administer sufficient i.v. fluid to bring the CVP up to 15 cmH$_2$O of water
  - if this does not bring up the blood pressure consider *inotropic support*
- Use the urine output to assess the response to the improved blood pressure (catheter)
- Rest the gastrointestinal tract with nasogastric intubation on free drainage

### Nursing observations to monitor the response

- Hourly urine output to aim at > 50 ml/h
- Hourly pulse
- Hourly blood pressure
- Hourly pain score
- 2-hourly oxygen saturations
- 2-hourly temperature (shock, central lines and the underlying disease can all lead to sepsis)
- Careful charting of input and output
- Continuous cardiac monitoring

In this man's case the initial urine output was 10 ml in the first 3 h, in spite of vigorous fluid replacement, and his blood pressure remained low. He was therefore started on i.v. dopamine at 5 μg/kg per min. His blood pressure responded, followed after 2 h by an increase in his urine output.

*When do we use dopamine, dobutamine and noradrenaline in patients with shock?*

The priority in shock is to maintain the circulation by normalising the blood pressure. The key to this is to give adequate i.v. fluids. This may require several litres in the first 24 h but if, after 2 or 3 L, the blood pressure remains low, the next stage is to use i.v. inotropes: drugs that directly increase the blood pressure and improve the blood flow to the kidneys.

**Which one to use?**

*Dopamine.* Dopamine is used in the range 2–20 mg/kg per min. At the lower dose it acts to improve kidney perfusion (although the clinical value of this is questionable), in the mid range it also begins to stimulate the heart, and at the higher doses it begins to constrict peripheral arteries to produce additional beneficial effects on the blood pressure. It is the most widely used 'general-purpose' inotrope. It is usual to start with the lower dose and increase accordingly.

*Dobutamine.* Dobutamine only stimulates the heart and tends to be reserved for cardiogenic shock.

*Noradrenaline.* In the range 0.5–5 mg/kg per min, noradrenaline has a marked effect on the peripheral vessels and will bring up the blood pressure, but it does not stimulate the heart. It is the drug of choice in septic shock.

### How to monitor their effectiveness

- The blood pressure
- The mental state (brain blood flow)
- The hourly urine output (kidney blood flow), which should be kept above 0.5 ml/kg per h
- The blood lactate levels (lactate levels fall as tissue perfusion improves)

There are two adverse effects that must be identified:

1. if the vasoconstrictor effect on the peripheral vessels is too strong, the patient can develop ischaemic tips to their fingers and toes, i.e. fixed blue/black discolouration
2. the cardiac stimulation can lead to marked tachycardia and then arrhythmias: these patients need close cardiac monitoring

## ENSURING ADEQUATE OXYGEN DELIVERY TO VITAL ORGANS: MAINTAINING THE OXYGEN SATURATION AND THE BLOOD PRESSURE

*Oxygen therapy*

The main indications for emergency oxygen therapy are:

- oxygen saturations of less than 90%
- systolic blood pressure of less than 100 mmHg
- respiratory distress (respiratory rate of more than 20 breaths/min)
- cardiac or respiratory arrest
- acidosis on blood gas results

There is understandable anxiety about the correct dose of oxygen in patients with COPD, but in general the problem in acutely ill medical patients is not giving too much oxygen, but in giving too little. *The aim, whatever the circumstances, should be to give sufficient oxygen to raise the oxygen saturation above 90%.* Oxygen is a drug and should be prescribed – the prescription should specify the mask, the flow rate and, in the case of the Venturi mask, the oxygen concentration. A target oxygen saturation should also be specified. The different techniques of oxygen administration are illustrated in Fig. 10.2.

### Oxygen masks

- **High-flow (Venturi) masks** – these give fixed percentages of oxygen from 24% to 60%, depending on the property of the individual mask and the flow rate that is used. Masks are colour-coded and the appropriate flow rate is clearly marked on each mask. Thus a green Venturi valve delivers

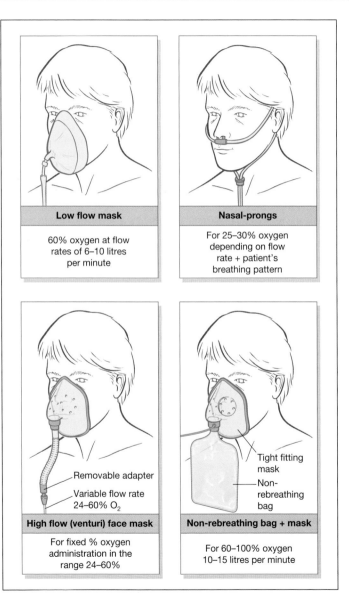

**Fig. 10.2** Techniques of oxygen administration

60% oxygen when the flow rate is 12 L/min, a blue valve delivers 24% when the flow rate is 2 L/min. Venturi masks are used when the oxygen concentration has to be precise, such as in the patient with unstable COPD (24% or 28%) or one with severe asthma (60%).

- **Low-flow masks** (simple oxygen masks, Hudson masks, MC masks) – these provide 60% oxygen at flow rates of 6–10 L/min, but underperform at rates of less than 5 L/min. These masks are suitable for most situations in which emergency oxygen is needed.
- **Nasal prongs** – the percentage of oxygen delivered by nasal prongs at 2 L/min is between 25% and 30%. Nasal prongs are less intrusive than masks and tend to be better tolerated in uncooperative patients, but oxygen delivery may be inadequate for a critically ill patient.
- **Non-rebreathing mask with reservoir bag** – Depending on their fit, these masks can administer from 60% to 100% oxygen with flow rates set at 15 L/min. Proper use requires some expertise because the mask must fit tightly, the reservoir bag must be filled before the patient starts to breathe and the flow rate requires adjustment to ensure the bag remains at least half full throughout the respiratory cycle. Non-rebreathing masks with reservoir bags are used in the critically ill to correct severe hypoxia.

### The blood pressure

There are two main reasons why the blood pressure can suddenly fall in the critically ill. First, the heart may start to fail as a pump – examples would be an acute myocardial infarction or the toxic effects of septicaemia. Secondly, there may not be enough fluid returning to the heart to fill it sufficiently; examples would be rapid blood or fluid loss or the sudden loss of vascular tone seen in overwhelming sepsis. Improving the circulation of the blood by restoring the blood pressure is as important as correcting the amount of oxygen contained in it. It is critical to ensure there is sufficient circulating volume to carry any additional oxygen to the tissues. If there is hypotension and evidence of inadequate tissue perfusion – notably oliguria, poor capillary refill and impaired conscious level – *an urgent challenge with 500–1000 ml of i.v. saline should be considered.*

### When is a central line used?

- To assess the state of the circulation from the central venous pressure
- To gain access to major veins:
  — when there is no peripheral access
  — for administration of irritant infusions or drugs, e.g. dopamine and amiodarone
- To insert a temporary pacemaker

**Inserting a central venous line: subclavian and internal jugular venous cannulation.** These are the two preferred sites for inserting central venous lines. Placement involves the Seldinger technique, in which the vein is first cannulated with a needle, through which is pushed a guide wire. The needle is removed, leaving the wire in place, and then the cannula is fed into the vein over the guide wire, which itself is then withdrawn. Success rates have improved and complications are less common with the use of portable ultrasound machines to locate the central veins before cannulation.

*The procedure*

1. Are the results of clotting studies available to the operator?
2. This is a sterile procedure: masks, gowns, drapes, gloves and full skin preparation are required.
3. 2% aqueous chlorhexidine is more effective as a skin disinfectant than povidone–iodine
4. The patient must be 20° head-down to prevent air entering the cannula (air embolus) during insertion.
5. The operator must check the trolley and packs before starting the procedure.
6. The infusion should be run through and ready.
7. If a multi-lumen catheter is inserted, the staff must be pre-briefed about its correct use.
8. Decide beforehand what dressings are to be used to secure the site.
9. Explain and reassure the patient (and the relatives) about the procedure:
   — the rationale for needing a central line
   — the fact that it is a routine method of monitoring/administering certain treatments
   — local anaesthetic will be used
   — the doctor will provide an appropriate level of information on the benefits and risks
   — it would be normal practice to obtain written consent if the patient is well enough.

*Complications.* The two main complications are puncturing the lung and puncturing an artery. Pneumothorax is much more common with cannulation of the subclavian vein. The approach is from below the clavicle and the route into the vein skirts the apex of the lung. There must *always* be a post-procedure chest film, which *must* be seen and interpreted by the person who put the line in or his or her designated deputy (lines tend to be put in at the end of work shifts). If a patient deteriorates acutely with breathlessness or hypotension immediately after the procedure, it is important to consider a pneumothorax. Arterial bleeding is more likely during internal jugular vein cannulation, as the carotid artery is adjacent to the point of entry. Such bleeding is not dangerous, but it will need 10 min firm digital pressure before it will stop.

**The central venous pressure.** The CVP is a simple measurement that gives important information about the overall state of the circulation, and specifically about the degree of hydration. The measurement is taken from the height of a vertical column of fluid that is in free communication with a central venous catheter (→ Figs 10.3 and 10.4). If the patient is lying flat, the reference point from which the measurement is made is in the mid-axillary line at a point vertically below the sternal angle. This coincides with the position of the right atrium.

The normal central venous pressure is from 0 to + 8 cmH$_2$O

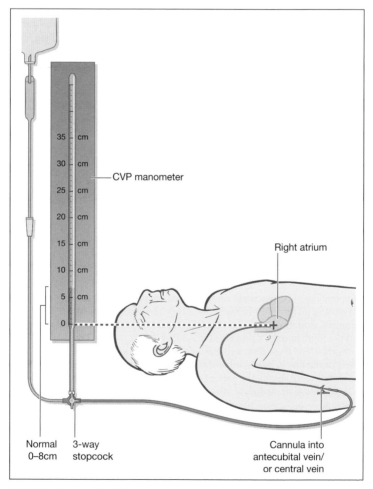

**Fig. 10.3** Measuring the CVP

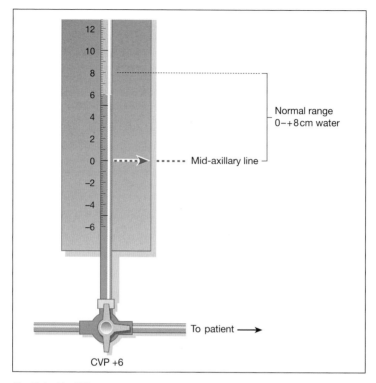

**Fig. 10.4**   The CVP manometer

The central venous pressure is abnormally high in congestive cardiac failure and in overtransfusion; it is too low in hypovolaemic and septic shock, in which values of –3 cmH$_2$O or less will be found.

In a sick patient with a low blood pressure, the CVP provides invaluable information on the fluid requirements, which may not be obvious from simple observation. In particular, patients who are septic tend to be dehydrated:

- they have a poor intake
- they have been sweating
- the respiratory rate is increased, so there is increased respiratory fluid loss
- patients with sepsis often have diarrhoea

In these patients, a fluid challenge can be given with confidence if there is a combination of hypotension and a low CVP. Conversely, if the blood pressure is low but the CVP is high, the cause may be cardiac and a fluid challenge would be inappropriate.

*Fluid challenge*

Hypovolaemia is the most likely cause of hypotension (systolic blood pressure < 90 mmHg) in the critically ill patient and in these circumstances, once the airway is secured and oxygen saturations are corrected, the circulating volume is expanded using relatively large amounts of fluid over a short period of time. The term 'fluid challenge' applies to the combination of aggressive volume expansion and a careful assessment of its effect on the patient. Either a crystalloid (500–1000 ml of isotonic saline or 5% dextrose) or a colloid (300–500 ml of polygeline [Haemaccel]) is given over 30 min and if necessary repeated. The response is evaluated using the vital signs, capillary refill, and urine output. The patient is observed for signs of fluid overload: overfilling of the neck veins (increased JVP), and new-onset breathlessness with wheezing and crackles (pulmonary oedema) at the lung bases.

## WHICH CRITICALLY ILL PATIENTS MAY NEED TRANSFER TO INTENSIVE CARE/HDU?

- **When there is a threat to the safety of the airway** – this may be due to a poor conscious level or due to a local inability to protect the airway, such as respiratory muscle weakness with a feeble cough.
- **When there has been a respiratory arrest** – these patients remain at marked risk until the underlying problem (pneumonia, asthma, etc.) has been treated.
- **A respiratory rate of less than 8 or more than 40 breaths/min** – extremes of respiratory rate indicate severe illness with impending cardiorespiratory arrest.
- **Oxygen saturations that remain less than 90% in spite of at least 50% oxygen by mask** – these patients will need extra respiratory support, possibly even intubation and ventilation of the lungs.
- **After a cardiac arrest** – particularly if the arrest was in the setting of a critically ill patient rather than as a 'simple' early complication of an acute myocardial infarction.
- **A pulse rate of less than 40 or greater than 140 beats/min in spite of treatment** – this can be evidence of circulatory failure, although clearly straightforward uncontrolled atrial fibrillation would not come into this category.
- **A systolic blood pressure that stays below 90 mmHg in spite of fluid replacement** – this suggests established shock and may need support with inotropic drugs.
- **An unexpected and sudden fall in the conscious level** – (a fall in GCS of more than 2 points). This may be a manifestation of falling cerebral blood flow due to persistent shock.
- **Increasing arterial carbon dioxide tension with acidosis** – deteriorating blood gases in spite of treatment is a warning of impending respiratory arrest

- Any patient giving cause for concern in whom there is a reasonable expectation of recovery

## SURVIVING SEPSIS

There is increasing concern about the rising incidence of severe sepsis as a cause of critical illness and the very high associated mortality – approaching 40% in the UK – some of which can be reversed with better early resuscitation, particularly in the first 6 h of admission. The key is to recognise:

- significant sepsis-induced tissue under-perfusion
- increased respiratory rate
- hypotension
- increased blood lactate levels

Once sepsis is recognised, initial therapy with aggressive fluid challenge, oxygen, early antibiotics and if necessary dobutamine/noradrenaline will significantly improve the outlook.

## ANAPHYLACTIC SHOCK

Anaphylaxis is the term used for a severe generalised allergic reaction. Allergic diseases in general are on the increase, and a growing number of acute anaphylactic reactions are now being seen – often in patients with a history of asthma.

The most common causes are:

- foods, especially nuts
- insect stings
- drugs, especially antibiotics, aspirin and ACE inhibitors
- latex allergy, especially in health-care workers

From 5 min to an hour after exposure, the patient develops a generalised reaction with swelling, redness and itch. In cases of oral ingestion in food allergy, the swelling usually starts in the mouth and tongue and progresses to upper airway obstruction. The time course depends on the route of exposure: it may take 30 min for latex to be absorbed sufficiently by the skin to trigger a reaction. Occasionally, the delay from exposure to reaction is as long as 6 h, or there may be an early reaction that clears, to be followed by a delayed reaction 1–2 days later.

The two potentially fatal complications are:

- airway obstruction (laryngeal obstruction and an asthmatic reaction; → Case Study 10.4)
- circulatory collapse (severe hypotension with syncope)

**CASE STUDY 10.4**  Acute anaphylaxis due to nut allergy

Ten minutes after finishing a bowl of cereal, a 30-year-old woman developed sudden itching and discomfort in her throat. Within a further few minutes there was a generalised itchy red blotchy rash and she started to wheeze. She felt faint and collapsed on the kitchen floor. Her husband dialled 999.

In casualty she was still wheezy and distressed, with a widespread urticarial rash. She was given i.v. piriton, hydrocortisone and nebulised salbutamol, and admitted to hospital.

On admission to the Acute Medical Unit, the following initial assessment was made:

### ABCDE: the safety of the patient

- The patient was drowsy, but responding to the spoken voice
- The face, lips and tongue were swollen and the voice was hoarse
- The patient was having difficulty in swallowing her saliva
- There was a loud harsh wheeze
- The oxygen saturation was 85% on air and respiratory rate was 35 breaths/min
- Pulse was 105 beats/min, with a lying blood pressure of 75/40 mmHg
- There was a widespread raised urticarial rash

The assessment was of acute anaphylaxis with impending upper airway obstruction (unable to swallow, swollen tongue, voice change). There was bronchospasm, hypoxaemia and circulatory collapse.

### Management

The patient already had venous access. High-flow 60% oxygen was given. Intramuscular adrenaline, 0.5 ml of 1:1000 (0.5 mg), was administered immediately. This was followed by i.v. chlorpheniramine and hydrocortisone. A litre of isotonic saline was given over 30 min, followed by 1 L over 1 h.

The recovery was uneventful, but the patient was referred on to the allergy service as a case of probable nut allergy, was fully assessed and advised appropriately before discharge. She now wears a Medicalert bracelet and carries an EpiPen to self-administer adrenaline should it be necessary.

---

### Box 10.3 – Emergency treatment of anaphylaxis

- Intramuscular adrenaline 0.5 ml of 1:1000 (0.5 mg or 500 μg)
- Intravenous chlorpheniramine 10 mg
- Intravenous hydrocortisone 200 mg
- Intravenous fluids
- Oxygen

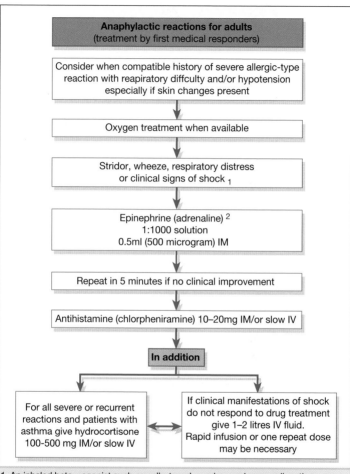

**Anaphylactic reactions for adults**
(treatment by first medical responders)

Consider when compatible history of severe allergic-type reaction with reapiratory diffculty and/or hypotension especially if skin changes present

Oxygen treatment when available

Stridor, wheeze, respiratory distress or clinical signs of shock 1

Epinephrine (adrenaline) 2
1:1000 solution
0.5ml (500 microgram) IM

Repeat in 5 minutes if no clinical improvement

Antihistamine (chlorpheniramine) 10–20mg IM/or slow IV

**In addition**

For all severe or recurrent reactions and patients with asthma give hydrocortisone 100-500 mg IM/or slow IV

If clinical manifestations of shock do not respond to drug treatment give 1–2 litres IV fluid. Rapid infusion or one repeat dose may be necessary

1. An inhaled beta$_2$-agonist such as salbutamol may be used as an adjunctive measure if bronchospasm is severe and does not respond rapidly to other treatment.
2. If profound shock judged immediately life threatening give CPR/ALS if necessary. Consider slow IV epinephrine (adrenaline) 1:10 000 solution. This is hazardous and is recommended only for an experienced practitioner who can also obtain IV access without delay. Note the different strength of epinephrine (adrenaline) that may be required for IV use.
3. If adults are treated with an adrenaline auto-injector, the 300 micrograms will usually be sufficient. A second dose may be required. Half doses of adrenaline (epinephrine) may be safer for patients on amitriptyline, imipramine or beta blocker.
4. A crystalloid may be safer than a colloid.

**Fig. 10.5** Algorithm for the emergency management of anaphylaxis

*Management of anaphylactic shock (→ Box 10.3, Fig. 10.5)*
*Intramuscular adrenaline.* Adrenaline is the most important part of the management and must be given early. It is important to be familiar with the different preparations of adrenaline and to understand that in anaphylaxis the preferred route is intramuscularly and *NOT* subcutaneous or intravenous – and that the dose is *NOT* 'one ampoule' but 0.5 ml of 1:1000 strength adrenaline.

*Intravenous adrenaline?* Severe bronchospasm, increasing upper airway obstruction or continuing hypotension are indications for the careful use of i.v. adrenaline. The adrenaline is diluted to 1:100 000 and infused at 10–20 mg/min.

*Oxygen.* The patients are hypoxic and shocked.

*Fluids.* Intravenous fluids and adrenaline should restore the blood pressure.

*Bronchodilators.* Patients can die from the asthmatic component of the anaphylactic reaction: treatment is with nebulised salbutamol or, in the critically ill, i.v. aminophylline.

*Antihistamines.* This will clear the rash and the itch.

*Steroids.* Steroids will not have an immediate effect, but will help any asthmatic component and prevent a prolonged or delayed response.

*Prevention.* There must be effective education in allergen avoidance and good control of any underlying asthma by optimising the use of prophylactic anti-inflammatory treatment with inhaled steroids. Many patients with food allergy are supplied with adrenaline auto-injectors (EpiPen) and trained in their use.

## ANSWERING RELATIVES' QUESTIONS IN SHOCK

*What do you mean by shock?* This is not the same as emotional shock. By shock, we mean a drastic change in the overall function of the body due to a fall in the patient's blood pressure. The kidneys are not producing enough urine to flush out waste products, and the brain is at risk of being starved of oxygen.

*What is the cause?* The most common cause is dehydration due to blood loss or loss of other body fluids. Two other common causes are shock complicating a heart attack and shock complicating an overwhelming infection.

*What else can go wrong?* The damage to some of the organs could become more serious. The kidneys and lungs are at particular risk and we are paying particular attention to these.

*How are you treating the main causes?* We are using drugs and intravenous fluids to try and keep the blood pressure up. The extra oxygen is to make up for the problems with the circulation. We are giving antibiotics to combat infection and we are replacing any lost blood or body fluids.

*How will we know that he is going to recover?* Within 24–48 h of starting treatment we should see a general improvement: less drowsiness, a better urine output and an increase in the blood pressure. Any fever should start to fall and you may see that we are easing off on the drugs and the intensity of the nursing observations.

*What can we do to help?* It is reassuring to have somebody familiar at hand particularly if, as commonly happens in shock, there is an element of confusion. Try and keep him calm. Keep the oxygen mask in place and explain what it is for. Keep visitors down to a few very close relatives, because for the first 48 h there will be a lot of clinical activity going on in the form of observations, changing drip bags, administering drugs and so forth.

# EMERGENCY BLOOD TRANSFUSION IN SHOCK

There are two main indications for transfusion on the Acute Medical Unit: acute blood loss and to improve oxygen transport in patients with anaemia.

- **Acute blood loss** – this is the most common indication and may require massive transfusion, with its associated risks
- **Improving oxygen transport in patients with anaemia** – this is of uncertain benefit in the acute situation unless the haemoglobin levels are particularly low – probably down to less than half normal

Transfusion is often regarded with suspicion by patients and their relatives. This has been exacerbated by the recent discovery that two patients have developed new variant CJD transmitted in blood from infected donors. Fortunately the risks associated with transfusion are surprisingly low. The chance of catching AIDS through transfusion is around 1 in a million. In fact they are 100 times more likely to be given the wrong blood (as a result of human error), but even this risk is extremely low. The most common reactions are minor febrile reactions and rashes that require symptomatic treatment and reassurance. The risks involved in blood transfusion are listed in Table 10.1.

It is important to reassure the patient and provide adequate information (if he is well enough to discuss it):

- indications for and purpose of the transfusion
- risks to the patient
- benefits to the patient
- the patient's right to refuse
- alternative treatments to transfusion
- a National Transfusion Service information leaflet should be given to the patient or relatives

**Table 10.1   Risks involved in blood transfusion**

| Risk / reaction | Risks per unit |
| --- | --- |
| Urticarial rash | 1 in 50 |
| Febrile reaction | 1 in 100 |
| Pulmonary oedema | 1 in 5000 |
| Wrong blood | 1 in 30 000 |
| Bacterial contamination | 1 in 50 000 |
| Hepatitis B | 1 in 100 000 |
| Hepatitis C | 1 in 200 000 |
| Major reaction | 1 in 600 000 |
| HIV | 1 in 3 000 000 |

## TRANSFUSION REACTIONS

*Clinical features and basic management*

It is important to monitor transfusion using a standard protocol. The patients must be told to report:

- shivering
- rashes
- flushing
- breathlessness
- loin and limb pains

The temperature, pulse and blood pressure are recorded before the start of the transfusion, after 15–20 min and at the end of delivery of each unit of blood. This information is recorded and dated separately from the routine observations. Most transfusion reactions start within 15 min of starting the blood, so the early observations are critical.

**Urticarial rashes.** Urticarial rashes may occur during transfusion. If the patient develops an acute allergic response to any protein in the donated blood product, urticaria, an intense itchy red eruption, will develop. It is more common with platelet transfusions or FFP than with whole blood. Urticaria is frightening for the patient, but not serious. The best treatment is i.v. chlorpheniramine 10 mg, an antihistamine. Provided that the reaction is not associated with major symptoms or changes in the pulse or blood pressure, the transfusion does not have to be stopped. The observations should be increased to hourly.

**Febrile reactions.** These may occur towards the end of a transfusion or within hours of its completion. The patient reacts against the white cells in the donated blood. It can be simply treated with paracetamol to bring the temperature down. If patients have had reactions before, they can be premedicated with antihistamines. Rarely, a patient can develop signs of septic shock during transfusion – hypotension, increased respiratory rate and a fever – which is due to bacterial contamination of the blood; platelet transfusions are the most likely to be contaminated.

**Pulmonary oedema.** This is not always due to overtransfusion – there is a form of acute transfusion-related lung injury that is a direct toxic effect of stored blood. The symptoms are the same as cardiac pulmonary oedema: increasing breathlessness, increased respiratory rate, tachycardia and hypoxia. Platelets and FFP are the most dangerous in this regard.

**Wrong blood.** Within the first few millilitres of the transfusion, a reaction may occur that is due to the patient rejecting the blood. Usually this is a case of AB blood being incorrectly given to an O group patient. It is vital to recognise this type of transfusion reaction.

*Nursing assessment to identify a severe transfusion reaction*
**When to suspect a reaction**

- Patient complains of symptoms
- The basic observations change (pulse, temperature and blood pressure)

**What action to take.** Any of the following may lead you to suspect a severe reaction:

- a reaction starts within minutes of the start of blood
- an error is discovered
- the patient develops acute loin or limb pain
- there is fever, hypotension and tachycardia

In this situation, it is imperative that you act.

1. Stop the blood and call a doctor.
2. Change the giving set and put up slow saline to keep the vein open.
3. Tell the blood bank and return the blood.
4. Start 15-min observations of pulse, blood pressure and temperature.
5. Observe volume and colour of any urine passed.

**Avoiding human error.** The most important risk in blood transfusion is that of simple human error leading to the administration of the wrong blood. The mistakes are predictable:

- when blood samples are taken for cross-matching they are mislabelled at the bedside
- the wrong blood is collected from the blood bank
- the blood is given to the wrong patient (identification bracelets must be fitted on admission)

It is important to work to defined protocols for taking blood for cross-matching, collecting the correct blood from the bank, receiving the correct blood on the ward and administering it to the correct patient.

*An example of good practice.* Take the transfusion request form to the patient.

1. Ask the patient to give their name and date of birth.
2. Confirm this with the identification bracelet.
3. Check these details and the hospital number with the form.
4. Take blood and then label the tube *at the bedside*, but not with an addressograph label.

Transfusion should start as soon as the blood is delivered to the ward. If blood has been out of the refrigerator for more than 30 min and is not about to be used, the hospital blood bank should be consulted and the blood returned.

The *bedside* check before the start of the transfusion is vital. There must be exact matches:

patient → blood transfusion compatibility report form → compatibility label on blood pack → prescription or fluid balance chart → medical notes

Keep the blood transfusion compatibility report form readily available during the transfusion, in case there is a reaction.

## MASSIVE BLOOD TRANSFUSION

Acute massive blood loss on the Acute Medical Unit is usually due to upper gastrointestinal bleeding. The term is usually used when a patient loses around half his blood volume (2–3 L) over 2–3 h. Surprisingly, there is a tendency to underestimate the total volume loss. Massive blood loss requires large-volume transfusions with cross-matched blood. In extreme life-or-death situations, blood from 'universal donors' – group O rhesus negative – can be used while awaiting the emergency cross-match (saline or polygeline [Haemaccel] may be used while awaiting blood).

The aim of emergency transfusion is:

- to normalise the blood pressure
- to maintain a urine output of at least 30 ml/h

Stored blood carries very little clotting factor, and so massive transfusion can lead to a clotting deficiency.

- Full clotting studies (platelet count, prothrombin time, KCCT and fibrinogen levels) must be checked before the start of the transfusion
- These are repeated after every 3 units of blood
- The prothrombin time and KCCT must be kept at no more than 1.5 times the normal value using FFP – probably 1 unit of FFP every 30 min for 4 units. (*Note*: FFP takes 30 min to thaw out)

- Platelets will need to be replaced after more than 20 units of blood
- Low fibrinogen levels will need correction with cryoprecipitate

Occasionally, rather than a clotting deficiency, massive transfusion triggers off spontaneous clotting within the small arteries and veins – this is DIC. There are five reversible factors that increase the risk of DIC and which are, to some extent, amenable to standard resuscitation measures:

- massive blood loss
- hypoxia
- hypovolaemia
- administration of excessively cold fluids
- failure to correct the clotting factors and platelets

# ACUTE RENAL FAILURE

To function, the kidneys require:

1. an adequate blood pressure
2. sufficient functioning glomeruli to filter the blood
3. intact renal tubules to reabsorb water and exchange electrolytes
4. an unobstructed urinary tract leading from the kidneys to the outside of the body

Fig. 10.6 summarises the basic mechanisms of acute renal failure.

In the Acute Medical Unit, problems with kidney function are commonly the result of an inadequate blood pressure – *pre-renal failure* – which occurs in the setting of acute fluid depletion. This will usually respond to fluid replacement.

Uncorrected pre-renal failure may progress to *acute tubular necrosis*. Acute tubular necrosis can also be the result of direct renal toxicity from drugs such as NSAIDs, from the products of acute muscle damage (rhabdomyolysis), and from sepsis.

Urinary tract *obstruction* is clearly important, because it is easy to treat and is a fully reversible cause of kidney failure.

Diseases of the glomeruli – acute *glomerulonephritis* – are rare causes of acute renal failure on the Acute Medical Unit, although they are important to recognise because the patients usually need specialist assessment and care.

While acute renal failure is an important clinical area, it is often handled with limited confidence on the Acute Medical Unit. Once a set of very abnormal kidney function tests comes back from the biochemistry laboratory, the tendency is to phone the renal unit and hope that they will take the problem over. This is unfortunate, because many of the cases are straightforward and will recover – with fluid replacement, with catheterisation, or simply with time – provided that immediate problems of electrolyte disturbance and fluid balance are addressed.

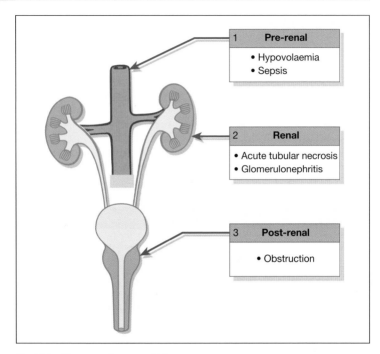

**Fig. 10.6**  The causes of acute renal failure

*Which patients are at particular risk from acute renal failure?*

- Patients with fluid depletion – severe diarrhoea, major upper gastrointestinal bleed
- Patients with septic shock
- Patients with a vulnerable blood supply to the kidneys – acute and chronic heart failure, vascular disease, hypertension
- Patients taking diuretics, NSAIDs, ACE inhibitors and those undergoing chemotherapy.
- Patients who already have chronic renal failure
- The elderly frail and those who have several medical conditions, particularly if those include diabetes and hypertension

*Illustrative case studies*
The following case studies (Case Studies 10.5–10.7) illustrate the typical presentation and immediate management of acute renal failure. The main features of emergency management of acute renal failure are summarised in Fig. 10.7.

## CASE STUDY 10.5  Rapid deterioration in severe pneumonia

A 34-year-old woman was admitted with a bilateral pneumonia. On admission, the temperature was 35.5°C, blood pressure 90/60 mmHg, pulse 100 beats/min and respiratory rate 15 breaths/min; the saturations were 90% on high-flow oxygen. On admission the WCC was $1.2 \times 10^9$/L, urea 10.7 mmol/L and creatinine 102 μmol/L. She was treated with fluids and antibiotics, but was markedly oliguric, passing less than 10 ml/h. Within 24 h her WCC had increased to $28.2 \times 10^9$/L, her urea had increased to 24.3 mmol/L and her creatinine was 259 μmol/L. Her respiratory rate increased to 25 breaths/min and she was transferred to the ITU with a view to ventilation.

## CASE STUDY 10.6  Renal tract obstruction

A 70-year-old woman was awoken in the early hours of the morning with severe constant pain in the right loin. This was described as being as severe as labour pain. Her pain persisted for 72 h, during which time she developed rigors and passed absolutely no urine. In the past she was known to have a chronically damaged left kidney from childhood infections.

She was admitted to hospital where she was found to be pyrexial and dehydrated, with a pulse rate of 110 beats/min and a blood pressure of 70/60 mmHg when lying. On palpating her abdomen, there was an enlarged tender right kidney. Investigations showed a high WCC ($15 \times 10^9$/L) and a low platelet count. There was mild renal insufficiency. An urgent ultrasound confirmed hydronephrosis (an obstructed kidney) due to a large stone blocking off the ureter.

She was treated with fluid replacement and i.v. antibiotics. Her subsequent management included an emergency nephrostomy to allow drainage of urine from the obstructed right kidney, followed some time later by surgical removal of the stone.

## CASE STUDY 10.7  Acute post-streptococcal glomerulonephritis presenting as oedema and cardiac failure

A 50-year-old man with a 2-week history of malaise was admitted because of swelling of his eyes and ankles. Three weeks previously he had had an acute sore throat.

On admission there was generalised oedema. His blood pressure was 202/114 mmHg. His ward urine testing was strongly positive for blood and protein. A subsequent MSU showed red cell casts.

His chest film showed mild pulmonary oedema. His creatinine was 128 μmol/L, urea 11.6mmol/L. The total 24-h urinary excretion of 1.14 g. His ASO titre was greater than 800 units/ml (indicative of a recent streptococcal infection).

He was treated with frusemide and fluid restriction. At follow-up 3 months later, his creatinine had fallen to 105 μmol/L, his urea to 6.9 mmol/L, and his blood pressure was normal. His urine testing showed microscopic haematuria.

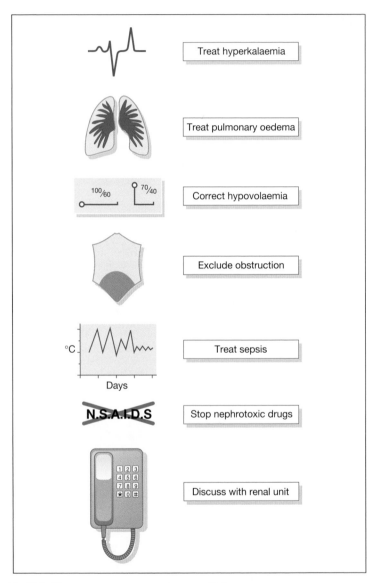

**Fig. 10.7** The emergency management of acute renal failure

## MANAGEMENT OF ACUTE RENAL FAILURE

Management follows the same principles that govern other medical emergencies:

1. ABCDE: ensure the immediate safety of the patient.
2. Complete a full clinical assessment.
3. Identify priorities and institute a management plan.
4. Provide the patient and the relatives with reassurance and an explanation.

### Ensuring the safety of the patient

The safety of the patient is established with attention to the airway, oxygenation and the circulation. There are two life-threatening complications that require urgent action: hyperkalaemia and pulmonary oedema.

**Hyperkalaemia.** Hyperkalaemia, or an increase in the serum potassium level, is the most serious complication of acute renal failure because it has a dramatic effect on the heart. Levels above 6.0 mmol/L lead to cardiac arrest. It is critical to measure and document serial changes in the potassium in any patient with established or threatened kidney failure. Hyperkalaemia produces characteristic changes on the ECG (peaking of the T waves and slurring of the QRS complexes) and, if these are present or the potassium level reaches 6.0 mmol/L, urgent action must be taken to protect the heart and to bring the potassium concentration down.

### Emergency management of hyperkalaemia

1. Give 10 ml of 10% calcium gluconate over 60 s and repeat until the ECG starts to improve. Calcium gluconate protects the heart, but does not reduce the potassium.
2. Give 10 units of neutral insulin solution (Actrapid) in 50 ml of 50% glucose over 5 min. This will reduce the potassium level by 2.0 mmol/L over 1 h.
3. Give 15 g of calcium resonium orally every 6 h. This takes 4 h to work.

**Pulmonary oedema.** This occurs because of the inability of the failing kidney to get rid of fluid. Pulmonary oedema is often triggered by over-enthusiastic i.v. fluid replacement in the critically ill, particularly if saline has been used and the CVP has not been monitored. The evidence for pulmonary oedema will be obtained from the initial assessment of a patient whose blood tests have shown kidney failure:

- low oxygen saturation
- increased respiratory rate
- unable to lie flat because of breathlessness
- in advanced pulmonary oedema, the patient is restless and confused

The management is the same as for other types of pulmonary oedema:

- sit the patient up
- administer high-flow 60% oxygen
- diuretics (often in high doses) and low-dose i.v. opiates

*Completing the clinical assessment*
**Assessing fluid balance:**

- What fluid has been lost?
  — a history of vomiting, diarrhoea, gastrointestinal bleeding?
  — is there internal fluid loss, as in acute pancreatitis?
- Is there any postural hypotension on sitting the patient up?
- What is the CVP?
- What is the urine output?

**Is there evidence of obstruction?**

- There may be a history of prostatism:
  — hesitancy in starting
  — poor stream
  — terminal dribbling
  — frequent small amounts.
- A distended bladder may be palpable.
- Sudden complete cessation of urine output or overflow with constant dribbling.
- Pain over the kidneys due to distension and back pressure.
- If the patient has a catheter – *is it blocked*? (gentle flush and aspiration with sterile water).

**What was the previous kidney function?**

- Examine old notes and laboratory reports.
- The GP's surgery may have results of prior renal function.
- A flow chart of results and their dates is invaluable.

**Is there a comprehensive drug list?** In particular:

- diuretics
- NSAIDs
- ACE inhibitors

**What does ward urine testing show?** Urine testing is usually negative in pre-renal failure. In acute tubular necrosis there is usually a combination of light to moderate proteinuria and microscopic haematuria. In acute glomerulonephritis, the characteristic findings are haematuria and heavy proteinuria. Send a spot urine sample for osmolality ('concentration')and urinary sodium. In hypovolaemia, the kidneys are trying to retain fluid and sodium to keep up the blood pressure – osmolality will be high (in excess of 450 mosmol/L) and sodium low (less than 10 mmol/L). The reverse is the case once acute tubular necrosis becomes established (osmolality less than 300 mosmol/L and sodium more than 20 mmol/L).

### Establishing a management plan

Assuming there has been emergency treatment of acute hyperkalaemia and pulmonary oedema, the priorities are:

- **To correct hypovolaemia** – if hypovolaemia is present, prompt fluid replacement should immediately increase the blood pressure and increase the urine output to more than 0.5 ml/kg per h. Depending on the frailty of the patient and their cardiac status, fluid replacement may require between 250 and 1000 ml of isotonic saline, aiming for a systolic blood pressure of 100 mmHg. If the urine output remains poor in spite of adequate hydration, a fluid challenge may be indicated.
- **To remove any obstructive component** – this will range from bladder catheterisation to percutaneous drainage of an obstructed kidney.
- **To stop any nephrotoxic drugs** – this relies on a full drug history, with details from both hospital and GP sources. The ward pharmacist will advise on nephrotoxicity and the need for dose modifications in the presence of renal failure.
- **To identify and treat sepsis** – sepsis is an important cause of renal failure and is easy to miss, especially in the elderly. Symptoms may simply consist of an abrupt change in health. Sites for 'hidden' sepsis include the perineum, the joints, the spine and the soft tissues, including infected bed sores. It is important to take at least two sets of blood cultures if sepsis is suspected: each set consists of 5 ml into each of two culture bottles – one aerobic and one anaerobic.

The management of pre-renal failure and acute tubular necrosis is outlined in Box 10.4.

---

| Box 10.4 – The management of pre-renal failure and acute tubular necrosis |
|---|

- Correct hypoxaemia
- Conduct emergency management of hyperkalaemia or pulmonary oedema
- Ensure the patient is well hydrated
- Administer a fluid challenge, usually 5% dextrose:
  - 1. 250 ml over an hour
  - 2. Watch urine output for next hour
  - — If output is less than 0.5 ml/kg per h:
  - 3. 5% dextrose 250 ml/h for 2 h
  - — If the output remains less than 0.5 ml per kg per hour, then consider:
  - 4. Dopamine 2.5 µg/kg per min and frusemide 50 mg/h

*Critical nursing tasks in acute renal failure (see box)*

> ## CRITICAL NURSING TASKS IN ACUTE RENAL FAILURE
>
> - **Prepare to start treatment for hyperkalaemia**
> - **Carry out basic management of pulmonary oedema**
> - **Identify sepsis: strong clues are fever, malaise, rigors and perhaps dysuria**
> - **Identify hypovolaemia:**
>   - **— symptoms of thirst and dizziness**
>   - **— signs of postural fall in blood pressure**
>   - **— low CVP**

*Important nursing tasks in acute renal failure*
### Confirm that the problem is not a simple outflow obstruction

- Enlarged tender bladder
- Blocked catheter

### Take a full history

- Any history to indicate hypovolaemia?
  - — severe diarrhoea
  - — vomiting
  - — bleeding
- Any history to suggest sepsis?
  - — dysuria
  - — rigors
  - — fever
- Any history to suggest obstruction?
  - — absolute anuria
- Past history
  - — chronic kidney disease
  - — diabetes
  - — hypertension
- Drug history
  - — NSAIDs
  - — ACE inhibitors
  - — diuretics

### Exclude rhabdomyolysis in prolonged immobility/coma

- Be aware of the possibility in coma, alcoholics and overdoses.
- Look for tense swollen legs and areas of bruising suggesting soft tissue damage. In rhabdomyolysis, the blood creatinine kinase level will be very high.

---

**IMPORTANT NURSING TASKS IN ACUTE RENAL FAILURE**

- ■ Confirm that the problem is not a simple outflow obstruction
- ■ Take a full history
- ■ Exclude rhabdomyolysis in prolonged immobility/coma
- ■ Check the urine
- ■ Ensure that there is a system for reviewing the abnormal urea and electrolyte results on the ward

---

**Check the urine**

- Appearance (e.g. a muddy appearance is typical of myoglobinuria – rhabdomyolysis)
- Dip for blood and protein
- Send for microscopy to look for casts (hyaline casts are from normal urinary constituents and occur in pre-renal failure because the urine is concentrated. Red cell casts indicate glomerulonephritis; granular casts indicate acute tubular necrosis)

**Ensure that there is a system for reviewing the abnormal urea and electrolyte results on the ward.** There should be flow charts that follow sequential tests in a critically ill patient. The most common cause for a delayed diagnosis of renal failure on the Acute Medical Unit is a failure to see and act on the abnormal results when they come back to the ward.

## ANSWERING RELATIVES' QUESTIONS IN ACUTE RENAL FAILURE

*What does acute kidney failure mean?* The kidneys filter impurities from the blood, so they need a constant stream of blood and an effective filtering mechanism. If anything too drastic happens to either mechanism, the kidneys become inefficient and eventually, as a result, impurities build up and poison the body – this is known as kidney failure.

*Will the kidneys recover?* The kidneys have good powers of recovery, particularly if they were working normally before this happened. We are checking previous hospital records and blood tests to see if the kidneys were completely normal up until the present illness. In many cases of acute kidney failure, the kidneys start to show signs of recovery within a few days of starting treatment.

*Why are you not sending him to a kidney unit?* The doctors use the unit for advice during the initial period of stabilisation. If the kidneys do not show the expected rate of recovery or if complications occur that could be more effectively dealt with in a kidney unit, we can transfer the patient at that stage.

*Have his drugs damaged the kidneys? Couldn't his own doctor have seen this coming?* Some drugs – especially diuretics and anti-inflammatories – can damage the kidneys or make them more vulnerable, particularly in older patients. It is not always easy to anticipate problems with the kidneys, and most people who take these drugs have no particular problem. You may want to discuss this with the doctors when the present episode is over and we can give you more information as to the exact cause of the kidney failure.

# SUDDEN COLLAPSE AND CARDIAC ARREST

It is important to understand the events that can precede and progress to a cardiac arrest.

- A respiratory arrest may lead to a cardiac arrest, and *vice versa*. In most arrest situations the term cardiorespiratory arrest is appropriate
- Most cardiac arrests occur as an early complication of myocardial infarction. These have the most successful outcomes
- However, cardiorespiratory arrest should also be viewed as an end-point in acute illnesses other than myocardial infarction. Examples include acute severe asthma, septicaemic shock and uncorrected acidosis. By recognising and treating them at an early stage, the risk of progressing to cardiorespiratory arrest can be reduced. Several studies have now shown that 'sudden death' on Acute Medical Units is often preceded by a period of potentially reversible deterioration – most notably unrecognised hypoxaemia and hypotension. Competent assessment and early intervention in the critically ill (Chapter One) should prevent this sequence.

*Common causes of the sudden collapse (→ Fig. 10.8)*
*Cardiac.* In 80% of cases, sudden pulseless collapse is due to ventricular fibrillation or ventricular tachycardia. In the remainder, the problem is a severe bradycardia or asystole. Pulmonary embolism is a classical cause of sudden severe collapse.

*Respiratory*

- Tension pneumothorax
- Aspiration/upper airway obstruction; this can cause a major deterioration, especially in coma
- Massive haemoptysis, usually as a terminal event in lung cancer

*Gastrointestinal.* A catastrophic bleed, usually from oesophageal varices. A ruptured abdominal aortic aneurysm.

*Anaphylaxis.* A characteristic setting with a recognised trigger, wheeze, oropharyngeal swelling and severe hypotension.

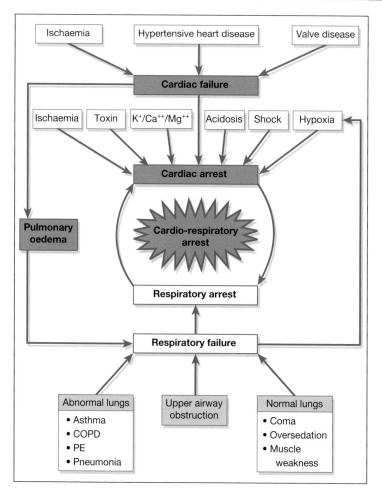

**Fig. 10.8** Cardiorespiratory arrest: an overview of causes and interactions

*Assessment of collapse*
What is the setting in which it occurred?

1. New patient just arrived on ward: this could be anything.
2. A patient admitted earlier in the day with unexplained breathlessness: pulmonary embolus.
3. A patient with known heart disease/chest pain: a major arrhythmia.

4. A patient admitted with deliberate self-harm: an arrhythmia or a respiratory arrest.

## Diagnosing cardiac arrest

Look at the patient and his monitor if it is available, but *treat the patient, not the monitor*. A patient who has collapsed with no apparent signs of life has had a cardiac arrest.

There are four common scenarios:

1. pulseless and collapsed with ventricular fibrillation or ventricular tachycardia – cardiac arrest
2. pulseless and collapsed with a flat trace – cardiac arrest
3. pulseless and collapsed but with an electrical rhythm (pulseless electrical activity or PEA) – cardiac arrest
4. flat trace but patient looks well – has an electrode come off?

If this is a pulseless cardiac arrest, the cause is almost certainly ventricular fibrillation or ventricular tachycardia. With immediate defibrillation, these patients have a 23% chance of survival. If ventricular fibrillation deteriorates into asystole or the initial rhythm is asystole (a flat trace) or PEA, the chances of survival decrease to 2%.

## THE CHAIN OF SURVIVAL

This is the term used to describe the sequence of events from prevention, in the form of the recognition and treatment of the critically ill patient, through early resuscitation integrating CPR and urgent defibrillation to the final link of effective post resuscitation care. The key to survival is the immediate recognition of a cardiac arrest and institution of BLS. The aim is to keep the patient alive and neurologically undamaged until defibrillation can be carried out.

## Basic life support

Basic life support describes the process of:

- the initial assessment of the collapsed patient
- the techniques to keep the airway open
- the use of expired air ventilation and chest compression – CPR

The equipment used in BLS comprises a simple airway and a face mask to facilitate mouth to mouth breathing.

If the cause of the collapse is a respiratory arrest, then BLS alone may succeed. In most cases, however, the patient has had a cardiac arrest, the rhythm is ventricular fibrillation (VF arrest) or pulseless ventricular tachycardia (VT) and *BLS is a holding operation until the defibrillator arrives and the process moves into that of ALS*. Advanced life support involves following established management algorithms for treating resistant arrhythmias and for maintaining ventilation with endotracheal intubation or other airway adjuncts.

*Providing immediate and effective BLS markedly increases the chances of success in a cardiac arrest:*

- *2 or 3 minutes' delay will halve the chances of survival*
- *3 or 4 minutes' delay will result in brain damage*
- *Interruptions to chest compression must be kept to an absolute maximum*

BLS must be started at the time of the arrest and, except during defibrillation, it must be continued throughout the resuscitation procedure until the return of a spontaneous circulation.

- Start BLS
- The primary helpers continue active resuscitation
- Secondary helpers may need to:
    - fetch the crash trolley
    - make the referral letter and the medical and nursing notes readily available
    - ensure laboratory results are fed back to the arrest team
    - put any recent X-rays up on the viewing box (is this a pneumothorax?)
    - see to other patients in the ward and move any patient if appropriate
    - make the paramedics' assessment documents available
    - send for any old hospital notes
    - handle the relatives: phone calls and direct contact

**Sequence of actions in BLS (→ Fig. 10.9)**

1. Ensure safety of rescuer and patient.
2. Shout for help. Check the patient and see if he responds: gently shake his shoulders and ask loudly, 'Are you all right?'
3. If he responds by answering or moving:
    - place him in the recovery position
    - check his condition (ABCDE), give oxygen, secure IV access and attach monitors
    - reassess him regularly
    If he does *not* respond:
    - turn the patient on to his back
    - open his airway by tilting his head and lifting his chin:
        - place your hand on his forehead and gently tilt his head back, keeping your thumb and index finger free to close his nose if rescue breathing is required
        - at the same time, with your fingertip(s) under the point of the patient's chin, lift the chin to open the airway
        - remove any visible obstruction from the patient's mouth, including dislodged dentures, but leave well-fitting dentures in place.

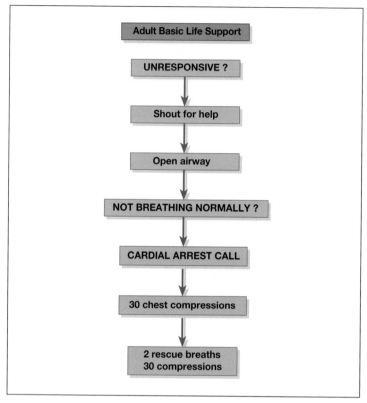

**Fig. 10.9**  The BLS algorithm

4. Keeping the airway open, look, listen and feel for normal breathing (occasional gasps, slow and laboured or noisy breathing are abnormal):
   — look for chest movements
   — listen at the patient's mouth for breath sounds
   — feel for air on your cheek
   — look, listen and feel for 10 s before deciding that breathing is absent.
5. If he is breathing normally:
   — turn him into the recovery position
   — check for continued breathing
   If he is *not* breathing normally:
6. Assess the patient for signs of a circulation and for signs of life:
   — look for any movement, including swallowing and coughing
   — check the carotid pulse
   — take no more than 10s to do this

| **Box 10.5 – Techniques of mouth to mouth ventilation** |
|---|

### The Laerdal Pocket mask (→ Fig. 10.10A)

Rescue breathing is usually started with a Laerdal Pocket mask, which is an acceptable and safe way to administer mouth to mouth ventilation until the self-inflating bag-mask and reservoir is available.

- The patient is approached from behind the head
- The thumbs and index fingers press and seal the mask onto the face
- The remaining fingers perform the jaw thrust to keep the airway open
- Blow through the inspiratory valve for 1 s and watch the chest rise
- Apply oxygen to the input valve at 10 L/min

### Guedel or oropharyngeal airway

The Guedel airway is used with head tilt and jaw thrust to ensure the airway remains patent. It will not be tolerated by a conscious patient. In the correct position it stops the tongue falling back and blocking the upper airway.

1. Select the size (from small 2, medium 3, or large 4) by matching an airway to the vertical distance between the incisors and the angle of the jaw.
2. Remove any loose material from the patient's mouth.
3. Insert the airway upside down and, when it is in position with the flat part between the patient's teeth, turn it the right way up.

### The self-inflating bag-mask and reservoir (→ Fig. 10.10B)

During resuscitation expired air alone supplies the patient with only 16% oxygen. This can be significantly enriched using a Laerdal mask, but only with a bag-mask and reservoir can the levels approach 100%. The technique, however, requires two people: one to secure a tight seal and maintain a clear airway using the Laerdal mask technique, and the other person, utilising both hands, to squeeze the bag. Ventilation at 10 breaths per minute can be continued without interrupting chest compression.

7. If you are *confident* that you can detect signs of a circulation within 10 s (ie this is a respiratory arrest):
   — start rescue breathing (Box 10.5), if necessary until the patient starts breathing on his own
   — every 10 breaths check for a circulation, take no more than 10 s each time
   — if the patient starts to breathe on his own but remains unconscious, turn him into the recovery position. Check his condition and be ready to turn him onto his back and restart rescue breathing if he stops breathing

If there are *no* signs of a circulation, or you are at all unsure:
   — start chest compression rather than initial ventilation (→ Fig. 10.11):
     - Place the heel of one hand in the centre of the victims chest (in the middle of the lower half of the sternum)
     - Place the heel of the other hand on top of the first hand.

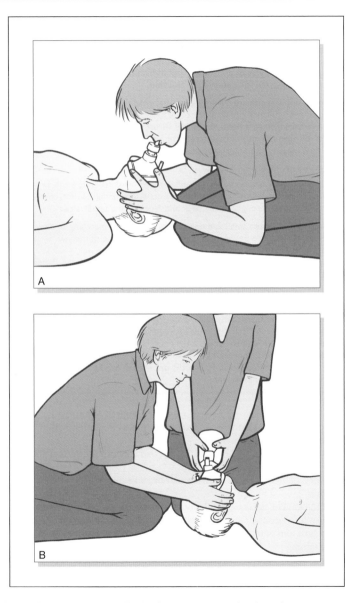

**Fig. 10.10**  Techniques for mouth-to-mask and two-person and mask ventilation

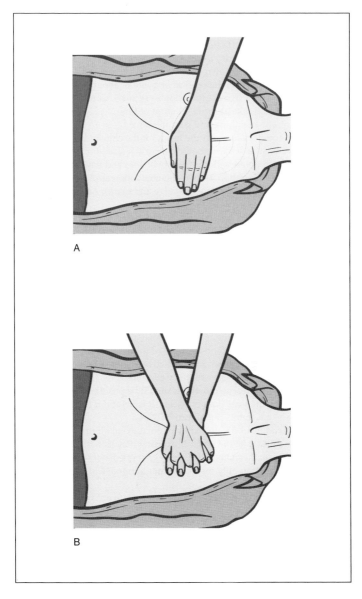

**Fig. 10.11** The correct hand position for cardiac massage

- Interlock the fingers of both hands. Ensure that pressure is not applied over the patient's ribs. Do not apply any pressure over the upper abdomen or bottom tip of the sternum
- position yourself vertically above the patient's chest and, with your arms straight, press down on the sternum to depress it 4–5 cm (1.5–2 in)
- release the pressure, then repeat at a rate of about 100 times a minute (a little less than two compressions a second). Compression and release should take an equal amount of time
— combine rescue breathing and compression:
  - after 30 compressions, tilt the head, lift the chin and give two effective breaths – these should be normal sized breaths (600 to 700 ml) each given without force over 1 second with an equal time allowed for expiration, (this recommendation applies to any form of CPR ventilation including bag valve and mark). Add supplemental oxygen as soon as possible
  - return your hands immediately to the correct position on the sternum and give 30 further compressions, continuing compressions and breaths in a ratio of 30:2
— when using two-person BLS, the following points should be noted:
  - when changing from single-person to two-person BLS, the second rescuer should take over chest compressions after the first rescuer has given two rescue breaths. During these rescue breaths, the incoming rescuer should determine the correct position on the sternum and should be ready to start compressions immediately after the second rescue breath has been given. It is preferable that the rescuers work from opposite sides of the patient.
  - a ratio of thirty compressions to two rescue breaths should be used. By the end of each series of thirty compressions, the rescuer responsible for rescue breathing should be positioned ready to give a breath with the least possible delay. It is helpful if the rescuer giving compressions counts out aloud: '1-2-3-4-5…'
  - chin lift and head tilt should be maintained at all times. Each rescue breath should take the usual 1 s, during which chest compressions should cease; they should be resumed immediately after inflation of the chest, waiting only for the rescuer to remove his or her lips from the patient's face.
8. Continue resuscitation until the cardiac arrest team arrives to assist.

**Notes on techniques of BLS** Box 10.6 summarises the key to initial resuscitation.

- Only a small amount of resistance to breathing should be felt during rescue breathing, and each inflation should take about 1 s
- The tidal volume to be achieved is about 600–700 ml in an adult, which is the amount normally required to produce visible lifting of the chest
- The rescuer should wait for the chest to fall fully during expiration before giving another breath. This should normally take about 1 s

---

**Box 10.6 – The key to initial resuscitation**

- Airway control: head tilt, chin lift and jaw thrust
- Effective use of a Laerdal mask or a bag and reservoir
- Effective bagging needs two people
- If gurgling: suction must be used (Yankauer) but only to oropharynx

---

- Once the airway is secured with an endotracheal tube or similar the lungs are ventilated at 10 breaths per minute without any pause in chest compression.

**Chest compression**

- *Any interruptions in chest compression lessens the chance of recovery and must be kept to an absolute minimum.*
- In an adult, the aim should be to press down approximately 4–5 cm and apply only enough pressure to achieve this.
- At all times the pressure should be firm, controlled and applied vertically. Erratic or violent action is dangerous.
- The recommended rate of compression is a rate, and not the number of compressions that are to be given in a minute; this will depend upon interruptions for rescue breathing.
- About the same time should be spent in the compression phase as in the released phase.
- As the chances are remote that effective spontaneous cardiac action will be restored by BLS without other techniques of ALS (including defibrillation), time should not be wasted by further checks for the presence of a pulse. If, however, the patient makes a movement or takes a spontaneous breath, the carotid pulse should be checked to see if the heart is beating; no more than 10 s should be taken to do this. Otherwise, resuscitation *should not be interrupted*.
- The presence of dilated pupils has, in the past, been variously used as a sign of cardiac arrest, failure of the circulation during resuscitation and the presence of established brain damage. This sign is unreliable and should not be used to influence management decisions before, during or after cardiopulmonary resuscitation.

**Recovery position.** When circulation and breathing have been restored, it is important to maintain a good airway and ensure that the tongue does not cause obstruction. It is also important to minimize the risk of inhalation of gastric contents.

For this reason, the patient should be placed in the recovery position (→ Fig. 10.12). This allows the tongue to fall forward, keeping the airway clear.

- Remove the patient's spectacles
- Kneel beside the patient and make sure that both his legs are straight
- Open the airway by tilting the head and lifting the chin

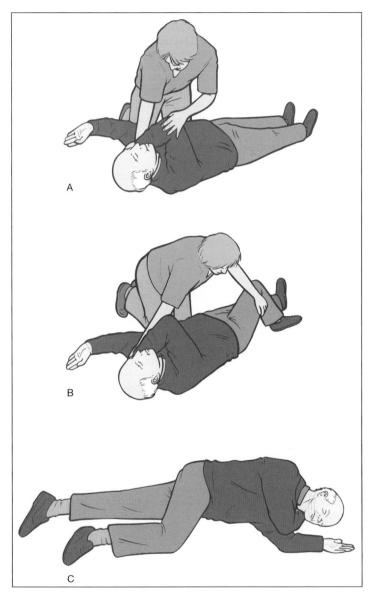

**Fig. 10.12** The recovery position

- Place the arm nearest you out at right angles to his body, elbow bent, with the palm of the hand uppermost
- Bring his far arm across the chest and hold the back of the hand against the patient's nearest cheek
- With your other hand, grasp the far leg just above the knee and pull it up, keeping the foot on the ground
- Keeping his hand pressed against his cheek, pull on the leg to roll the patient towards you onto his side
- Adjust the upper leg so that both the hip and knee are bent at right angles
- Tilt the head back to make sure the airway remains open
- Adjust the hand under the cheek, if necessary, to keep the head tilted
- Check breathing regularly and ensure that oxygen is being administered

### What the team leader of an arrest team should want to know from the ward nursing staff

- How, when and where the arrest occurred.
- Was there a witnessed account?
- What was the time from collapse to BLS?
- What was the initial rhythm?
- What is the time from arrest to defibrillation?
- Were there any special circumstances, e.g. tricyclic overdose/hypothermia?
- What is the DNAR status?
- Is there any equipment malfunction?

### Problems to avoid and look for during cardiopulmonary resuscitation

- Ensure suction and wide-bore rigid suckers (Yankauer) are available
- Correct ampoules and drug doses
- Good i.v. lines that will not 'tissue', especially with sodium bicarbonate (all i.v. drug boluses should be followed by a 20 ml N saline flush)
- Avoid letting fluids 'run through'
- Avoid injury to the patient's limbs and eyes from malposition and spillage
- Avoid staff electrocution
- Avoid burns to the patient during defibrillation – move oxygen masks or nasal cannulae at least a metre away from the patient's chest

One member of staff should be recording the events:

- timing of events
- number of shocks and strength
- administered drugs – dose and timing
- equipment problems

*After basic life support*

Although BLS is a holding measure that keeps the patient alive, it must be continued throughout the resuscitation attempt, except when a patient is undergoing defibrillation. Once the arrest team arrives the situation can be reviewed, with the first priority being to analyse the heart rhythm from the ECG/monitor.

In a cardiac arrest, the heart rhythm falls into one of two categories:

1. Shockable rhythms: ventricular fibrillation and pulseless ventricular tachycardia (VF/VT). Patients in this group need immediate defibrillation.
2. Non-shockable rhythms: asystole (a straight line) and electrical complexes, but with no palpable pulse (Pulseless Electrical Activity – PEA, previously known as electromechanical dissociation – EMD). This group needs emergency drugs and continuing CPR.

**Defibrillation strategy**

Once VF/VT is recognised immediately give one shock (150–200 J bi-phasic defibrillator or 360 J monophasic defibrillator)

Do *not* wait to check the rhythm or feel for a pulse but *immediately* re-start chest compression.

Continue CPR for two minutes in the ratio 30:2 and then check the monitor

If there is still VF/VT give a second shock (150–360 biphasic, 360 monophasic) and restart CPR immediately

After two minutes recheck the monitor and if there is still VF/VT give 1 mg of adrenaline IV followed immediately by a third shock and further CPR. If after two further minutes of CPR VF/VT persists give 300 mg of amiodarone as an intravenous bolus followed by a fourth shock.

Regardless of the rhythm adrenaline is given every 3–5 minutes (i.e. immediately before alternate shocks) until there is return of a spontaneous circulation. If, during CPR, the patient shows signs of life and the monitor shows an organised rhythm – check the pulse and if it is present start post resuscitation care, if not continue CPR. Do not interrupt a two minute spell of CPR if there is an organised rhythm but no signs of life – continue CPR and only check the pulse at the end of the two minutes.

*Technical points in defibrillation.* For maximum success, the shocks must be applied without delay. If left, ventricular fibrillation deteriorates into asystole or PEA, which have a much worse prognosis. Effectively, defibrillation 'stuns' the heart, stops all electrical activity and, if successful, the heart re-starts with the natural pacemaker taking over to produce a normal rhythm. During CPR the time between stopping chest compression and administering the shock must be cut to the absolute minimum to maximise the chance of success.

The correct defibrillation electrode (or paddle) positioning is critical – one is placed to the right of the upper sternum below the clavicle while the other is placed in the mid-axillary line approximately level with V6 ECG lead – avoiding breast tissue in a woman (→ Fig. 10.13).

Automated External Defibrillators (AEDs)

Early defibrillation after the recognition of cardiac arrest and the immediate institution of basic life support is the key to improved survival. This has been facilitated by the introduction of the Automated External Defibrillator which can:

- analyse the heart rhythm and either advise a shock or the resumption of 30:2 CPR
- provide spoken or visual directions on administering a shock or deliver a shock automatically
- prompt immediate resumption of CPR after the shock
- time the two-minute CPR cycle and then prompt to assess the rhythm, respiration and pulse

AEDs have played a major role in increasing the speed of response to cardiac arrest and increasing the number of people who can now successfully perform defibrillation.

**Asystole and PEA.** These non-shockable rhythms are treated with CPR, initially 30:2 but once the airway is secure continuous compressions at 100 per minute without pausing during ventilation at 10 breaths per minute. Adrenaline 1 mg is given as soon as there is IV access and continued every 3–5 minutes of CPR. Atropine 3 mg IV is given, once only, for asystole and for slow PEA (<60 per minute).

It is possible to make an erroneous diagnosis of asystole if the monitoring equipment fails or a lead becomes disconnected. Of equal importance is the risk

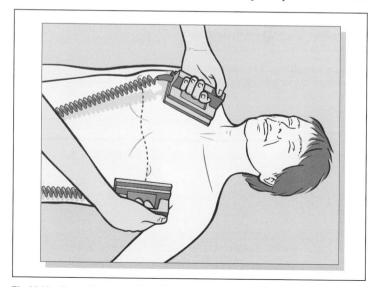

**Fig. 10.13**   The paddle positions for defibrillation

of diagnosing spurious asystole after unsuccessful defibrillation when monitoring is done through the defibrillator paddles. The shock can adversely affect the conducting properties of the gel pads so that the monitor shows a straight line (which can be misinterpreted as asystole) for sufficient time to critically delay the next shock. Rather than rely on 'through the paddles' monitoring, chest leads and a monitor are the preferred way to assess the response to each shock. The value of through the paddles monitoring is to obtain a rapid look at the rhythm which is present when the arrest team first arrives on the scene.

**Fine VF or asystole?**
If there is doubt about whether the rhythm is asystole or fine VF manage the patient as a non-shockable rhythm. Do not attempt defibrillation – continue chest compressiion and ventilation.

**Precordial thump?**
A single precordial thump can be tried in a witnessed and monitored cardiac arrest and is most likely to be successful in the first few seconds after collapse particularly in VT but also occasionally in VF. The bottom edge of a fist is brought down sharply from about 20 cm above the lower half of the sternum.

**The uses of adrenaline in the collapsed patient.** Adrenaline is used in cardiac resuscitation and in the treatment of acute anaphylaxis. It increases the efficiency of resuscitation by:

● increasing flow of blood in the heart muscle
● increasing flow of blood through the brain
● sustaining a falling blood pressure

There are two strengths of adrenaline: 1:1000 for intramuscular administration in anaphylaxis and 1:10 000, ten times weaker, for i.v. administration in cardiac resuscitation and in severe unresponsive

**Table 10.2   Administration of adrenaline (epinephrine)**

|  | Strength | |
| --- | --- | --- |
|  | *1:10 000* | *1:1000* |
| Concentration | 1 g       in   10 000 ml<br>1 mg     in   10 ml | 1 g       in   1000 ml<br>1 mg     in   1 ml |
| Indications | Cardiac arrest | Acute anaphylaxis |
| Route | Intravenous | Intramuscular |
| Dose | 1 mg (10 ml) | 0.5 mg (0.5 ml) |
| If repeated: | Every 3–5 min | At 5 min |

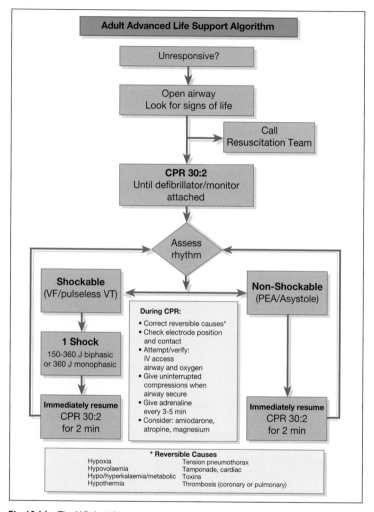

**Fig. 10.14** The ALS algorithm

anaphylaxis. Details of adrenaline administration are given in Table 10.2. Fig. 10.14 shows the ALS algorithm.

### Treatable causes of cardiac arrest: 4H and 4T

During cardiac resuscitation, it is vital that the team consider and correct any reversible causes of the cardiac arrest. For example, a patient with acute asthma may suffer an acute cardiorespiratory arrest during an attack as a result of a tension pneumothorax. A patient with a huge gastrointestinal bleed may arrest due to sudden hypovolaemia – in addition to BLS, this patient will need emergency fluid replacement.

*Hypoxia.* Hypoxia is the most easily preventable cause of cardiac arrest. The aim in any acutely ill patient is to monitor the oxygen saturations *and keep the oxygen saturation above 90%*. In the patient with COPD who has collapsed, the issue of controlled oxygen therapy is now irrelevant – in the emergency situation high concentrations of oxygen are needed as an immediate life-saving measure.

*Hypovolaemia.* Sudden, severe fluid loss in the form of blood (gastrointestinal bleed or massive haemoptysis) or body fluid (diarrhoea or DKA) will lead to hypotension and cardiac arrest. The key is to recognise that the low blood pressure is due to fluid depletion rather than a problem with a sick heart, and take appropriate action.

*Hypothermia.* Cardiac arrest can complicate severe hypothermia. Cardiopulmonary resuscitation must be continued until the patient's temperature is brought back up above 35°C or the efforts are judged by a senior medical member of the team to be fruitless.

*Hyperkalaemia and hypokalaemia.* A very high serum potassium, characteristically complicating acute renal failure, and a very low potassium, as may be seen in excessive diuretic treatment, can lead to cardiac arrest and must be addressed urgently. Intravenous calcium chloride is used for hyperkalaemia, hypocalcaemia and in overdose with calcium channel blockers (eg nifedipine). Intravenous magnesium can be life saving in serious arrythmias due to magnesium deficiency – seen in over-diuresis and with some chemotherapy regimes.

*Tension pneumothorax.* Characteristically, this gives a picture of PEA: a rhythm on the monitor but no palpable pulse. Unless the pneumothorax is recognised and treated, resuscitation will be unsuccessful.

*Therapeutic accident.* The common cause in this category is tricyclic poisoning after self-harm. Even very protracted resuscitation can be successful, and it is one of the few situations in which i.v. sodium bicarbonate can have a life-saving effect.

*Tamponade.* Cardiac tamponade occurs when there is a build-up of fluid under pressure in the pericardial sac – it compresses the heart and drastically reduces the cardiac output to an extent that it can lead to sudden PEA. Resuscitation will be unsuccessful unless the fluid is also drained off.

*Thromboembolism (Pulmonary embolism).* The classic cause of sudden death on the medical ward, massive pulmonary embolus can, in fact, be a reversible cause of cardiac arrest. It is likely that, in patients who survive, the cardiac massage acts to break up or dislodge clot that is sitting in the pulmonary artery and preventing blood from leaving the right side of the heart.

### When to stop the resuscitation procedure
Legally, the most senior doctor present has this responsibility. However, he or she should consider other views within the team. Survival becomes less likely with time. but many patients have recovered from prolonged resuscitation, particularly after:

- drowning
- electrocution
- hypothermia
- tricyclic drug overdose

It is almost impossible to predict brain damage from the state of the patient during the arrest and, in particular, fixed dilated pupils are not a reliable guide. If the patient is oxygenated and undergoing efficient BLS, the repeated failure of defibrillation and appropriate cardiac drugs will eventually form the basis of the decision to stop resuscitation.

## DEALING WITH THE RELATIVES OF A VICTIM OF CARDIAC ARREST

This is a task for an experienced member of the ward team, preferably the nurse who was with the patient nearest to the time of the arrest. No matter how distressed and distracted the relatives appear, it is likely that every detail of the day's events will be etched on their minds forever.

Find out who you are addressing and if any key member such as a spouse is missing. You may need to gather clinical information from the relatives as well as providing them with news. Explain the situation in straightforward terms and do not be embarrassed if your comments sound like platitudes – it is far better to use everyday language that is clear and unambiguous than revert to medical jargon:

Thirty minutes ago John's heart suddenly stopped and we put out an emergency call. The doctors and nurses are doing everything they can to try and get it started again. The situation is critical and we do not know if he is going to survive.

I am really sorry to have to give you this terrible news: John's heart stopped suddenly at 5pm. We were there within seconds and tried everything we could to get it started again. We worked on him for an hour, but it was absolutely hopeless; we could not get a heart beat back and he died at 6.15pm. It happened with no warning and from the moment his heart stopped John will have known nothing about it. At the end it was very peaceful, and I am sure that he did not suffer.

You must let and encourage the family to see the body. Try not to have the family, however well intentioned, 'protect' a wife or husband from seeing the body – it may be their last chance to say goodbye and they will come to value that moment. They must be allowed the chance to say an unhurried goodbye, to touch the body, to show their distress and to express their grief.

It is unlikely that you will know what to say, and silence is often as good as anything. Keep in mind that, to the ward staff, this is another episode in a very crowded day – but to the family it is a life-changing event.

## ANSWERING RELATIVES' QUESTIONS IN CARDIAC ARREST

*What has happened?* The heart suddenly stopped beating, but we have been able to 'kick start' it using a small electric shock. The episode was short-lived and we were able to restore a normal heartbeat, probably before any further damage could be caused. The bruising or red marks on the chest are due to manoeuvres we had to perform to keep the blood pumping during the period when the heart had stopped. There will be pain and tenderness in this area for a few days.

*Has the heart been damaged?* It is too early to judge the extent of the damage. Good signs will be a return of the blood pressure to normal and successful withdrawal of all the intravenous drips and drugs.

*Has there been a heart attack?* We will only know from tests on the heart and blood, which we will get back once he has recovered. It is possible to have a cardiac arrest from a sudden electrical fault without having an actual heart attack.

*Has there been any brain damage?* We cannot tell at present. The confusion/drowsiness/coma is not uncommon after a cardiac arrest and does not necessarily mean there is any permanent damage. The brain can go through a short-lived period of 'hibernation' after a cardiac arrest and still recover completely. We will only know if this is the case here after a period of time has elapsed (usually at least 24 h).

*Is he on a life-support machine?* The mask gives extra oxygen and must be kept in position for the next 24 h. If the condition deteriorates and the oxygen mask alone is insufficient, we can use a life-support machine. This will take over all the breathing functions and pump air directly into the patient's lungs through a tube. If this is needed, the patients are moved to the ITU, put to sleep, and then kept heavily sedated while they are on the machine.

## THE AFTERCARE OF PATIENTS WHO UNDERGO SUCCESSFUL CPR

Some patients are traumatised by the events associated with successful cardiopulmonary resuscitation. The physical effects – chest bruising, defibrillation burns, and even rib fractures – require simple explanation and symptomatic treatment. The psychological effects are more enduring:

- 'near death experiences'
- acute anxiety
- loss of confidence
- fear of a second arrest
- recurrent nightmares

For the first time in their life, the patient has become aware of his own mortality. The key to their immediate management is:

- give an honest account and explanation of the events that took place
- listen to the patient's concerns
- give firm reassurance
- consider offering other forms of help – discussion with the doctors, the priest and the clinical psychologist

# 'DO NOT ATTEMPT RESUSCITATION' – DNAR

It is important to try and differentiate between the natural process of dying and a sudden cardiorespiratory arrest from which a patient can be rescued. If the patient has a physical illness from which there is no likelihood of recovery and if it is clear that before admission the patient's life was nearing its end – then resuscitation would seem futile. Common examples of the latter include patients with cancer who are bed-bound and can no longer take oral medication and patients with worsening heart failure in spite of repeated admissions and optimisation of their drug regimen. Conversely, cardiac arrest as an early complication of an acute myocardial infarction is worth an attempt at resuscitation in virtually all situations.

The distinction may not be obvious in every case, and so it is important that decisions concerning resuscitation are made by a senior member of the medical team – ideally, but not always, the consultant. It is also essential to understand that a mentally competent adult can refuse consent to medical

> **CASE STUDY 10.8**   55-year-old man who declines resuscitation and dies peacefully
>
> A 55-year-old man with lung cancer had undergone palliative chemotherapy and came in with marrow failure and septicaemia. In spite of antibiotics, he deteriorated. He asked the staff, in the presence of his family, to have no more tests or any 'messing about'. Although weak and drowsy he understood the situation exactly. Subcutaneous morphine and haloperidol were used to control his pain and breathlessness. The decision not to resuscitate was formally posted in his nursing and medical notes. He died peacefully.

treatment (including resuscitation), even if that decision would lead to the person's death.

*Communication and explanation*
Communication is of paramount importance in this area. Discussions must be held with all the relevant parties, which may also involve the patient. It is important to provide patients with a realistic assessment of the likely outcome of a cardiac arrest (the benefits versus the burdens). Many patients, for example, would decline resuscitation if they were given a 50% chance that the outcome would include severe cognitive or functional impairment. DNAR decisions must be clearly documented, with the underlying reasons, in the nursing and medical notes, and the status of each patient on the ward communicated at handover (→ Case Study 10.8).

The on-call team must be included in the communication. There is little point in having a detailed discussion at 17.00 h, only for the arrest team to attend at 03.00 h and be faced with a ward team who are not aware of the resuscitation status of their patients.

*When in doubt: resuscitate.*

*A DNAR protocol*
**It is important to work to a protocol.**  There should be a standard way to review and record DNAR decisions in the notes. Any DNAR notice that has been posted should be kept under regular review, as the status of the patient may alter as their medical condition changes.

**When a DNAR decision is appropriate**
- When resuscitation would not be successful
- When resuscitation is against the patient's wishes (expressed when the patient was competent to do so)
- When resuscitation would not be in accord with an Advanced Directive

- Where successful resuscitation is likely to be followed by a length and quality of life that would be an intolerable burden to the patient. This is the most common reason for not performing resuscitation, and is the most difficult area in which to make decisions

*Important points about DNAR*

- In any discussions, do not exclude close friends and family members. Particularly in the case of patients with learning disorders and the young chronic sick, the professional carers from long-stay institutions and nursing homes may consider themselves as 'family' and must be included in the discussions.
- It can be helpful to 'anticipate' cardiac arrests or sudden deterioration so that some early discussion can be had with relatives. Patients with advanced disease, say with COPD or severe cardiac failure who survive 'near misses', can be asked if they want to be involved in future discussions concerning resuscitation should the same thing happen again.
- It should be made clear to everyone – staff, patient and relatives – that a DNAR decision is *NOT* the same as withdrawing all forms of care. The priority in these patients remains medical treatment, nursing care and, if the situation deteriorates, ensuring the patient is kept comfortable and free of pain.

## ANSWERING RELATIVES' QUESTIONS ABOUT 'DO NOT RESUSCITATE' DECISIONS

*Does this decision mean that all treatment will now be withdrawn?* No, it does not mean this at all. Resuscitation means starting urgent life-support measures if the heart stops – the aim is to restore a normal heart beat. We do this if there is a reasonable chance of restoring the patient to his previous health without suffering side-effects or damage as a result of the cardiac arrest and subsequent resuscitation. After considering this, and as a result of our discussions with you, we have decided that either resuscitation would not work or it would leave the patient in an intolerable situation. However, we can still treat other complications apart from a cardiac arrest – infection, congested lungs, low blood pressure – and we can still ensure effective symptom control if there is pain, distress or breathlessness.

# BEREAVEMENT ON THE ACUTE MEDICAL UNIT

Bereavement on the Acute Medical Unit is an important and difficult problem:

**CASE STUDIES 10.9** Bereavement

## CASE 1

A 75-year-old woman with known ischaemic heart disease, severe airflow obstruction and myelodysplasia was diagnosed as having an advanced squamous carcinoma of the lung. There had been full involvement by a consultant chest physician and the lung cancer specialist nurse. The patient had her own patient-held record.

The patient was admitted after a period of deterioration with dehydration and sepsis. She initially responded to i.v. antibiotics. Unfortunately, at 03.00 h the patient became acutely distressed, hypotensive and confused. She died over a period of 20 min. The relatives came to the ward after the patient had died.

Several months after the event, despite extensive counselling, the daughter was still extremely distressed. She felt guilty, having promised that her mother would die at home and that, if it was necessary, she would take her out of hospital. Previous members of the family had died in unexpected circumstances on their own. In addition, she had 'chivvied' her mother along during her final illness to encourage her not to give up. She felt guilty about this.

## CASE 2

A 55-year-old woman with known advanced breast cancer previously treated with chemotherapy and radiotherapy was admitted for 'terminal care'. The lesion was fungating, she had a pleural effusion and could not move at all in bed without the help of two nurses. Her husband did not leave her side. She was started on subcutaneous opiates and moved onto another ward which, in the information sheet for the Acute Medical Unit, is described as a 'recovery ward'. She died suddenly from a pulmonary embolus at 05.00 h a few days later. Weeks later, her husband came back to the hospital with a number of complaints.

- He had not realised that she was dying
- If she was dying, why had she been moved to a 'recovery ward'?
- When was she last seen alive and by whom?
- Why was her usual medication cut down?
- Did she die alone, and why was he not called in?

We had talked to this man on several occasions at the bedside. We had not appreciated that, in his distress, he had not taken in the most fundamental issue about his wife's illness. He needed to know everything about the final few hours when he was not there with her. He was still inconsolable months later, because of the way in which we had failed to communicate effectively with him.

- the deaths will be sudden
- the relatives will have had little warning
- the ward will be busy and staff time will be at a premium

However, if bereavements are handled sensitively, relatives are more likely to come to terms with their loss and the risks of subsequent abnormal grief reactions will be reduced. Two examples of the common problems encountered after bereavement are given in Case Studies 10.9.

There are a number of problems surrounding sudden death in hospital, particularly regarding the actual sequence of events. Relatives need to know what went on, who was present, whether the patient asked for his next of kin, whether there were any nurses present and whether the doctors had been called. It is extremely important that the actual events are covered in detail at the time of the death, because only then can the relatives start to come to terms with the situation. It is common for relatives to mull over the events surrounding the death. Even months later, they may have several unanswered questions.

### Critical nursing tasks when dealing with the bereaved

**Ensure effective communication with relatives.** Ensure that communication with the relatives of very sick patients remains the utmost priority on the ward.

### Make sure the facts are correct

- Make *absolutely sure* that you have the facts correct:
  — that the patient in question has died
  — that you are dealing with that patient's relatives
  — that you know their names and relationships
  — that the relatives you are talking to include the next of kin.

### Find out the likely cause and mode of death

- Find out from the doctors the likely cause of death.
- Speak to those who were with the patient in his final moments: the relatives will need to know these details. Sometimes relatives will ask to speak to the night shift who were involved.

### Give the relatives time with the deceased

- Ensure the relatives have an unhurried and private time with the deceased.

### CRITICAL NURSING TASKS WHEN DEALING WITH THE BEREAVED

- Ensure effective communication with relatives
- Make sure the facts are correct
- Find out the likely cause and mode of death
- Give the relatives time with the deceased
- Ensure liaison with the patient's GP

- Give the relatives enough time:
  — to absorb the news and recover from the initial shock
  — to express their distress
  — to ask questions.

**Ensure liaison with the patient's GP.** Ensure that the ward lets the patient's GP know of the death.

*Important nursing tasks when dealing with the bereaved*
**Establish the need for coroner involvement or post-mortem.** Establish from the doctors whether they:

- will need to inform the coroner/procurator fiscal
- would like to seek permission for a post-mortem

**Help the relatives with practical details.** Ensure the relatives understand the process of:

- death certification
- handling the deceased patient's possessions
- the help that bereavement officers and the undertakers will give

**Understand the role of the coroner and death certification.** Make sure you understand the role of the coroner and know before dealing with the relatives whether (and when) a death certificate can be issued.

**Be sensitive to distress among staff.** Be sensitive to distress among junior members of the nursing and medical team after a bereavement. For staff, a series of deaths and the associated feelings of inadequacy/failure that they engender may leave them vulnerable and stressed.

---

### IMPORTANT NURSING TASKS WHEN DEALING WITH THE BEREAVED

- Establish the need for coroner involvement or post-mortem
- Help the relatives with practical details
- Understand the role of the coroner and death certification
- Be sensitive to distress among staff

---

## FURTHER READING

### RESUSCITATION

A Joint Statement from the British Medical Association, Resuscitation Council (UK) and Royal College of Nursing 1999 Decisions relating to cardiopulmonary resuscitation. Available from the Resuscitation Council: http://www.resus.org.uk/

Field D, Kitson C 1986 Coping with death: the practical reality. Nursing Times 19 March: 33–34

Project Team of the Resuscitation Council (UK) 1999 Emergency medical treatment of anaphylactic reactions. Journal of Accident and Emergency Medicine 16: 243–247

**TRANSFUSION**

British Committee for Standards in Haematology, Blood Transfusion Task Force 1999 Guideline: the administration of blood and blood components and the management of transfused patients. Transfusion Medicine 9: 227–238S

**OXYGEN THERAPY**

Bateman NT, Leach RM 1998 ABC of oxygen: acute oxygen therapy. British Medical Journal 317: 798–801

Murphy R, Mackway-Jones K, Sammy I et al 2001 Emergency oxygen therapy for the breathless patient. Guidelines prepared by the North West Oxygen Group. Emergency Medicine Journal 18: 421–423

Woodrow P 1999 Pulse oximetry. Nursing Standard 13 (42): 42–47

**SEPSIS**

Dellinger PR, Carlet JM, Masur H et al 2004 Surviving Sepsis Campaign guidelines for management of severe sepsis and septic shock [Review]. (Erratum in: Crit Care Med 2004 32 (6): 1448. Correction of dosage error in text.) Crit Care Med 32: 858–873

**WEBSITES**

Resuscitation Council (UK) Guidelines 2005: http://www.resus.org.uk/
European Resuscitation Council Guidelines 2005: http://www.erc.edu/new/

# EMERGING PROBLEMS: OUTBREAKS AND DELIBERATE RELEASES – SARS, TOXINS AND BIOLOGICAL AGENTS

## INTRODUCTION

This chapter considers the possibility that the Acute Medical Unit has to deal with the outbreak of an infectious disease or with an act of bioterrorism – the deliberate release of a biological agent or toxin. Such an occurrence, although unlikely, has very serious implications for the personal safety of the hospital staff. In spite of infection control measures, many of the fatalities in the SARS outbreak were among the nursing and medical staff on the acute units. SARS is a typical example of spread by air-borne transmission for which specific protective measures are required as soon as a suspected case occurs.

## HOW INFECTION SPREADS

- close contact with unrecognised infected persons
- infectious respiratory secretions – cough and sneeze
- true air-borne transmission ('aerosol')
- faecal and oral transmission
- contact with contaminated body surface (shaking hands)
- touching contaminated external surfaces

The possibility of an outbreak of an unfamiliar infection or of disease caused by bioterrorism cannot deflect the ward staff from basing all their initial management of seriously ill patients on the principle of probability: common things occur commonly. Thus an outbreak of severe pneumonic illness is more likely to be due to *Legionella* from say a faulty cooling tower (as in a 2003 outbreak in Montpellier) than from SARS or an air-borne terrorist release of plague. A patient with progressive paralysis is far more likely to be suffering from the Guillain–Barré syndrome than from botulism, and a haemorrhagic rash more likely to be meningococcal septicaemia than Ebola virus.

Nonetheless, there is an issue of early recognition because, in their initial stages, these rare infections and toxins share clinical features with more commonplace conditions. The fact that deliberate infections and mass poisonings have taken place in recent years means further attacks are likely. Staff should therefore remain vigilant and plans must be in place. Previously, the responses to outbreaks and toxic releases have been characterised by:

- inadequate preparations
- late recognition
- poor communications

It is critical that the most up-to-date information is to hand. Local expertise will be limited, although there is increasing experience with strict respiratory protection through its use in multi-drug-resistant TB. Fortunately, international experience and guidelines are freely available electronically through several important websites.

The minimum knowledge that is required is:

- how to recognise an outbreak alert (using SARS as an example)
- the broad nature of the most likely bioterrorist threats (anthrax, botulism, plague, smallpox, tularaemia, viral haemorrhagic fevers and the nerve gas, sarin).
- how to protect the health of the staff

There are several basic principles involved.

- An awareness of new threats and the emergence of novel infections/agents
- An appreciation that there will be no previous personal experience with cases
- The need for immediate up-to-date information from the internet
- The need to review protocols and procedures in the light of new information
- The skills of infection control in highly contagious patients
- The need for timely communication
- The rapid involvement of designated staff and resources

# SEVERE ACUTE RESPIRATORY SYNDROME

SARS is uncommon, but it provides an important lesson in how an Acute Medical Unit may have to deal with the emergence of a new and highly infectious disease.

In February 2003, a doctor from the southern Chinese province of Guangdong became ill while staying at a Hong Kong hotel. Twelve other guests became infected, of whom seven had rooms on the same floor. These index cases moved on – spreading SARS to Vietnam, Singapore, Canada, Ireland and the US. By mid April it had infected almost 3500 people in 27 countries, causing widespread panic. By May 2003, scientists had identified the infecting organism as a coronavirus (now known as SARS-CoV), which is normally an animal virus but which had crossed species to man. By July, the outbreak was over, having infected more than 8000 people and with an 11% mortality rate.

SARS is spread like TB or influenza, in droplet form, but in spite of infection control measures, 25% of the cases occurred in exposed health-care workers.

The implications of making a tentative diagnosis are so profound in terms of isolation measures and public health protection that it is vital to be aware of the precise diagnostic criteria (case definition).

## Case definition of SARS
**Possible case.** A patent who is ill enough to be in hospital with a high fever (> 38°C) *and* coughing, difficulty with breathing or dyspnoea *and* with chest

X-ray changes of pneumonia who, within 10 days before the onset of symptoms:

- has been in an area that has been designated by the World Health Organisation to be a zone of potential re-emergence of SARS (currently mainland China and Hong Kong)

  *or*

- has been in close personal contact with a probable case of SARS

**Probable case**

- Patients with a clinical diagnosis of SARS (possible cases) in whom preliminary laboratory tests are positive

**Confirmed case**

- Probable case in whom further tests are positive

### Management of a possible case of SARS

Patients with suspected SARS are likely to be severely ill and have the clinical picture of acute pneumonia. While confirmation of the diagnosis is awaited, they should be treated along conventional guidelines for severe pneumonia, *but with the additional need for strict infection control.*

Detailed guidance for infection control in possible cases of SARS should be available through a local protocol and can also be found at the Health Protection Agency website.

The patient should wear a surgical mask – within the constraints imposed by their oxygen requirements – and should be nursed in a negative-pressure single room. All health-care workers entering the room must comply with infection control:

- neck-to-heel gowns and gloves – to be left in the room before leaving
- a respirator mask conforming to EN149:2001 FFP3, such as the 3M mask: 1873 V
- cap and goggles or visor – to be removed, with the mask, once outside the room
- boots
- strict hand washing in alcohol – before and after leaving the room

### Surgical masks versus particulate respirators

*Surgical face masks* are designed to prevent droplet emission and to act as a barrier to splashes of liquid. They will capture microorganisms in the exhaled breath, but do not protect against air-borne infection; for this an appropriate respirator is needed. *Respirators* are high-filtration masks that prevent inhalation of sub-micron sized particles. They do not filter the wearer's expired air. To be used safely and to maintain a high filtering efficiency, the respirator must be fitted correctly, with a less than 10% leak.

Some procedures increase the risk of droplet spread and must be avoided:

- nebulisers
- high-flow oxygen
- humidifiers
- physiotherapy
- bronchoscopy
- CPAP and NIV
- tracheal suction

Fig. 11.1 gives an overview of the initial pathway for a potential case of SARS. Fig. 11.2 summarises the strict infection control measures that are required. The clinical management of SARS is the same as for severe community acquired pneumonia, with fluid replacement and i.v. antibiotics. High-flow oxygen, above 6 L/min, is to be avoided, as it increases the risk of droplet spread; administer 30–40% oxygen using a Ventimask. Oral prednisolone (40–60 mg daily) in severe cases probably improves the prognosis. Daily chest films are essential for monitoring these patients, because the pneumonia characteristically progresses with alarming speed. There is a high chance of the patients needing ventilation – particularly if they are elderly or have co-morbidity. Close liaison will be needed with the ITU, and probably with a designated Regional Centre.

## OTHER EMERGING INFECTIONS

SARS is only one example of new infectious diseases that have profound implications for Public Health. In August 1999, eight similar cases of encephalitis were admitted to hospitals in the Northern Queens district of New York. Four of the individuals were paralysed and needing ventilation. All eight usually spent their evenings out of doors in the vicinity of breeding sites for *Culex* mosquitos, which were suspected to be spreading a virus. Subsequent investigations of a substantial number of bird deaths in the area and of the patients identified the offending organism: West Nile Virus. The lessons from the successful recognition of this disease include:

- an awareness of the importance of clustering of cases
- the value of good communication
- excellent cross-professional working

More recently, in 2003, a virulent avian flu virus broke out in South East Asia. The virus, the H5N1 strain of bird flu, crossed the species barrier from domestic duck to man and killed 20 people in Thailand and Vietnam. Many believe that a major flu pandemic from this type of source is inevitable. SARS and influenza spread in the same way, so that similar infection control measures would be required.

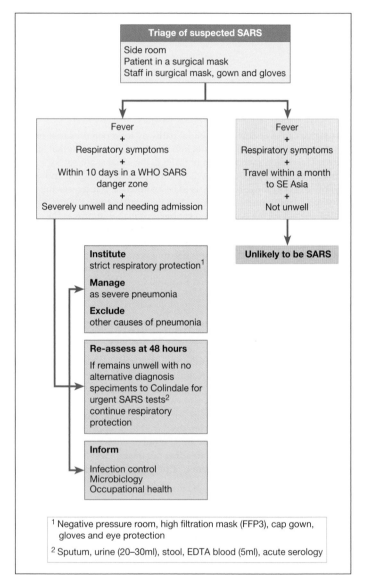

**Fig. 11.1** The initial pathway for a potential case of SARS

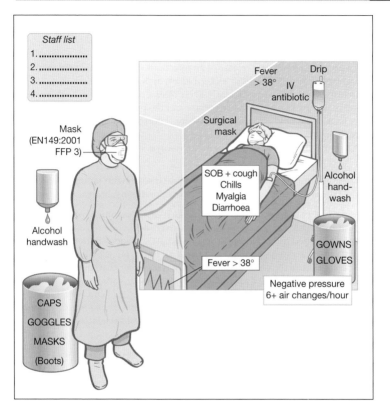

Staff list
1. ...................
2. ...................
3. ...................
4. ...................

Mask
(EN149:2001
FFP 3)

Alcohol
handwash

CAPS
GOGGLES
MASKS
(Boots)

Fever
> 38°

Drip

IV
antibiotic

Surgical
mask

SOB + cough
Chills
Myalgia
Diarrhoea

Alcohol
hand-
wash

Fever > 38°

GOWNS
GLOVES

Negative pressure
6+ air changes/hour

**Fig. 11.2**  The strict infection control measures that are required for a potential case of SARS

## UNUSUAL ILLNESSES – DELIBERATE RELEASE OF INFECTIOUS AND CHEMICAL AGENTS

In 1979, at least 66 Russian people down-wind from a weapons research facility died of inhalation anthrax after an accidental release of anthrax spores into the atmosphere. Iraq has admitted deploying anthrax in missiles, and in the USA in 2001 there were 11 cases of inhalational anthrax, including five deaths after malicious dissemination of anthrax spores via the postal service.

## DELIBERATE RELEASE OF INFECTIOUS AGENTS

### General principles

The effects of a deliberate release of an infectious or biological agent may be recognised only when cases of *unusual illness* appear on the Medical Admitting Unit. This is particularly likely after a covert release, as there will be no mass Emergency Service response and the presentation of the cases may have a less obvious pattern – the connection between them may not be immediately apparent.

An unusual illness may present in three ways:

- a diagnostic puzzle
- an illness 'out of place' – such as a tropical disease with no travel history
- the failure of a 'conventional' illness to respond to usual treatment

Obviously an outbreak, or clustering, of such cases has much more significance than a single incident, but in covert deliberate release the cases may be admitted to hospital with no immediately obvious pattern. Ideally, vigilance and awareness should be high at all times, but the likelihood of a deliberate release remains so low that there is a danger that, over time, the possibility is forgotten.

*It may therefore be advisable to have named members of the Ward Staff whose responsibility it is to keep themselves up-dated on current risks and infection control measures, to liaise with other appropriate departments and to maintain a file of information on the ward giving relevant protocols, contact details and websites.*

There are four important areas in the management of potential cases:

1. **Awareness and recognition**.
2. **Communication**.
3. **Decontamination and containment**.
4. **Seek early advice**.

### Awareness and recognition

Cases will not necessarily come in well-defined clusters, even if there is common exposure. Their presentation may be staggered or delayed from the time of exposure.

There are several warning signs of a potential outbreak:

- the receipt of a prior warning or threat
- people with a similar disease or syndrome presenting at the same time
- a number of cases of unexplained disease or death
- a familiar illness occurring in an unusual setting within a community
- illness affecting a key sector of the community
- a familiar disease with an unusually high death rate
- disease with an unusual geographic or seasonal distribution
- unusual, atypical, genetically engineered, or antiquated strain of agent

- simultaneous outbreaks of similar illness in separate areas
- unusual transmission routes, e.g. by aerosol, food or water
- animal deaths or illness that precedes or accompanies human illness or deaths
- illness only among people in proximity to common ventilation systems

**Taking the correct samples for screening for infections and toxins.** The samples for screening for infectious diseases should contain at least two sets of blood cultures. Two 10-ml samples of clotted blood are also required for serology and biotoxin measurements. Two 10-ml EDTA blood samples are needed for sophisticated molecular identification studies. A 20-ml sample of urine in a preservative-free bottle should also be sent.

To identify chemical toxins from high risk cases, 'Toxiboxes' are situated in Casualty and should be used for handling and transporting samples to the laboratory. The Toxibox has the containers and packaging to send the following samples:

a) 10 ml of blood in a plastic lithium tube
b) 5 ml of blood in a glass lithium tube
c) 4 ml of blood in an EDTA tube
d) 300 ml of urine in a preservative-free bottle

The samples require careful handling; they need to be marked 'high risk'. Each bottle is bagged separately. Blood forms, in separate bags, are attached to each matching bottle. Once the laboratories have been alerted, the samples are delivered urgently, by hand.

## Communication

There will have to be excellent lines of communication locally with Occupational Health, Control of Infection, Laboratory Service and, if an outbreak is confirmed, with Regional and National Bodies. There will inevitably be health and safety priorities that will be the responsibility of the local Occupational Health Department. The local Health Protection Unit, which is part of the National Health Protection Agency, will co-ordinate other aspects of management. This will include informing the police of a suspected outbreak, obtaining expert medical opinions and overall incident control.

## Decontamination and containment

The principles are to prevent further harm, to optimise treatment and, of paramount importance, to protect the health-care staff from harm (*if there is any doubt, action must always be taken to protect the staff*). For outbreaks in which *biological* agents are involved, the principle is the adoption of infection control – single rooms, the use of Universal Precautions and, when suspicion is high, specialised respiratory protection.

**Universal Precautions.** It is not always possible to identify people who may spread infection to others, therefore precautions to prevent the spread of infection must be followed at all times. These routine procedures are usually called 'Universal Precautions', and are designed to prevent exposure to potentially infectious blood and body fluids, and to avoid injury by sharp objects.

- Practice good basic hygiene, with regular hand washing
- Cover wounds or skin lesions with waterproof dressings
- Avoid contamination of person and clothing with blood/body fluids
- Disposable gloves and aprons should be worn when attending to dressings, performing aseptic techniques or dealing with blood/body fluids
- Handle and dispose of sharps safely
- Avoid puncture wounds, cuts and abrasions in the presence of blood
- Avoid using sharps if possible
- Protect eyes, mouth and nose from blood splashes
- Know what to do if there is a sharps injury or blood-splash incident
- Clear up blood spillages promptly and disinfect surfaces
- Dispose of contaminated waste safely
- Know how to deal with soiled linen
- Clean, disinfect and sterilise equipment as appropriate

**Specialised respiratory protection.** Where there is a risk of the air-borne spread of serious infection (e.g. MDTB, SARS, viral haemorrhagic fever), strict respiratory precautions are needed to minimise the risk to staff:

- negative pressure rooms with 6–9 air exchanges per hour
- staff wearing gloves, disposable gowns, caps, boots and eye protection
- high-specification masks
- ammonia, phenol and alcohol-based disinfectants
- hourly surface and floor wipes with diluted bleach (1 in 49 dilution of 5.25% sodium hypochlorite)
- alcohol-based hand washes
- initial visiting restrictions
- all gowning and de-gowning carefully supervised:
  — gowns and gloves left inside room
  — eye protection, mask and cap left outside

For outbreaks in which *chemical* exposure is involved, the initial management is centred on initial decontamination, which is the responsibility of the ambulance service and will take place in a designated area. It would be highly unusual for decontamination to take place on a ward, as it is a highly specialised and hazardous operation.

*Seek early advice*
It is of critical importance to maintain a list of up-to-date websites and contact telephone numbers on the Medical Admitting Unit.

## POISONING WITH BIOLOGICAL AGENTS

*Examples of potential pathogens and initial symptoms*

This section gives a brief clinical overview of what experts believe to be the most likely terrorist agents. Websites are available for more detailed information.

**Anthrax.** Influenza-like symptoms followed 2–4 days later by the rapid development and progression of severe respiratory failure and shock. Mortality rates in inhalation anthrax are extremely high, but specific treatment combines ciprofloxacin, vancomycin and rifampicin. Steroids may also help.

**Plague.** Severe myalgia, sore throat and headache merging into a severe pneumonic illness with copious bloody sputum. Specific treatment is with gentamicin, ciprofloxacin and doxycycline.

**Botulism.** The patient remains alert, with no sensory loss, but develops a rapidly descending flaccid paralysis due to blockage of nerve impulses to the muscles. There is no fever. Specific treatment is with an antitoxin, but the key is supportive care, which often includes ventilation.

**Smallpox.** Two to three days of severe fever, headache and malaise, followed by a deeply seated rash spreading and progressing from the mouth and face to the trunk, limbs, palms and soles. Treatment is supportive. Specific treatment is probably ineffective, but the antiviral drug cidofovir can be tried.

**Tularaemia.** A pneumonic illness with flu-like features or a septicaemic illness with severe shock. Specific treatment is with gentamicin.

**Ebola virus.** Fever, abdominal pain and bloody diarrhoea followed by bleeding from the nose, the gastrointestinal tract and into the skin. Treatment is supportive.

**Lassa fever.** Fevers, shivering attacks and severe tonsillitis, followed by disturbed conscious level, respiratory distress and abdominal distension. Treatment is supportive.

Table 11.1 summarises the features of and responses to poisoning with biological agents.

**Table 11.1 Poisoning with biological agents**

| Disease | First symptom | Severe pneumonia | Clinical picture | Rash | Staff prophylaxis | Control of infection |
|---|---|---|---|---|---|---|
| Anthrax | Fever | Yes | Rapid deterioration over 1–6 days | Yes | Antibiotics | No isolation, G, A, HW |
| Plague | Fever | Yes | Rapid deterioration over 1–6 days | Yes (H) | Ciprofloxacin | SR, G, GN, E, HW, FFP3 |
| Botulism | No | No | Sudden descending flaccid paralysis | No | Not needed | No isolation, G, A, HW |
| Smallpox | Fever | No | Fever ++, systemic symptoms ++, abdominal pain | Yes (H) | Immediate vaccination | SR*, G, GN, E, HW, FFP3 |
| Tularaemia | Fever | Yes | Variable rate of deterioration | Yes | Not needed | SR, G, GN, E, HW, FFP3 |
| VHF | Fever | No | Rapid deterioration, abdominal pain, diarrhoea | Yes (H) | Nil | SR*, G, GN, E, HW, FFP3 |

A, apron; E, (eye protection) goggles; FFP3, particulate filter respirator for staff (see SARS section)/surgical mask for patient; G, gloves; GN, fluid-resistant gown; (H), haemorrhagic rash; HW, hand washing ++ (alcohol); SR, side room, which should be at negative pressure; SR*, side room in a designated centre; VHF, viral haemorrhagic fevers (Lassa fever, Ebola, etc.)

## POISONING WITH NERVE AGENTS

In 1994 and 1995, the Aum Shinrikyo religious cult released the neurotoxin, sarin gas, in terrorist attacks in Japan. The second attack was in the Tokyo subway, where plastic bags of dilute sarin were punctured with umbrella tips. The released vapour was directly absorbed through the skin and lungs; other people were then indirectly exposed from initial victims' contaminated clothing. In total, 1000 passengers were injured, of whom 12 died. The hospitals were overwhelmed; many staff members were secondarily exposed because there was no chemical-resistant personnel equipment (butyl rubber gloves and boots), there were no decontamination facilities, and ventilation in the treatment areas was poor. The antidotes, atropine and pralidoxime, were soon exhausted. Another 4000 people reported to hospital – many had nothing wrong with them and were not actually exposed.

There are five organophosphorous nerve agents, but there is most experience with sarin, which is a highly volatile vapour that acts predominantly after inhalation but is also absorbed through the skin. In the event of a deliberate release, victims should arrive at hospital having already been decontaminated, so that only standard hospital precautions would be necessary for personal staff protection. The Acute Medical Unit would be receiving moderately ill patients, not those in need of immediate ITU care, for whom the main objectives will be antidote administration and the treatment and monitoring of any respiratory difficulties.

Nerve agents act by blocking the enzyme, acetylcholinesterase, which normally works as a break on nerve impulse transmission. The clinical effects are therefore due to an overload of nerve traffic throughout the nervous system. The antidotes – atropine and related drugs – act by unblocking the enzyme and reducing the flow of traffic.

For clinical purposes, the three important effects are due to overactivity in the parasympathetic nerves – the nerves that oppose the sympathetic nervous system – and hence the signs of nerve agent poisoning are the 'opposite' of the fight or flight reaction:

Bradycardia – pulse rate of less than 40 beats/min
Bronchospasm – severe wheeze
Bronchorrhoea – excessive airway and lung secretions

This overactivity is reversed by atropine and two related drugs: pralidoxime and obidoxime. Their effectiveness as antidotes can be monitored by the improvement in these three features.

- Overactivity in the nerves to the respiratory muscles leads to respiratory distress and, ultimately, respiratory arrest.
- Overactivity in the brain leads to coma and convulsions. Convulsions can be prevented with diazepam.

The management after initial decontamination can be summarised by ABC:

1. **A**ntidote administration
2. **B**reathing support
3. **C**oma and convulsion care

### Antidote administration

*Atropine* is an effective but short-lived antidote that is given intramuscularly every 5 min until the pulse rate increases above 80 beats/min. Pralidoxime and obidoxime have a slower onset, but are long acting. When given i.v., they are effective for around 4 h. Intravenous diazepam prevents convulsions and other signs of muscular overactivity, particularly muscular twitching.

The front-line emergency services may have already administered antidotes using the *Autoject (Combo Pen) L4 A1*, which contains a single-dose combination of atropine, pralidoxime and a form of diazepam. It is given intramuscularly into the lateral aspect of the thigh every 5–15 min, depending on the improvement in the 'three Bs', to a maximum of three doses.

### Breathing support

Death from nerve agent poisoning is usually due to respiratory failure. The mainstay of management is based on high concentrations of oxygen, and nasopharyngeal suction to keep the upper airway clear of the excessive secretions.

Signs of improvement will be:

- less wheeze
- an increasing pulse rate
- reduced airway and nasopharyngeal secretions

### Coma and convulsion care

This comprises the standard management and monitoring of a reduced level of consciousness, and the immediate treatment of any convulsions with i.v. diazepam.

## KEY NURSING SKILLS IN OUTBREAKS AND DELIBERATE RELEASES

- Core skills in infection control
  — Understanding the routes by which infection spreads
  — Strict adherence to and proper use of Universal Precautions

- Supervision of twice-daily cleaning and disinfection of room (particularly touched surfaces, e.g. bed rails, TV controls)
- Advanced skills in the use of Personal Protective Equipment
  - The use of high-filtration respirator masks, including the use of a fit-test
  - Ensuring there is consistency in the use of Personal Protective Equipment by all team members
- Core nursing skills in the assessment of the critically ill patient
  - Initial assessment using the generic ABCDE approach
  - Monitoring of the critically ill with impending respiratory failure
  - Supporting the patient and their family
- Advanced communication skills for nursing patients in isolation
  - Dealing with fear and anxiety in a victim of a 'dreaded' illness
  - Minimising the bars to communication imposed by protective clothing
  - Minimising the impact of the illness on the patient's well-being
- Disease-specific nursing problems
  - Ensuring that a system exists for early recognition and immediate infection control
  - Minimising high-risk procedures
  - Reducing possible transmission from the time of the first clinical encounter
  - Designating 'clean' and 'dirty' areas for isolation materials
- Dealing with the individual threat to personal health
  - The issue of 'working quarantine'
  - The concept of 'cohort nursing' – logging health-care personnel
  - Limiting and educating visitors
- Participating in a strong management system
  - The best systems for controlling an outbreak are those that have been tested
- Using information systems on the internet
- The supervision and protection of relatives and visitors

## CONCLUSION

From the personal testimony of health-care professionals involved with the SARS outbreak in China, Hong Kong and Toronto, it is clear that nursing large numbers of critically ill patients with a highly infectious disease places a major burden on the health-care system. It also presents a huge personal challenge to individual members of the staff. Inevitably, if the problem recurs the Acute Medical Assessment Units will be in the front line and will have to cope. It is the responsibility of Acute Unit staff to be aware of the current threats and to be up to date on their management: to understand the issues of effective infection control, to institute them immediately any suspicion is raised, and to ensure that health personnel are not put at unnecessary risk. There are many sources of advice once the diagnosis is made, but the key is a high index of suspicion and appropriate levels of vigilance.

## FURTHER READING

### WEBSITES

An algorithm for potential cases of SARS and avian flu:
http://www.hpa.org.uk/infections/topics_az/avianinfluenza/pdfs/Algorithm.pdf

Information about specific substances or agents that could be used in terrorist attacks:
http://www.dh.gov.uk/PolicyAndGuidance/EmergencyPlanning/DeliberateRelease/fs/en

SARS: Department of Health website:
http://www.dh.gov.uk/PolicyAndGuidance/HealthAndSocialCareTopics/SevereAcuteRespiratorySyndrome/fs/en

SARS: Health Protection Agency website:
http://www.hpa.org.uk/infections/topics_az/SARS/Guidelines.htm

WHO website: Guidance for hospital infection control in SARS:
http://www.who.int/csr/sars/infectioncontrol/en/

# INDEX